# Clinical Workbook for Speech-Language Pathology Assistants

# Clinical Workbook for Speech-Language Pathology Assistants

Robert Kraemer, PhD, CCC-SLP
Jacqueline Bryla, SLPA

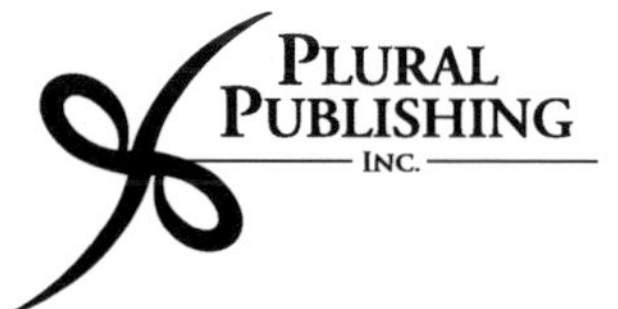

PLURAL PUBLISHING INC.

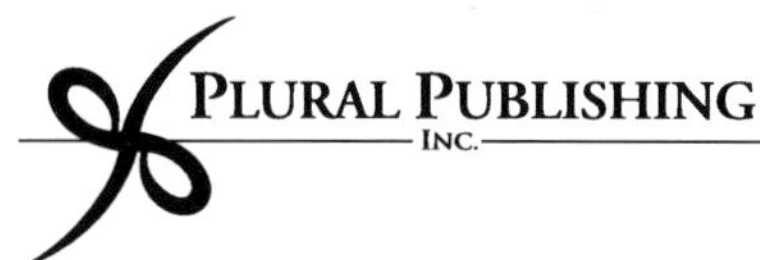

5521 Ruffin Road
San Diego, CA 92123

e-mail: info@pluralpublishing.com
Website: http://www.pluralpublishing.com



Typeset in 11/14 Palatino by Flanagan's Publishing Services, Inc.
Printed in the United States of America by McNaughton & Gunn
20 19 18   2 3 4 5



ISBN-13: 978-1-59756-890-6
ISBN-10: 1-59756-890-2

# CONTENTS

# FOREWORD

The ability to clearly and competently communicate is often taken for granted by those without a communication disorder. This basic skill, as complex as it is, is crucial for academic, social, emotional, and financial well-being. For those who struggle communicating, dedicated and well-trained speech-language pathologists (SLPs) and speech-language pathology assistants (SLPAs) are ready to help.

This workbook is a must for any beginning or experienced SLP and/or SLPA who works with children with communication needs. Within these chapters, you will find a gold mine of evidence-based lessons many with current, state-of-the-art applications (apps). The authors have devised lessons that are easy to follow and that allow for creative freedom. As a fan and user of many of the apps included in this workbook, I can vouch for their utility and effectiveness. And, most important, they are engaging for both the client and SLP/SLPA!

As sole or coauthor of 16 books, I am enthusiastic about the addition of another fantastic resource. As a part-time itinerant SLP who works in the public schools with preschoolers, elementary children, and teenagers, I am especially happy to see a practical, hands-on resource that we all can use to serve students on our ever-growing caseloads. This workbook is a shining example of "Monday morning," helpful resources that we can all begin using at once. Because the complexity of our students' needs is increasing and paperwork can be so time-consuming, I welcome practical resources to make our jobs easier.

This workbook should be a required text in every SLPA course and on the shelf of every practicing SLPA (and SLP, for that matter).

I hope you find this book as essential and timely as I. Congratulations on your decision to join one of the most amazing and rewarding professions today.

—Celeste Roseberry-McKibbin, PhD, CCC-SLP
Professor
Department of Speech Pathology and Audiology
California State University Sacramento
Sacramento, CA

As speech-language pathologists, it is important to remain committed to our roles as leaders and experts, bringing together interdisciplinary knowledge, clinical expertise, and evidence-based practice. Whether we are working with a physical deck of articulation cards, paper-based resources created by expert clinicians, or a fun new articulation software application (app), we transform toys into tools. However, in the ever-increasing arena of cutting-edge research and apps, it is becoming more and more difficult to identify quality over trendy.

This is one of the main reasons why I created YappGuru, an online resource for professional development in special education. Through our work together at YappGuru, Jackie Bryla has shared her expertise in the integration of technology and practical application. As a result of a genuine passion in this area, she consistently updates others on new apps.

In addition to providing extensive information based on common disorders and target skills, *Clinical Workbook for Speech-Language Pathology Assistants* provides guidance, including corresponding objectives, technology tools, and step-by-step guides, on directing the session. This workbook is a creative, timely, effective, and well-organized resource for our industry and one I'm sure clinicians will find as an asset to their toolbox reflecting current and practical tools combined with strategies and specific tips for implementation.

—Mai Ling Chan, MS, CCC-SLP
CEO and Co-Founder of YappGuru

# ACKNOWLEDGMENTS

We gratefully acknowledge the thoughtful suggestions, support, encouragement, and guidance of the many individuals who made this project possible.

We gratefully acknowledge Felice Clark, Jenna Rayburn, Mia McDaniel, Lauren LaCour, Katie Lambert, and Viola Dean for use of their materials shown in many of the activities. We are also thankful to the following: Terry Kappe, Lauren Enders, and Sharon Stanley for adding their expertise and knowledge for Chapter 6 (AAC for Complex Communication Needs); Amy Prince and Amber Ladd for their contributions in Chapter 3 (Communicative Intent); and Nancy Barcal and Hannah Lee for their work in Chapter 8 (Voice and Fluency Disorders).

We are indebted for the unending support and encouragement of our friends and colleagues: Celeste Roseberry-McKibbin, PhD, for providing inspiration and the necessary "gentle push" off of the proverbial ledge; Mai Ling for always checking in and sending those much-needed messages of support; and Robert Pieretti, PhD, and Heather Thompson, PhD, for their constant encouragement.

We also thank these students who helped in various ways: Sarah Mohalley, Adrienne Mowry, and Sharon Shultz-Sundman.

A special thanks to Helen Wagner and Angela Moorad for their time and effort in providing essential feedback.

A big thank you also goes out to all the app developers who provided permission to republish screen images throughout this workbook as well as the many parents who consented to have images of their wonderful (and patient) children be a part of this workbook.

We want to thank Plural Publishing for supporting our project and helping us navigate the many steps in creating and publishing this workbook.

Finally, a heartfelt thanks to our families for their patience and love throughout this endeavor.

# CONTRIBUTORS

This workbook would not exist without the amazing contributions from the following individuals. Their contributions are deeply appreciated.

**Amber Ladd, MA, CCC-SLP, BCBA**, Talk Team, Fresno, California

**Amy M. Prince, MA, CCC-SLP, BCBA**, Talk Team, Fresno, California

**Felice Clark, MS, CCC-SLP**, The Dabbling Speechie, Roseville, California

**Hannah Lee**, Graduate Student, Granite Bay Speech, Roseville, California

**Katie R. Lambert, MS, CCC-SLP**, The Reading Speechie, Rancho Cordova, California

**Lauren S. Enders, MA, CCC-SLP**, Assistive Technology Augmentative Communication Consultant, Bucks County, Pennsylvania

**Lauren LaCour, MA, CCC-SLP**, Busy Bee Speech, Baton Rouge, Louisiana

**Mia McDaniel, MA, CCC-SLP**, Putting Words in Your Mouth, Prairieville, Louisiana

**Nancy Barcal, MA, CCC-SLP**, Granite Bay Speech, Roseville, California

**Sharon Stanley**, Augmentative-Alternative Communication Specialist, Elk Grove Unified School District, Elk Grove, California

**Terry H. Kappe, MA, CCC-SLP**, Augmentative Communication Specialist, Temple City, California

**Viola Dean, MS, CCC-SLP**, Miss V's Speech World, Lincoln, California

*In loving memory of Lisa Cabiale O'Connor (1937–2012), whose dedication, commitment, and perseverance contributed to implementing speech-language pathology assistant (SLPA) programs; teaching and mentoring SLPA students; and serving on the California licensing board for 13 years, which pushed forward the concept of assistants and led to ensuring integrity and quality in addressing the topic of SLPAs within the American Speech-Language-Hearing Association structure and throughout the United States.*

# 1

# Introduction

Whether working as a speech-language pathologist (SLP), speech-language pathology assistant (SLPA), or enrolled in SLPA coursework, this workbook will save you time when creating treatment activities. The activities presented in this workbook are tried and true and, as such, have been carefully thought out before being considered for inclusion in the text. All of the activities are presented using clear and concise verbiage. So, if you are someone being exposed to the profession for the first time, you will be able to easily grasp the purpose of the activity and conceptualize its implementation. This is a critical process for untrained students as well as newly trained SLPAs in ensuring the activity chosen meets the needs of the client (and the therapy session). For ease of implementation, each activity is explained with detailed, step-by-step instructions and supporting photographs. Aside from Chapter 1, the workbook has a chapter dedicated to common communication needs of clientele. For SLPs, SLPAs, and SLPA students seeking information on SLPA scope of practice and ethics please, refer to Ostergren (2014).

What makes this workbook unique is that it is the first workbook of its kind with activities that employ applications (apps). In addition to the apps, each chapter includes examples of basic treatment objectives in order to guide the clinician when choosing a treatment method for a corresponding treatment need. The apps presented in this workbook are adaptable for individual or group sessions and include their corresponding Uniform Resource Locator (URL) and Quick Reference (QR) codes. For activities that do not rely on apps, we have provided the links to http://www.teacherpayteacher.com products and/or symbol images software. The QR codes have been generated using QR Code Generation (http://goqr.me/). Essential resources are listed in many of the lessons with links to video tutorials and access to additional resources to support these lessons. This workbook is especially advantageous for itinerant SLPAs/SLPs in that the majority of the activities are contained within the technology, lightening the load of materials, toys, and decks of cards one often must drag from site to site.

Although the activities in this workbook rely on many of the popular apps used today, it would be impossible to include the tens of thousands that would also support many of these activities. We suggest you embark on an app journey and find those that may fit not only these activities but guide you in developing enriching lessons and activities for your clients. SLPAs should also be aware of the option to purchase discounted apps during local, state, and national conferences and conventions (i.e., ASHA Annual Convention). In addition, apps are also advertised during various "awareness" months (i.e., Autism Awareness Month, Better Hearing and Speech Month, etc.). The focus of the chapters is as follows:

1

## CHAPTER 2. SPEECH SOUND DISORDERS: ARTICULATION, PHONOLOGY, AND APRAXIA

This chapter includes activities addressing the needs of clients with articulation and phonologic disorders as well as apraxia of speech (AOS). This chapter has 11 activities ready for use with clients requiring speech sound disorder therapy.

## CHAPTER 3. COMMUNICATIVE INTENT

This chapter includes activities addressing the needs of clients who struggle with intentional communicative intent, replacing off-task communication behavior with a functional communication system. This chapter has five activities ready for use with clients struggling with communicative intent.

## CHAPTER 4. LANGUAGE DISORDERS

This chapter includes activities addressing both receptive and expressive language disorders. Several of the activities can be used interchangeably between receptive and expressive language needs, allowing flexibility for clinicians to address these needs in clients who struggle in both areas. This chapter has eight activities ready for use with clients having language impairments.

## CHAPTER 5. SOCIAL LANGUAGE AND PRAGMATICS

This chapter includes activities addressing social language needs. This chapter has six activities ready to use with clients who struggle with aspects of social language.

## CHAPTER 6. AAC FOR COMPLEX COMMUNICATION NEEDS

This chapter includes activities addressing complex communication needs of clients who require augmentative and/or alternative communication (AAC) systems. AAC systems can vary from "no tech" to "high tech" in nature, from paper icons to iPad apps. This chapter has five activities ready to use with clients with complex communication needs. This chapter has five activities ready to use with clients requiring AAC support.

## CHAPTER 7. LITERACY

This chapter includes activities addressing pre-, early, and school-age literacy needs. Key components of literacy include phonologic awareness, print concepts, alphabet knowledge, and literate language. Activities in this chapter can also be used—with some slight modifications—on clients with language impairments. This chapter has 12 activities ready to use with clients with literacy needs.

## CHAPTER 8. VOICE AND FLUENCY DISORDERS

This chapter includes activities addressing the needs of clients with voice and/or fluency disorders. This chapter has nine activities ready to use with clients with voice or fluency needs.

## CHAPTER 9. BEHAVIOR MANAGEMENT TECHNIQUES

This chapter includes behavior management activities for clients needing visual schedules and/or motivation/reinforcement in order to participate in therapy sessions. This chapter has four activities addressing visual supports and six suggestions addressing motivation and reward.

Thank you for adding this workbook to your clinical "tool kit." We hope you find these lessons and activities helpful as you embark on an amazing journey in an amazing profession.

## REFERENCE

Ostergren, J. A. (2014). *Speech-language pathology assistants: A resource manual.* San Diego, CA: Plural.

# 2

# Speech Sound Disorders: Articulation, Phonology, and Apraxia

Speech sound disorders (SSDs) include articulation disorders, phonologic disorders, and childhood apraxia of speech (CAS). As a school-based speech-language pathology assistant (SLPA), chances are you will work extensively with children having an SSD. As you may recall from your coursework, articulation disorders are SSDs due to physical deficits in the articulatory system. This can be due to a motor movement problem or to a malformation of the articulatory system. Articulation disorders are marked by consistent errors, most commonly substitutions, omissions, distortions, and additions. A majority of children you will work with will have a problem producing the /r/ sound. Phonologic disorders are those of linguistic processing and occur when there are phonologic rules in place, which alter the output based on those rules. This means that phonologic errors present in a variety of ways and may be more difficult to identify initially. Phonologic errors generally appear very inconsistent, especially compared to errors of articulation disorders. Children with phonologic disorders are often stimulable. For example, if you take a sound out of context making any phonologic rule inapplicable, the client has the ability to produce the sound. Finally, CAS is a neurologic disorder of motor programming without any paralysis, weakness, or incoordination. CAS is best identified by articulation and linguistic deficits, most notably disruptions in stress and prosody. Speech will often sound monotone and might have frequent vowel errors. Consonants are produced inconsistently, which could lead to frustration on the child's and listener's part. The activities included in this chapter will help you address the array of SSDs children present on your caseload. As you become familiar with these activities, you will begin to gain confidence working with clients with SSDs and, under the guidance of your supervising speech-language pathologist (SLP), can develop your own therapy materials to fit the therapy goals established by the SLP.

## ACTIVITIES FOR ARTICULATION

### Objectives

The following are some sample objectives for articulation therapy. These objectives are merely samples and do not fully represent all possibilities. In addition, the lessons below do not align with these sample objectives.

1. Client will produce initial /r/ at the word level in 9 out of 10 opportunities across three consecutive data collection points.

2. Client will produce /r/ at the sentence level in a variety of positions in 9 out of 10 opportunities across three consecutive data collection points.

3. Client will produce r-blends at the phrase level in initial, medial, and final positions in 9 out of 10 opportunities across three consecutive data collection points.

### Activity 1

Articulation Station PRO by Little Bee Speech for all ages working on articulation.

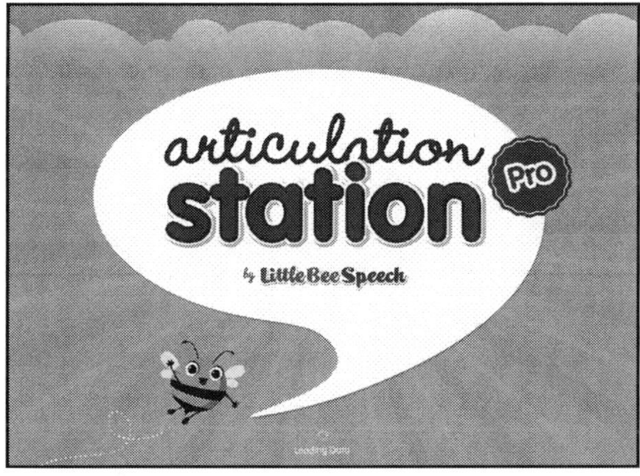


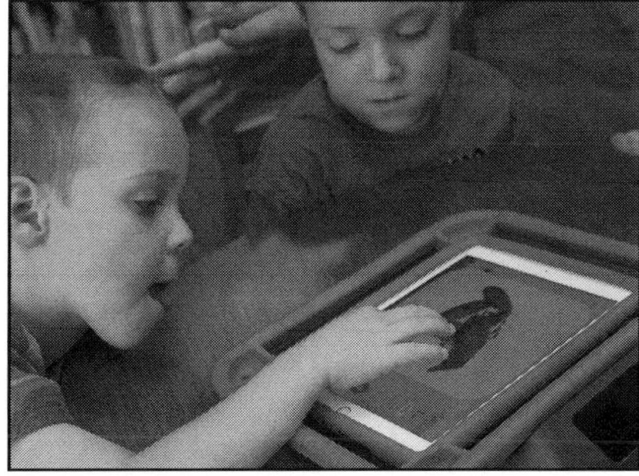

**FIGURE 2–1A.** Little Bee Speech articulation station main screenshot. Reproduced with permission of Little Bee Speech Co. Apps.

**FIGURE 2–1B.** Jason and Dillon Allen.

Articulation Station PRO is a comprehensive articulation IOS app for the iPad that provides multiple activities for targeting 22 phonemes that can be practiced at the word, phrase, sentence, and story levels presented in six varying activities. Articulation Station offers the ability to record client responses, which is helpful for self-monitoring, as well as an option to customize word lists for specific clients. This app is appropriate for both individual and small group articulation sessions working on one or more phonemes. Articulation Station offers an in-depth tutorial video within the app, which is very helpful for the new user to gain familiarity.

<table>
<tr><td>To make for more effective and efficient therapy sessions, enter specific client data (e.g., initials or names), create therapy groups, and customize settings as needed in the app prior to the therapy session.</td></tr>
</table>

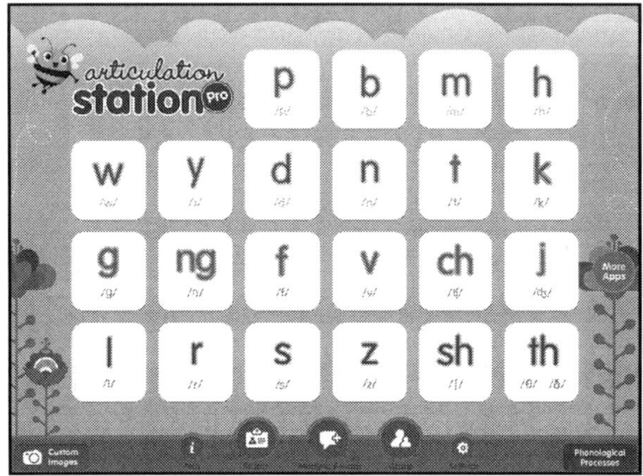

**FIGURE 2–2A.** Little Bee Speech phoneme screenshot. Reproduced with permission of Little Bee Speech Co. Apps.

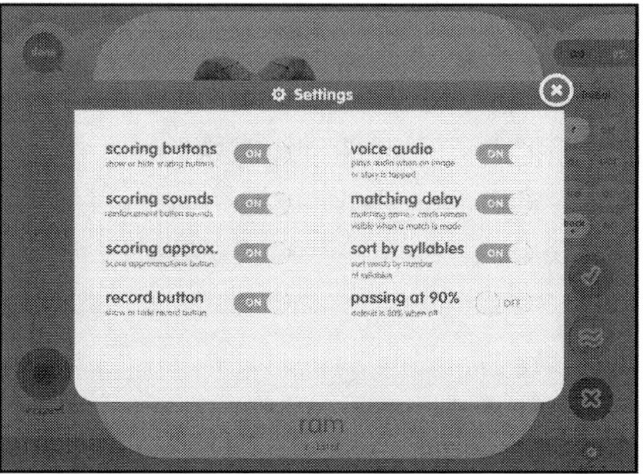

**FIGURE 2–2B.** Little Bee Speech settings screenshot. Reproduced with permission of Little Bee Speech Co. Apps.

To download Articulation Session PRO or the free version, visit http://littlebeespeech.com

**FIGURE 2–3.** Little Bee Speech QR code.

### *Individual Session*

Step 1:  With the client sitting aside or across from you, model the target sound and confirm the client is able to approximate the sound. *NOTE:* SLPA should take initial direction from the supervising SLP in regard to client's ability to produce approximation.

Step 2:  Explain that the client will be using an app during this session to help with working on his or her specific sound.

Step 3:  Open the app Articulation Station and proceed.

    a.  Select the phoneme (i.e., /r/) on the selection screen for an individual session and then proceed.

    b.  Select the appropriate level (word, phrase, sentence, or story).

    c.  Select the stimuli for the level chosen (flashcards, matching, rotating, unique, Level 1, Level 2).

    d.  Select the appropriate position (initial, medial, final) and modify the word list if needed.

    e.  Tap "Begin" to proceed with stimuli.

    f.  Select the appropriate score button on the right-hand side of the screen.

Step 4:  Upon completion of presented stimuli, press the "Done" button and SAVE the scored data to the appropriate client.

Step 5:  Share saved data as appropriate (print or email).

### Small Group Session

Step 1:  With the client sitting aside or across from you, model the target sound and confirm the client is able to approximate the sound. *NOTE*: SLPA should take initial direction from the supervising SLP in regard to the client's ability to produce approximation.

Step 2:  Explain that the client will be using an app during this group session to help with working on his or her specific sound(s).

Step 3:  Open the app "Articulation Station" and proceed.

    a.  Select the clients who belong to a therapy group session by pressing "Group" at the bottom of the screen, checking the clients to be added to the group session, and tap "Begin." *NOTE*: Clients should be set up in the app prior to the session as this may take some time.

    b.  Select the targeted client at the top of the screen (the client tab will change to RED).

    c.  Select the appropriate level (word, phrase, sentence, or story).

    d.  Select the stimuli for the level chosen (flashcards, matching, rotating, unique, Level 1 or 2).

    e.  Select the appropriate position (initial, medial, final) and modify the word list if needed.

    f.  Tap "Begin" to proceed with stimuli.

    g.  Select the appropriate score button on the right-hand side of the screen.

    h.  Repeat steps b through g for all clients within the group therapy session.

Step 4:  Upon completion of presented stimuli to all clients, press the "Home" button in the upper left corner of the screen to return to the Home screen.

Step 5:  Press the "Done" button and SAVE the scores from the group session.

Step 6:  Share saved data as appropriate (print or email) for the client file.

> Something to consider: It may be appropriate to offer choices for clients who are working on multiple phonemes (/k/, /g/) and allow them to choose which phoneme to begin with.

## Activity 2

Fun with /R/ by Virtual Speech Center Inc. for elementary school-age and above.

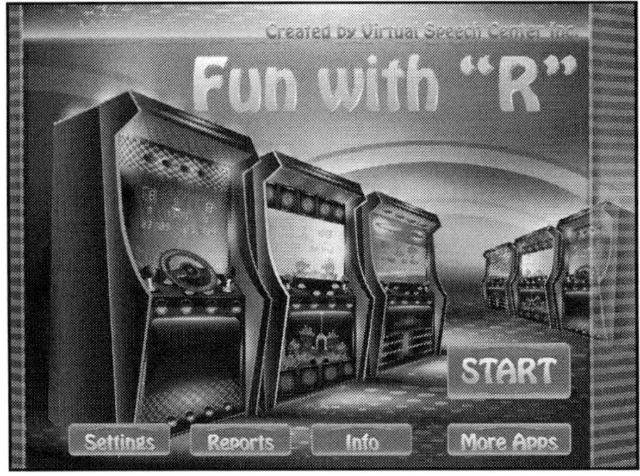


**FIGURE 2–4A.** Virtual Speech Center Fun with R main screenshot. Reproduced with permission of Virtual Speech Center.

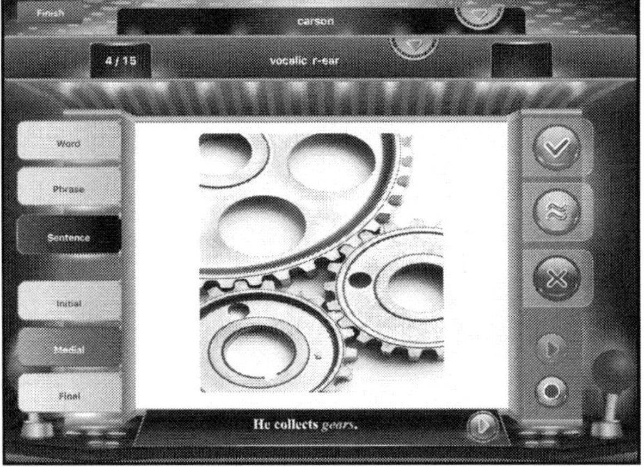


**FIGURE 2–4B.** Virtual Speech Center r-earscreen. Reproduced with permission of Virtual Speech Center.

Fun with /R/ is an app for targeting both prevocalic and vocalic /r/. The app has built-in motivational games for keeping clients highly engaged. Use this app for targeting and collecting student data for all positions of /r/. A customization setting within the Fun with /R/ allows for adding your own images and words and further individualizing the session for your clients.

> To make for more effective and efficient therapy sessions, enter specific client data (e.g., initials or names), customize settings, and select phonemes within the app prior to therapy session time.

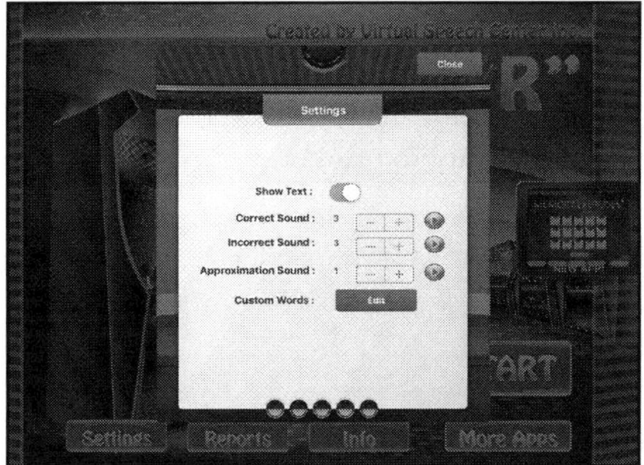

**FIGURE 2–5A.** Virtual Speech Center settings screenshot. Reproduced with permission of Virtual Speech Center.

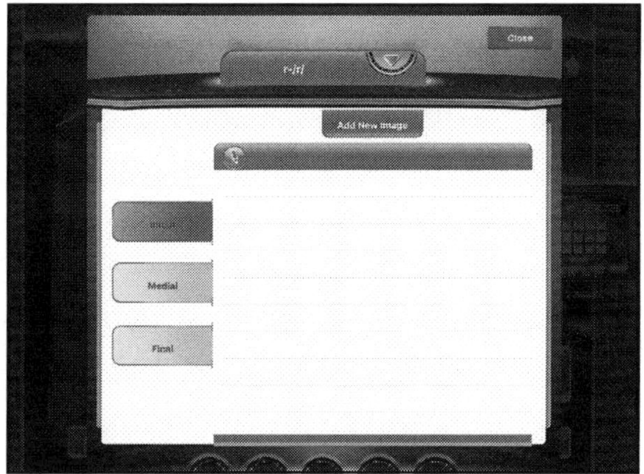

**FIGURE 2–5B.** Virtual Speech Center new image screenshot. Reproduced with permission of Virtual Speech Center.

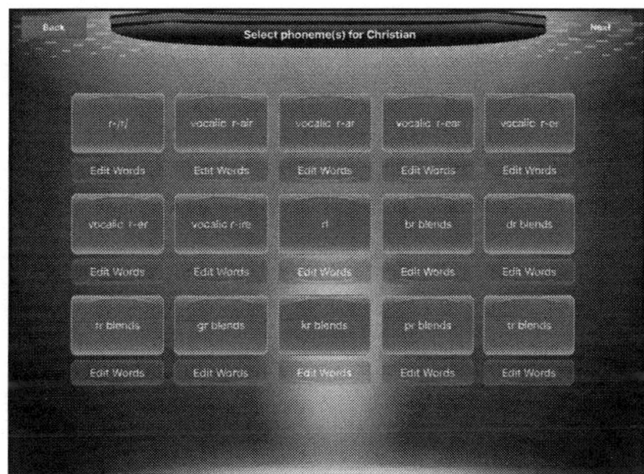

**FIGURE 2–5C.** Virtual Speech Center phoneme screenshot. Reproduced with permission of Virtual Speech Center.

To download Fun with /R/ and for other speech and language information, visit https://www.virtualspeechcenter.com

**FIGURE 2–6.** Virtual Speech Center QR code.

### Individual Session or Small Group Session

Step 1:  With the client sitting aside or across from you, model the target sound and confirm the client is able to approximate the sound. *NOTE*: SLPAs should take initial direction from the supervising SLP in regard to the client's ability to produce approximation.

Step 2:  Explain that the client will be using the Fun with /R/ app on the iPad during this session to help with working on his or her specific /r/ sounds.

Step 3:  Open the app Fun with /R/ and proceed.

    a.  Tap "START" to begin.

    b.  Select one or more students for the individual or small group therapy session. *NOTE*: Clients should be set up in the app prior to the session as this may take some time.

    c.  Select one of the stimuli game choices (Flashcards, Memory Game, Bingo Game) for the session.

    d.  Select the phoneme(s) and edit words if needed for each student (name will appear at the top of the screen), and press "Next," located at the top right corner for additional students.

    e.  Select the "level and position" for the student located on the left side of the screen.

    f.  Students will tap (Memory and Bingo Games) or swipe (Flashcards) to present stimuli on screen.

    g.  Tap the arrow located next to the phoneme to change phoneme during the session for those students working on multiple vocalic /r/ sounds (ear, ire, or, ar, etc.).

    h.  Tap the appropriate score button and continue with presenting the stimuli for the student.

    i.  Select the record button for an option to allow your students to record responses for self-monitoring.

    j.  Select the arrow next to student name to change the student for small group therapy sessions.

    k.  Select the "Finish" button in the upper left corner of the screen to complete the session.

    l.  View or email scored data for student(s) file.

> Something to consider: It may be appropriate to offer choices for clients who are working on multiple /r/ phonemes and allow them to choose which phoneme to begin with.

## Activity 3

Interactive Articulation Practice /s, l, r/ BLEND Flip Books by The Dabbling Speechie.

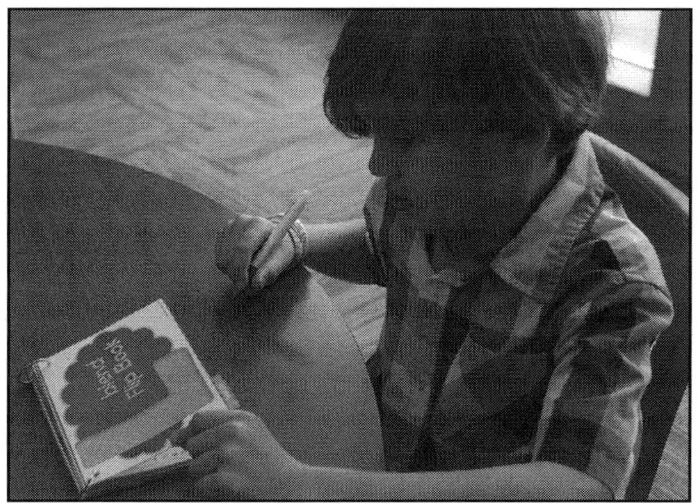

**FIGURE 2–7A.** Riley Clark flipbook.

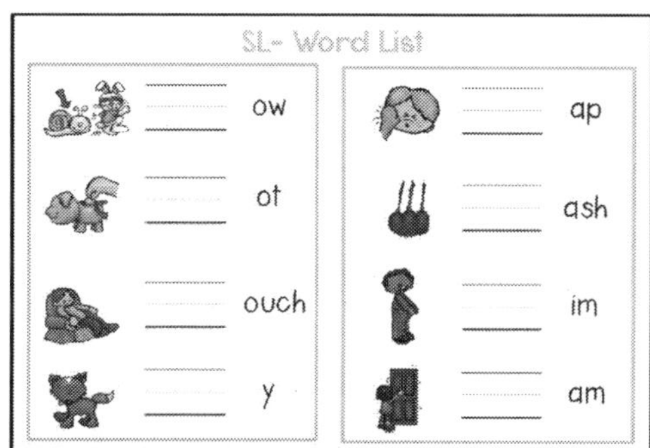


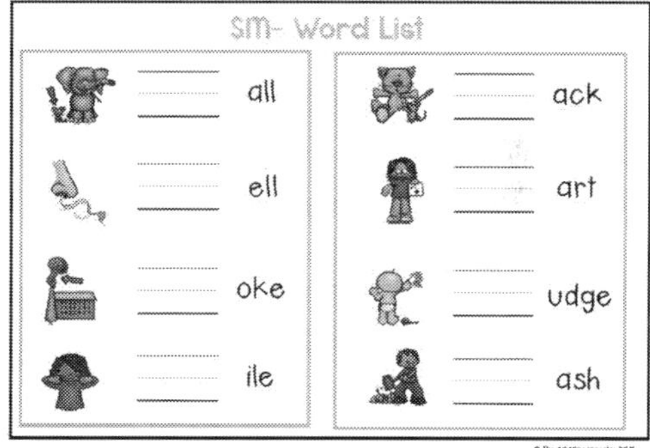


**FIGURE 2–7B.** Dabbling Speechie Felice Clark flipbook page. Reproduced with permission of The Dabbling Speechie.

The /s, l, r/ blend flipbooks by The Dabbling Speechie is an articulation activity intended for pre-K, kindergarten, and first-, second-, and third-grade clients. SLPAs should use judgment and guidance provided by the supervising SLP for other clients for whom this may be appropriate. The flipbook allows for practice at the word and phrase level for /s, l, r/ blends.

To download the /s, l, r/ blend flipbook, visit https://www.teacherspayteachers.com/Product/Interactive-Articulation-Flip-Books-For-slr-Blends-1753791

**FIGURE 2–8.** Dabbling Speechie QR code.

> This activity is to be printed on cardstock and laminated for durability and to be used with a dry-erase marker for interactivity. Cut book pages, hole punch, and then fasten pages with binder rings. Prepare the flip book material prior to session time.

### Individual Session or Small Group Session

Step 1:  With the client sitting aside or across from you, model the target sound and confirm the client is able to approximate the sound. *NOTE*: SLPA should take initial direction from the supervising SLP in regard to the client's ability to produce approximation.

Step 2:  Explain that the client will be using this interactive flipbook to help with working on blend sounds having /s, l, r/.

Step 3:  Begin with the individual client or first client in group therapy session. Choose the appropriate blend (/s, l, r/) phoneme flipbook for the client and turn to the appropriate page (Word or Phrases and specific blends /st, sn/).

Step 4:  Give the flip book to the client with a dry-erase marker.

Step 5:  Model words or phrases for the client if needed.

Step 6:  Have the client repeat the model or say words/phrases and fill in missing information using a dry-erase marker to add interactivity.

Step 7:  Score data session in the client file.

Step 8:  Repeat Steps 3 through 8 for small group therapy sessions that include multiple clients.

### Essential Resources

The Dabbling Speechie offers a variety of speech and language activities. To download a free /l/ phoneme flip book activity, visit https://www.teacherspayteachers.com/Product/Interactive-Articulation-Flip-Books-For-L-FREE-Resource-with-editable-slides-2034328

**FIGURE 2–9.** Dabbling Speechie FREE L QR code.

## Activity 4

Articulation practice combined with language and auditory memory skills for clients who have difficulty producing the following speech sounds: /s, z, r/, s-blends, r-blends, l-blends, "sh," "ch," and "th" for ages 6 years and older.

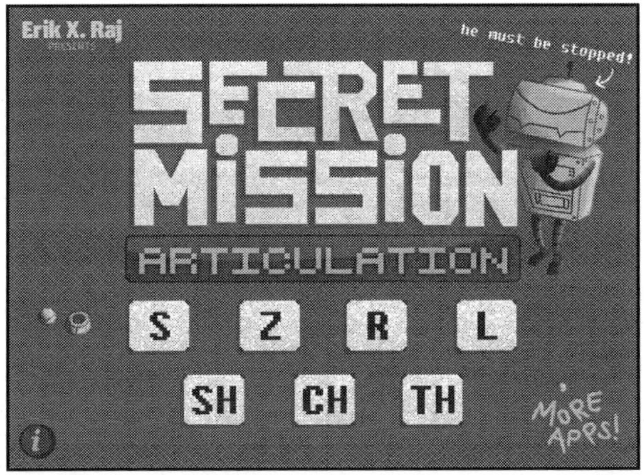


**FIGURE 2–10A.**  Erik X. Raj secret mission main screenshot. Reproduced with permission of Erik X. Raj, PhD, CCC-SLP, http://www.erikxraj.com

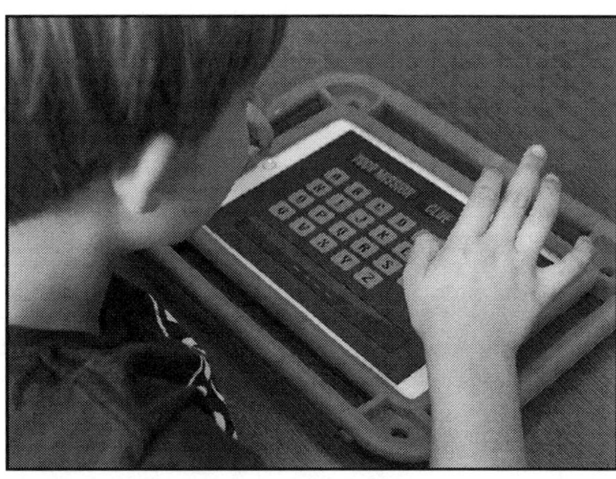

**FIGURE 2–10B.**  Riley Clark secret mission.

Secret Mission Articulation by Erik X. Raj is a unique speech therapy game that challenges players to guess a hidden word by choosing from different letters on an alphabet board. This word-guessing game features a comprehensive collection of over 600 sound-specific articulation words. In addition, it contains over 100 hilarious secret missions that players/clients can participate in.

To download Secret Mission Articulation, view demos, or other fun creative and motivating activities, visit http://erikxraj.com

**FIGURE 2–11.**  Erik X. Raj QR code.

### *Individual or Small Group Session*

Step 1:  With the client sitting aside or across from you, model the target sound and confirm the client is able to approximate the sound. *NOTE:* SLPAs should take initial direction from the supervising SLP in regard to the client's ability to produce approximation.

Step 2: Explain that the client will be using this interactive articulation app to help with working on his or her targeted speech sounds.

Step 3: Open Secret Mission Articulation.

Step 4: Tap on the appropriate speech sound for the client.

Step 5: Tap on "YOUR MISSION" to hear the secret mission presented or tap on "CLUE" to have a text box display the clue.

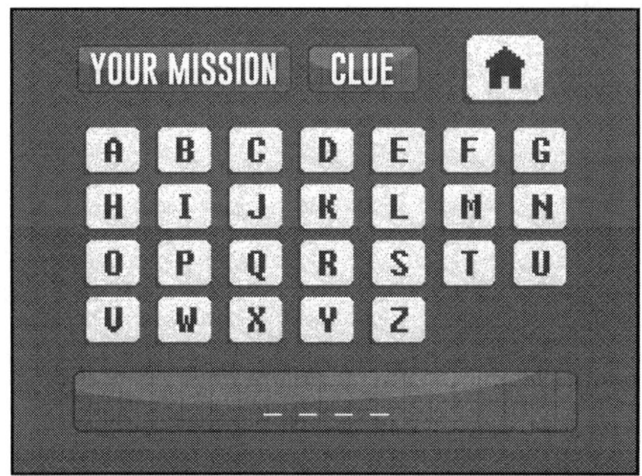


**FIGURE 2–12A.** Erik X. Raj mission Clue 1 screenshot. Reproduced with permission of Erik X. Raj, PhD, CCC-SLP, http://www.erikxraj.com

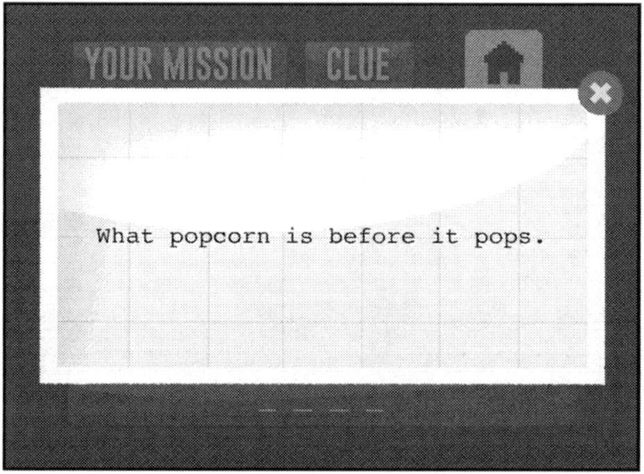


**FIGURE 2–12B.** Mission and Clue 2 screenshot. Reproduced with permission of Erik X. Raj, PhD, CCC-SLP, http://www.erikxraj.com

Step 6: Tap on the letters to fill in the missing password for the secret mission. Use this opportunity to have the client repeat the word several times or use it in a sentence. Take client data as needed.

Step 7: Tap "ENTER" when finished to listen to the word, see the clue again, or guess another password with the same speech sound.

Step 8: To change speech sounds or to allow another client to have a turn, tap the "Home" icon to return to the sound choices.

## ACTIVITIES FOR PHONOLOGY



### Objectives

The following are some sample objectives for phonology therapy:

1. Client will discontinue the phonologic process of stopping 9 out of 10 times.

2. Client will discontinue the phonologic process of fronting 9 out of 10 times.

3. Client will discontinue the phonologic process of initial consonant deletion 9 out of 10 times.

### Activity 1

Phono Learning Center App by Smarty Ears for ages pre-K, kindergarten, and those clients working on various phonologic processes. Advanced target activities for clients 8 years of age and older.

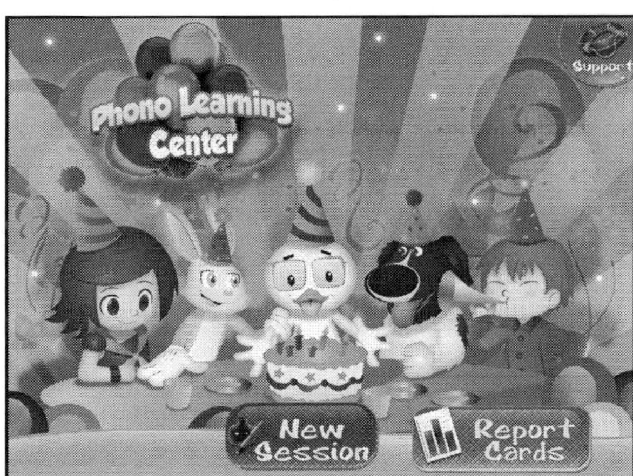


**FIGURE 2–13.**  Smarty Ears phono main screenshot. Reproduced with permission of Smarty Ears, LLC. All rights reserved.

Phono Learning Center by Smarty Ears, LLC is an evidence-based Cycles technique used specifically for those children who are unintelligible due to a sound system disorder that is authored by Mary Huston, MS, CCC-SLP. Phono Learning Center is a multiplayer app that is appropriate for individual and small group therapy sessions that target error patterns with a built-in Cycles approach and has the ability to customize to meet client objectives. Phono Learning Center has four engaging built-in games that present the stimuli. A "HomeWork" selection also offers the ability to "Share" with clients or caregivers by printing or emailing.

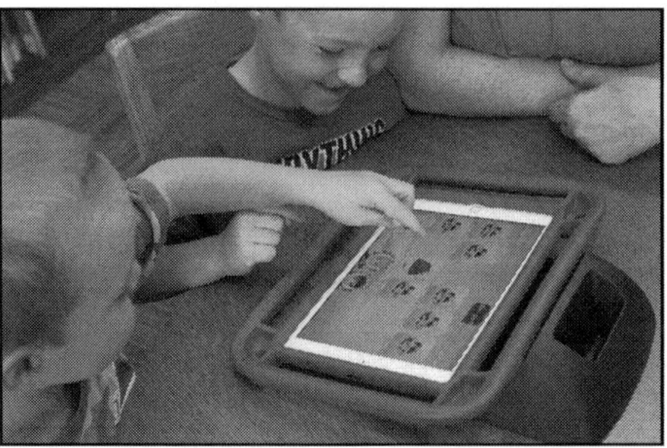

**FIGURE 2–14.**  Jason and Dillon Allen phonocenter.

To make for more effective and efficient therapy sessions, set up specific client data (e.g., initials or names), choose individualized targets, and customize settings within the app prior to the therapy session. *NOTE:* SLPAs should always select settings and a targeted approach with SLP guidance and supervision.

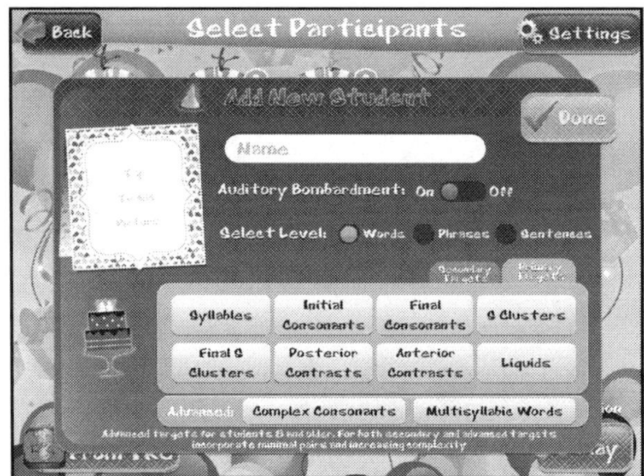

**FIGURE 2–15A.**  Smarty Ears phono Settings 1 screenshot. Reproduced with permission of Smarty Ears, LLC. All rights reserved.

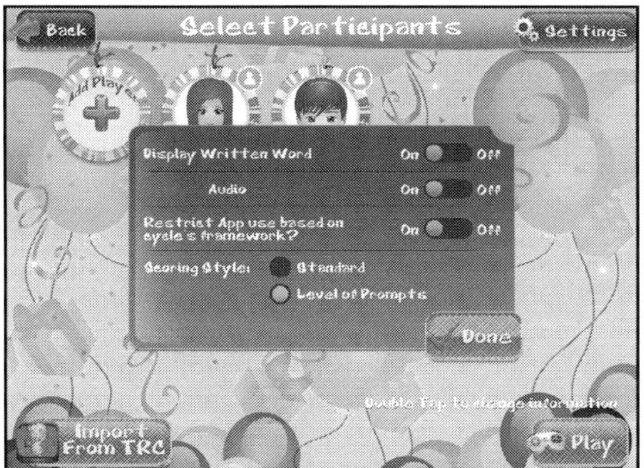

**FIGURE 2–15B.**  Smarty Ears phono Settings 2 screenshot. Reproduced with permission of Smarty Ears, LLC. All rights reserved.

To download Phono Learning Center, visit http://smartyearsapps.com

**FIGURE 2–16.**  Smarty Ears QR code.

### *Individual Session or Small Group Session*

Step 1:  With the client sitting aside or across from you, model the target sound and confirm the client is able to approximate the sound. *NOTE:* SLPAs should take initial direction from the supervising SLP in regard to the client's ability to produce approximation of the target sound.

Step 2:  Select one or more clients to participate in the session. *NOTE:* Clients should have been previously added and set up in the app prior to the session as this may take some time.

Step 3:  Tap the client's name (or avatar) at the bottom of the screen and press "Play" in the bottom right corner of the screen to begin the session for the client. All clients chosen in Step 2 will appear at the bottom of the screen.

Step 4:  Tap to choose a game (Balloon, Matching, BasketPaper, Puzzle) for presenting stimuli for this session.

Step 5:  Tap the appropriate "score button" in the top right corner of the screen to score client data for this session.

Step 6:  Repeat Steps 3 through 5 for additional client in therapy session.

Step 7:  Tap "Done" in the upper left corner of the screen to terminate the therapy session or the switch game.

Step 8:  View "Report Cards" for saved session data by tapping the client's name (or avatar) and "Share" information as appropriate for client file.

## Activity 2

PhonoPix–Full for helping remediate clients with several speech sound errors.

PhonoPix–Full by Expressive Solutions LLC is an IOS app with recorded audio, voice recording, and a data-scoring feature. PhonoPix–Full uses minimal pair decks to help clients differentiate between their production and a correct production. Included in the app are 10 decks with 40 minimal pairs in each for a total of 400 pairs. The following phonologic processes are addressed: prevocalic voicing, word final devoicing final consonant deletion, fronting, marked blend reduction, unmarked blend reduction, gliding, stopping, backing, and initial consonant deletion.

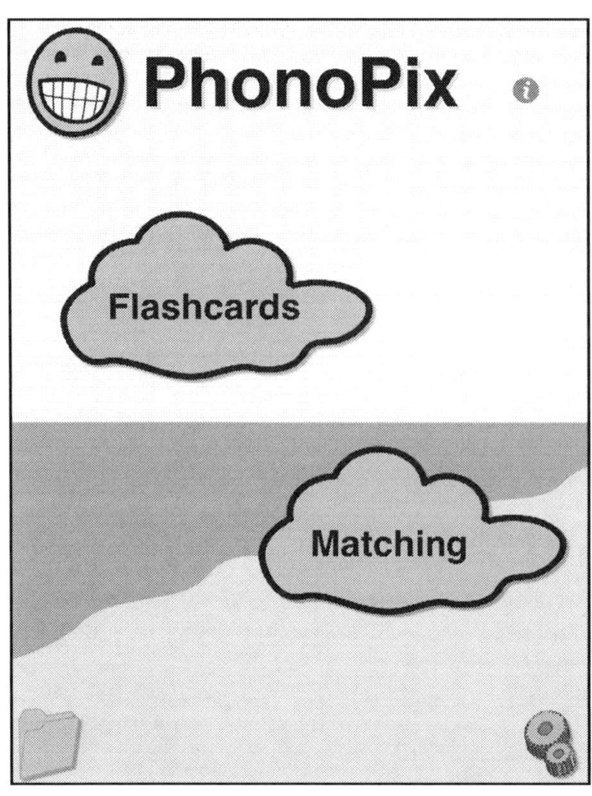



**FIGURE 2–17A.** Expressive Solutions phonopix main screenshot. Reproduced with permission of Expressive Solutions, LLC.

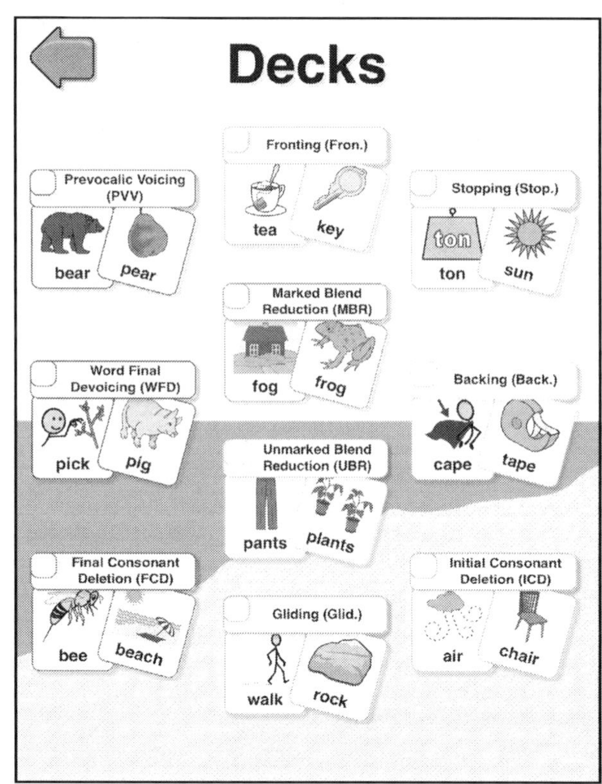



**FIGURE 2–17B.** Expressive Solutions phonopix decks screenshot. Reproduced with permission of Expressive Solutions, LLC.

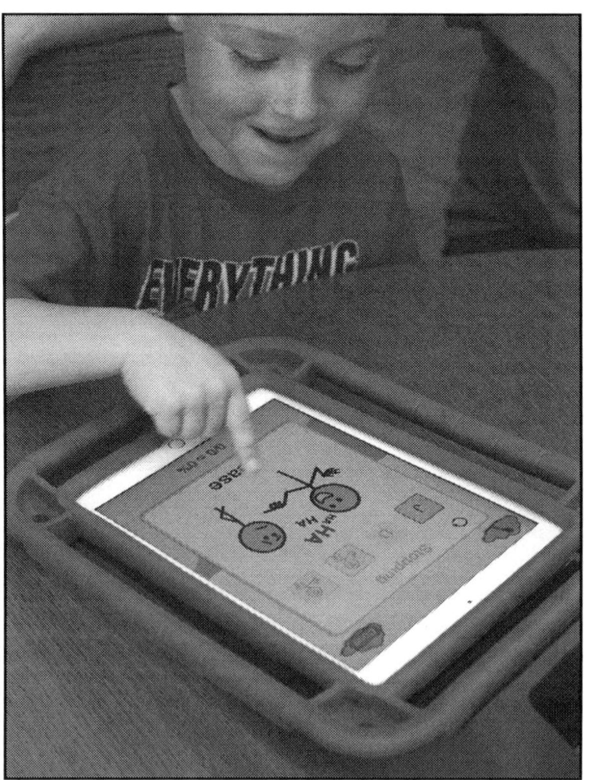

**FIGURE 2–17C.** Jason Allen phonopix.

To download PhonoPix–Full, visit http://expressive-solutions.com

**FIGURE 2–18.** Expressive Solutions QR code.

To make for more effective and efficient therapy sessions, enter specific client data (e.g., initials or names), and customize settings within the app prior to therapy session time.

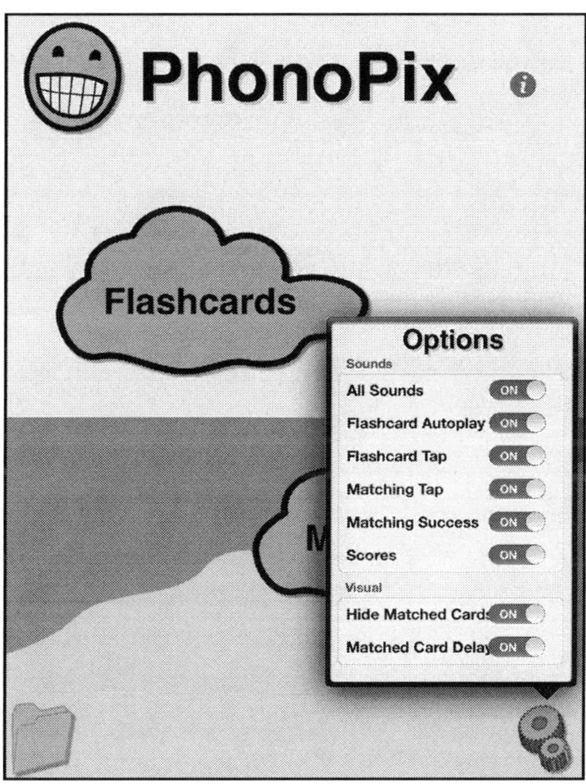


**FIGURE 2–19.** Expressive Solutions settings screenshot. Reproduced with permission of Expressive Solutions, LLC.

### *Individual Session or Small Group Session*

Step 1:  With the client sitting aside or across from you, model the target sound and confirm the client is able to approximate the sound. *NOTE*: SLPAs should take initial direction from the supervising SLP in regard to the client's ability to produce approximation.

Step 2:  Open the app PhonoPix–Full and proceed:

   a.  Select stimuli (Flashcards or Matching) for presenting to the client.

   b.  Select the phonologic process deck for each targeted error and press "Start." Deck options include prevocalic voicing, fronting, stopping, word final devoicing, marked blend reduction, backing, unmarked blend reduction, final consonant deletion, gliding, or initial consonant deletion.

   c.  Select the appropriate beginning or ending sounds based on the phonologic process deck(s) selected above and press "Start" to advance screen.

   d.  Tap the grayed-out images to add up to four client names for this session and press "Done." Grayed-out images will be replaced with client initials or photographs depending on initial setup. *NOTE:* Clients should be added and set up prior to the therapy session.

   e.  Select the box with the first client's name and have the student repeat the model or say images for the minimal pair.

   f.  Press the round arrow button on the upper left corner of the screen to flip over the card to present the matched minimal pair for the target objective.

   g.  Press the appropriate score image to score the client's production.

   h.  Tap the client's initials to move to the next client for a small group therapy session and repeat Steps f and g.

   i.  Tap "Done" to finish the therapy session and save scored data and enter or email for the client's file.

> Expressive Solutions LLC also offers two articulation IOS apps, ArtikPix, with free access to /h/, /w/, /j/, and "th" phonemes and ArtikPix Levels with free access for the "th" phoneme.

## Activity 3

Final Consonant Deletion for /p, b, t, d, k, g/ by Miss V's Speech World for ages preschool through second grade.

This activity includes 341 racecar-themed CVC flashcards to target the phonologic process of final consonant deletion (FCD). Each card contains the word in addition to a racecar visual that encourages students to add the word final sound (get to the finish line!).

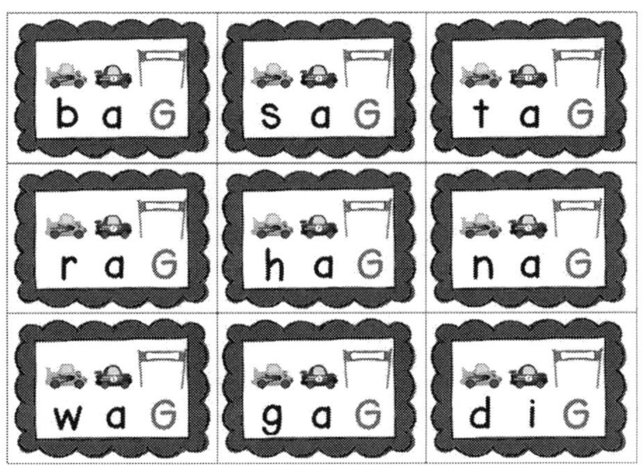

**FIGURE 2–20A.** Miss V's Speech World screenshot. Reproduced with permission of Miss V's Speech World.

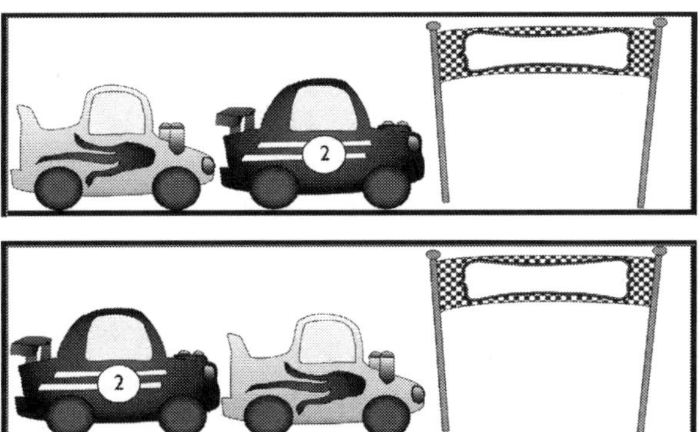

**FIGURE 2–20B.** Miss V's Speech World racecar visual. Reproduced with permission of Miss V's Speech World.

To download the final consonant deletion activity, visit https://www.teacherspayteachers.com/Product/Final-Consonant-Deletion-Racecar-themed-visual-CVC-flashcards-341-cards-874918

**FIGURE 2–21.** Miss V's Speech World QR code.

For a more effective and efficient therapy session, this activity can be printed on cardstock and laminated for durability prior to the therapy session.

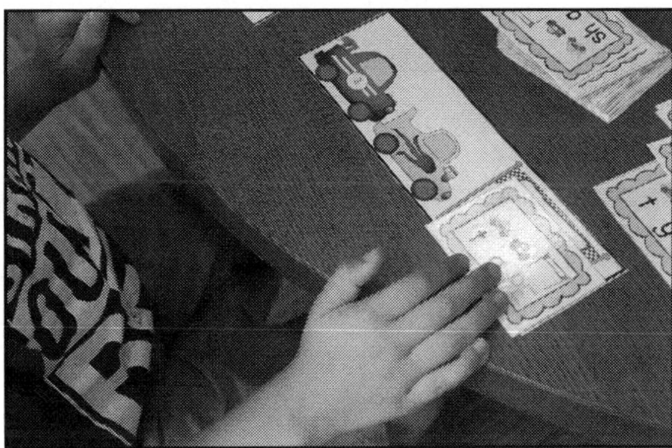

**FIGURE 2–22.** Riley Clark racecar.

### Individual or Small Group Session

Step 1:  With the client sitting aside or across from you give an explanation of what the intended therapy lesson will be (i.e., "Today we are using a fun racecar activity to practice speech sounds"). *NOTE:* SLPAs should take initial direction from the supervising SLP in regard to the client's ability and targeted objectives. Model for the client using a sample word flashcard and then placing it on the racecar visual card.

Step 2:  Give each client participating in the session a racecar visual card.

Step 3:  Choose the appropriate sound deck that targets the client objectives and goals (i.e., /p, b, t, d, k, g/).

Step 4:  Show the card to the client while modeling the word and placing emphasis on the final consonant that tends to be left off. If an additional cue is needed, tap or point to the finish line to represent the final consonant phoneme (i.e., /g/ for hog or /d/ for dud).

Step 5:  Allow the client to repeat the modeled word and place the card on the finish line.

Step 6:  Record data as required and needed in the client file.

Step 6:  If working in small groups, repeat Steps 4 through 6 for each client.

### Essential Resources

Miss V's Speech World offers many speech and language activities. Visit https://www.teachers payteachers.com/Store/Miss-Vs-Speech-World for more low-cost and free activities

**FIGURE 2–23.** Miss V's Speech World QR code.

# ACTIVITIES FOR APRAXIA

## Objectives

The following are some sample objectives for apraxia therapy:

1. Client will reduce instances of the simplification process of bilabialization at the word level 9 out of 10 times.

2. Client will use a slower and more rhythmic rate of speech when producing short phrases and/or sentences 9 out of 10 times.

3. Client will produce CCVC syllable shapes at the word level 9 out of 10 times.

## Activity 1

Providing opportunities for repetition of sound sequences with Word FLiPS for the iPad app by Super Duper Publications (2013), which engages clients with high interest technology.

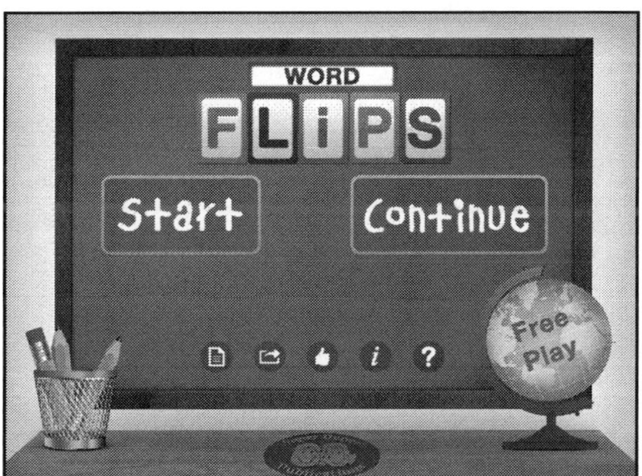


**FIGURE 2–24.** Super Duper word flips main screenshot. Reproduced with permission of Super Duper Publications.

Word FLiPS app is appropriate to use for clients with limited speech, unintelligible speech, and/or childhood apraxia of speech. Teach functional vocabulary words (i.e., hi, go, bye) while practicing up to three repetitions of sound sequences. Older or more verbal clients can practice a variety of sequences, such as "tie-tea-shoe" as a warm-up to practicing sentences. CV (consonant vowel) words can be combined to form other words (i.e., "tie-knee" can be combined form the word "tiny").

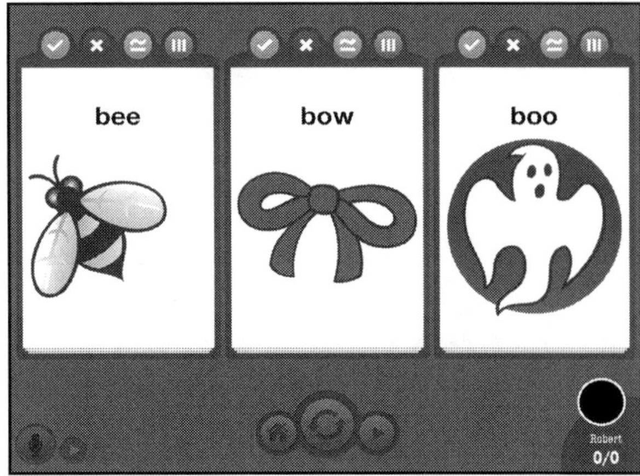


**FIGURE 2–25A.**  Super Duper 3 card flip screenshot. Reproduced with permission of Super Duper Publications.

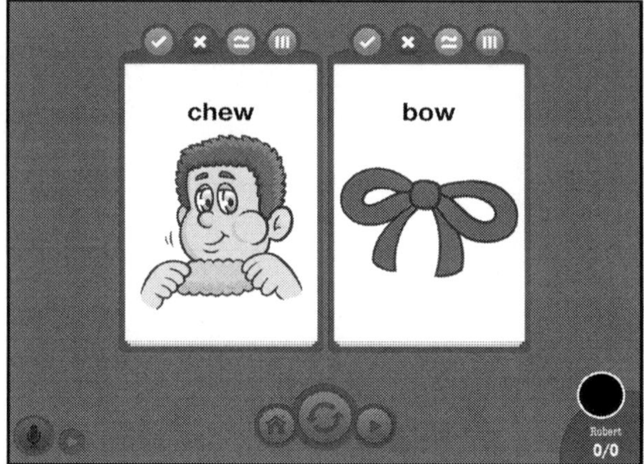


**FIGURE 2–25B.**  Super Duper 2 card flip screenshot. Reproduced with permission of Super Duper Publications.

Word FLiPS includes many features that allow for customizing individual flipbooks for clients of all abilities:

- Chooses words according to articulatory placements: bilabial, alveolar, velar, and palatal.

- Chooses words according to syllable structure: CV, CVC, CVCV, or CUSTOM.

- Chooses all words (including nonsense words) or only the suggested "real" words.

- Includes audio of all syllables.

- Free Play mode gives the ability to flip through the cards or randomly generate syllable combinations.

- Records a client's productions and replays audio clips.

- Tracks data for each syllable in a production or for the entire production.

- Keeps track of data for all clients.

- Emails, prints, and shares session results.

To download Word FLiPS, visit https://www.superduperinc.com

**FIGURE 2–26.**  Super Duper QR code.

For a more effective therapy session setup, always set up client target objectives within the app prior to therapy session time. Setting up a client is done one time only, and the target objectives can be modified as needed.

## *Task Setup*

Step 1: Tap "Start" on the home screen and the Settings screen will appear.

   a. Tap the "New Player" to add the client name or initials.

Step 2: Begin to create the client's flipbook.

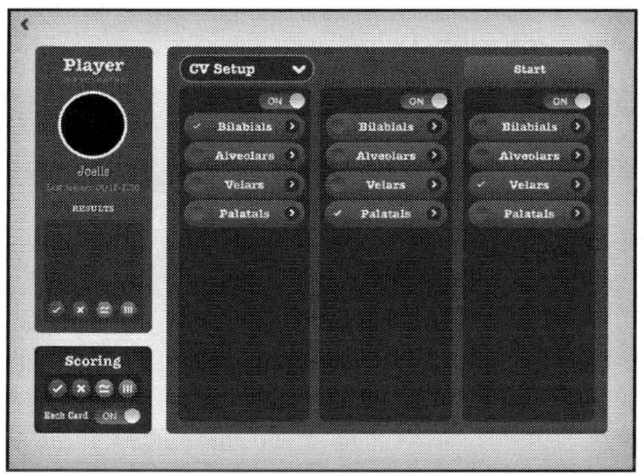

**FIGURE 2–27A.** Super Duper CV setup screenshot. Reproduced with permission of Super Duper Publications.

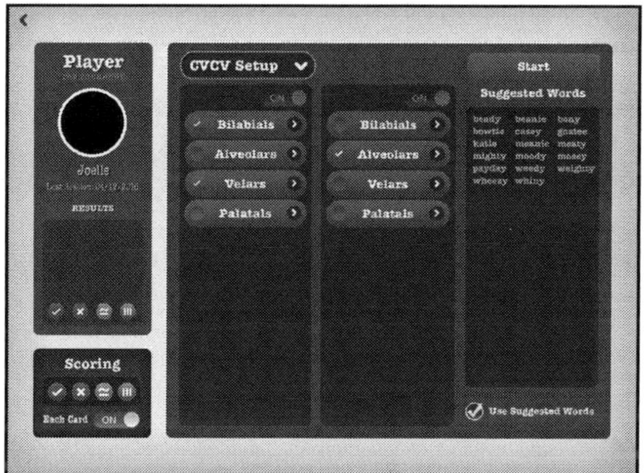

**FIGURE 2–27B.** Super Duper CVC setup screenshot. Reproduced with permission of Super Duper Publications.

   a. From the CV Setup drop-down menu, choose the syllable shape that targets the client's objective (i.e., CV, CVC, CVCV or customize a syllable shape). If CVC or CVCV are chosen, a list of suggested words will appear in the right column. Check "Use Suggested Words" to only use real words, keeping "Use Suggested Words" unchecked will allow nonsense words to appear in the activity.

   b. Tap On in each column to activate or deactivate the cards in the columns.

   c. Choose the place of production (i.e., bilabials, alveolars, velars).

   d. Choose to score Correct, Incorrect, Approximated, and/or Cued (prompted) responses by tapping the symbols in the scoring box. To turn off any or all of the score symbols, tap on the symbol and it will be darkened to indicate it is off.

   e. Choose to have each syllable sound (i.e., bee+moo, bye+she) scored by keeping the "Each Card ON" or turn "Each Card OFF" to only score for the set of syllables that produces a real or nonsense word (i.e., beemoo, byeshe).

Step 3:  Use the "FREE PLAY" option on the home screen to flip through cards without a specific client setup or to randomly generate syllable combinations. This is an excellent option for a warm-up exercise.

Step 4:  View detailed reports and session details from the home screen by tapping the document icon.

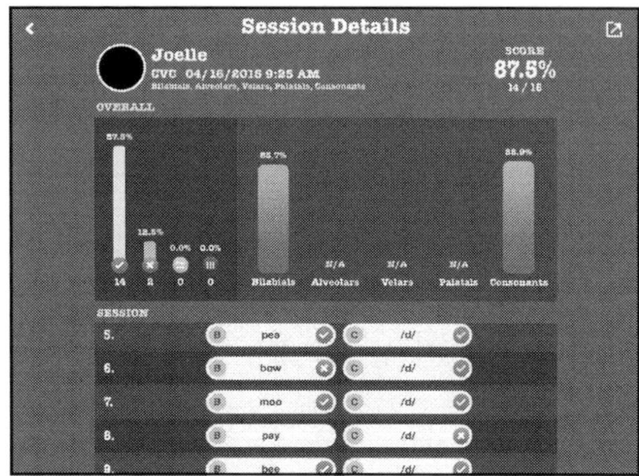

**FIGURE 2–28A.** Super Duper session detail screenshot. Reproduced with permission of Super Duper Publications.

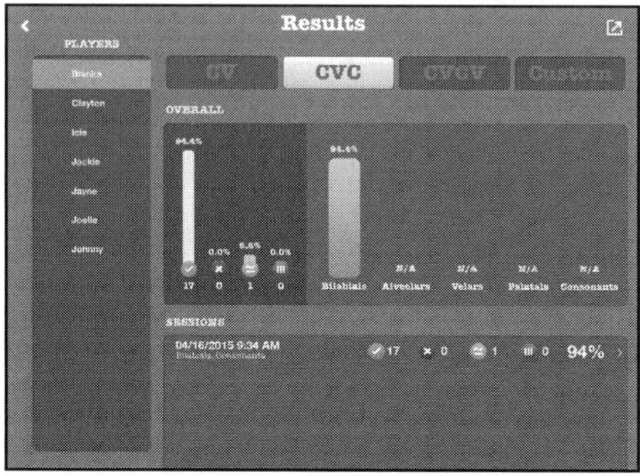

**FIGURE 2–28B.** Super Duper results screenshot. Reproduced with permission of Super Duper Publications.

### *Individual Session*

Step 1:  With the client sitting aside or across from, you explain the intended therapy lesson (i.e., "Today we are using a fun app call word flips to practice speech sounds and syllables"). *NOTE:* SLPAs should take initial direction from the supervising SLP in regard to the client's ability and targeted objectives.

Step 2:  Open the Word FLiPS app and choose the appropriate player (client) and tap "Start."

Step 3:  If an audio cue is needed for the client, tap the individual syllables to hear the audio for a specific card, and tap the ">" button to hear the audio of the sequence of cards. *NOTE:* To have the SLPA or SLP model the syllables and sounds or to remove the audio cues, turn off/down volume on the tablet.

Step 4:  Swipe the cards (syllable/sound) individually to flip the cards manually or use the circular arrow button to change the card (syllable/sound) sequence. Use this opportunity to allow the client to swipe the cards AFTER he or she has tried the card sequence and it has been scored.

Step 5:  Tap the record microphone icon to record the client if appropriate. Tap a second time to stop the recording. Often clients like to hear their recordings. This is also an excellent tool for those clients who are able to self-monitor.

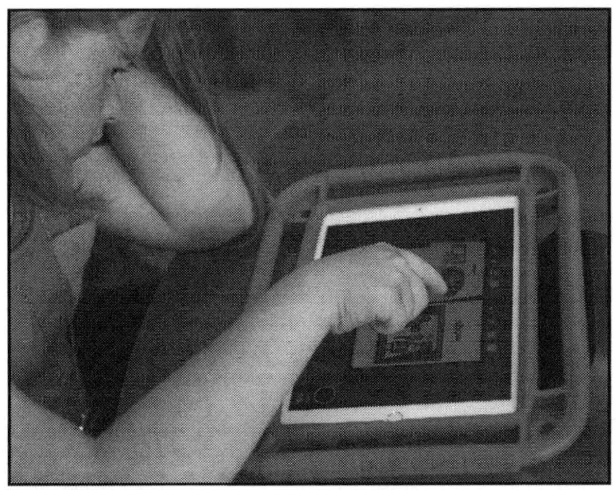

**FIGURE 2–29.** Elizabeth Giese word flips.

Step 6: Track data as needed. If scoring was set up during task setup, tap the appropriate scoring symbol for scoring and viewing results after the therapy session.

Step 7: Results can be viewed by tapping the "paper" icon on the home screen and choosing the appropriate client's results. Overall results are displayed and individual session results can be accessed by tapping the date of the session. Results also may be printed or emailed when the tablet is connected to Wi-Fi.

## Activity 2

Apraxia Ville app to present a variety of sounds and words while collecting data for clients.

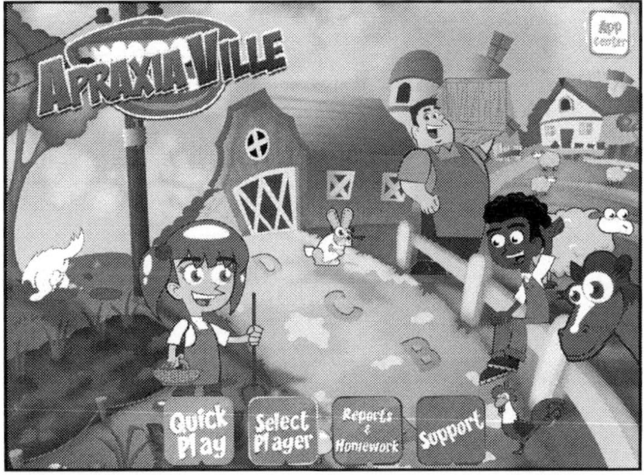


**FIGURE 2–30.** Smarty Ears Apraxia Ville main screenshot. Reproduced with permission of Smarty Ears, LLC. All rights reserved.

Apraxia Ville by Smarty Ears is a comprehensive application to help children with childhood apraxia of speech and severe speech sound disorders. Features include customizing targets, video modeling of consonants and vowels, word targets by syllable structure (CV, CVC, VC, etc.), and the ability to allow clients to monitor productions while following visual prompts. Use with a single client or multiple clients working on different targets in the same session. There are three activity areas from which to select: The Sound Windows focusing on sound production, The Farm House focusing on single-word production, and The Words Farm focusing on multiple-word production. A key component to working with Apraxia Ville is the built-in homework pages that are available to print or share via email.

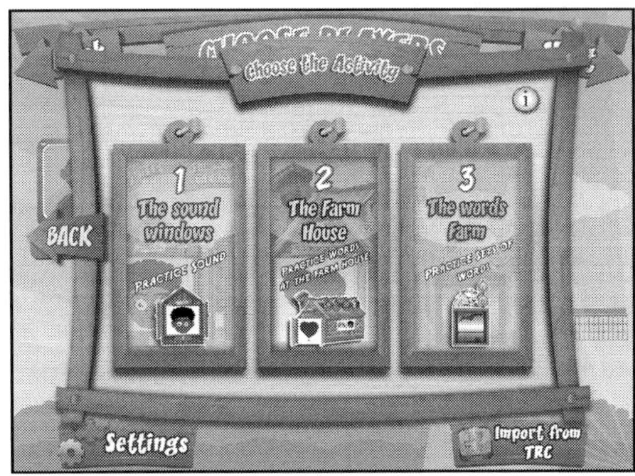

**FIGURE 2–31A.** Smarty Ears Apraxia Ville play area screenshot. Reproduced with permission of Smarty Ears, LLC. All rights reserved.

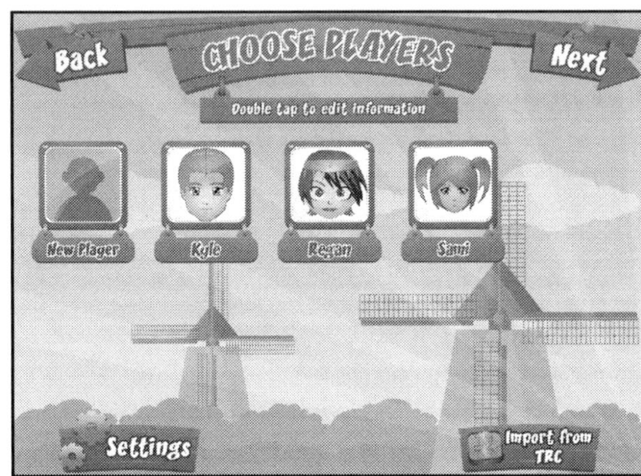

**FIGURE 2–31B.** Smarty Ears Apraxia Ville add player screenshot. Reproduced with permission of Smarty Ears, LLC. All rights reserved.

To download Smarty Ears Apraxia Ville, visit http://smartyearsapps.com

**FIGURE 2–32.** Smarty Ears QR code.

### Task Setup

Step 1:  Create client (player) profiles within the app.

   a.  Add client name or initials.

   b.  Choose a stock avatar or add a photo image to represent the client. *NOTE:* At times, it may be appropriate and fun for the client to have input and choose the representative avatar.

Step 2: Modify the word pool if needed by tapping on the settings (gear icon) on the main screen. *NOTE:* The date format for sessions results may be modified in this area as well as an on/off audio instruction cue.

a. Tap "Modify word pool" to display the original word and edit screen.

b. Choose the appropriate sound(s) for the therapy session.

c. Choose the syllable structure (CV, CVC, CCVC, etc.) and deselect or select words that are appropriate for therapy session.

d. Choose specific words by tapping "Deselect All" and tapping to the right of each word to display a "check mark" for the word desired or tap the "check mark" to uncheck. Words are selected when a "check mark" appears next to the word.

e. Add custom words by tapping "edit" and then "+" at the top of the screen to display the "Add Custom Images" screen. This screen allows for uploading the image from your photo library; naming the image; selecting syllable structure, phoneme, and word types; and recording audio for the word. To save custom words, tap "Add" to be returned to the word pool screen, and then tap "Done." Custom words will be saved and appear at the bottom of each word list within the word pool. Repeat Steps c and d above to select the custom word and have it appear in the word pool.

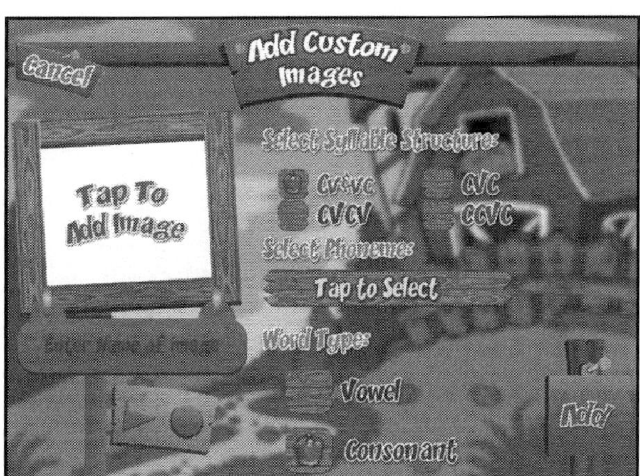


**FIGURE 2–33A.** Smarty Ears custom images screenshot. Reproduced with permission of Smarty Ears, LLC. All rights reserved.

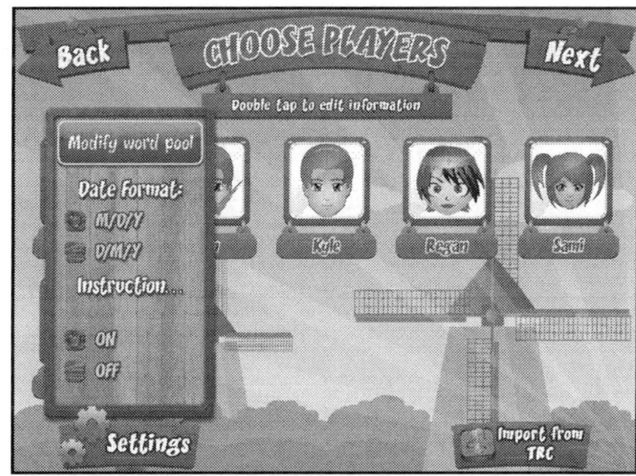


**FIGURE 2–33B.** Smarty Ears modify word pool screenshot. Reproduced with permission of Smarty Ears, LLC. All rights reserved.

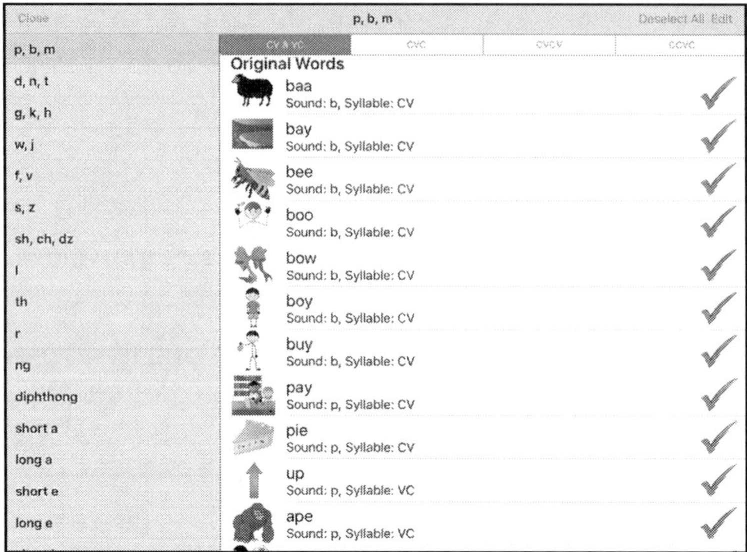

**FIGURE 2–33C.** Smarty Ears original word/edit screenshot. Reproduced with permission of Smarty Ears, LLC. All rights reserved.


### Individual or Small Group Session

Step 1:  With the client sitting aside or across from you, model the target sound and confirm the client is able to approximate the sound. *NOTE*: SLPAs should take initial direction from the supervising SLP in regard to the client's ability and targeted objectives.

Step 2:  Open the Apraxia Ville app and proceed:

    a.  Tap "Select Player."

    b.  Select one or more players for the therapy session and tap "Next."

Step 3:  With the client sitting aside or across from you, give an explanation of what the intended therapy lesson will be (i.e., "today we are using a fun app called Apraxia Ville to practice sounds, syllables, and words"). *NOTE*: SLPAs should take initial direction from the supervising SLP in regard to the client's ability and targeted objectives.

Step 4:  Select one of the three activities to target client objectives:

    a.  The Sound Windows activity is not directly attached to any player and can be used for a warm-up activity and sound practice for individual clients or groups. Change the consonant or vowel by tapping on it and selecting the one to be targeted. Tap the "face" to watch and hear an animation of the sound. Slide the apple across the bar to watch a silent animated production of the sound. Tap the camera icon to switch the view so the clients may view themselves making the targeted sound. Data should be collected separately and as needed as there is not automatic scoring for this activity.

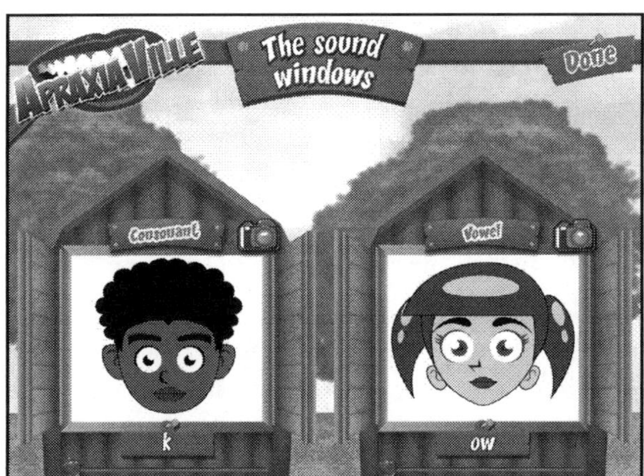

**FIGURE 2–34A.** Smarty Ears sounds window screenshot. Reproduced with permission of Smarty Ears, LLC. All rights reserved.

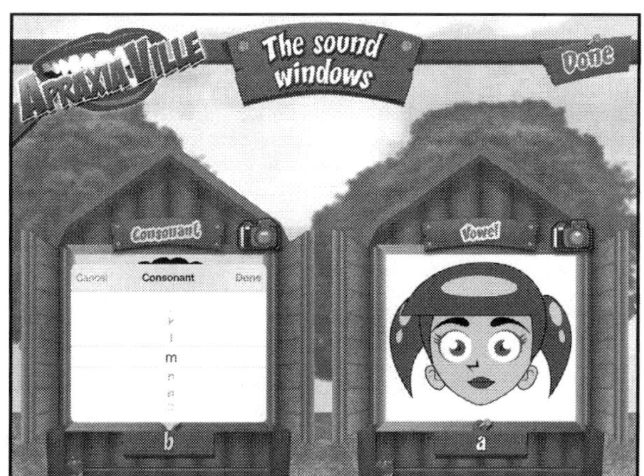

**FIGURE 2–34B.** Smarty Ears sounds window customized screenshot. Reproduced with permission of Smarty Ears, LLC. All rights reserved.

b. Choose "The Farm House" to work on single-word production. Choose the "Syllable Structure" (i.e., CV, VC, CCVC, Bisyllabic, etc.) and the "sound groups" (i.e., consonant groupings and vowels) for the specific client's objectives. *NOTE*: The client's avatar or photo will be displayed. Tap "Next." If more than one client was initially selected for this session, repeat for setup of each client. Score appropriately by tapping on the score icons above the client name/avatar (green/correct, yellow/approximation, red/incorrect). For clients requiring additional support, tap the "Window CUES" to set the specific sound and watch and listen to an animated view of the sound production. Tap the red record button to begin a recording, and tap again to end the recording. Use the green play arrow to listen to the recording for self-monitoring. *NOTE:* Wait until the word "recording . . . " flashes on the screen to begin talking.

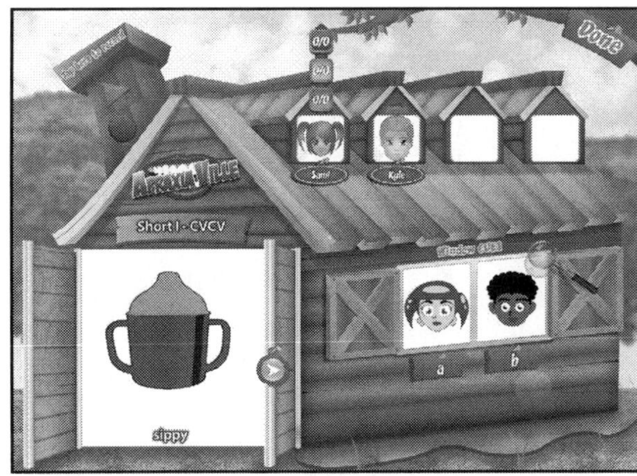

**FIGURE 2–35A.** Smarty Ears farmhouse Screenshot 1. Reproduced with permission of Smarty Ears, LLC. All rights reserved.

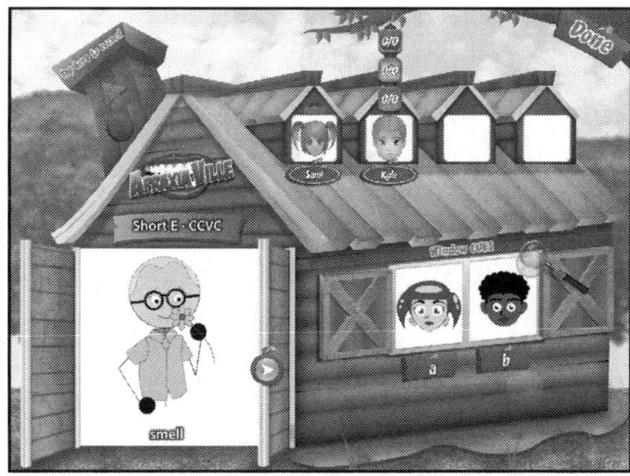

**FIGURE 2–35B.** Smarty Ears farmhouse Screenshot 2. Reproduced with permission of Smarty Ears, LLC. All rights reserved.

c.  Choose "The Words Farm" for multiple-word production. Choose 2 or 3 to indicate the number of words to appear for this activity. *NOTE:* The number of words will remain constant for all clients within a small group. Choose the "Syllable Structure" (i.e., CV, VC, CCVC, Bisyllabic, etc.) and the phoneme (i.e., consonants and vowels) for the specific client's objectives for each word placement. If working in small groups, move between clients by tapping the arrow next to the avatar. Score appropriately by tapping on the score icons (green/correct, yellow/approximation, red/incorrect). Tap the red record button to begin a recording, tap again to end the recording, and use the green play arrow to listen to the recording for self-monitoring. *NOTE:* Wait until the word "recording . . . " flashes on the screen to begin talking.

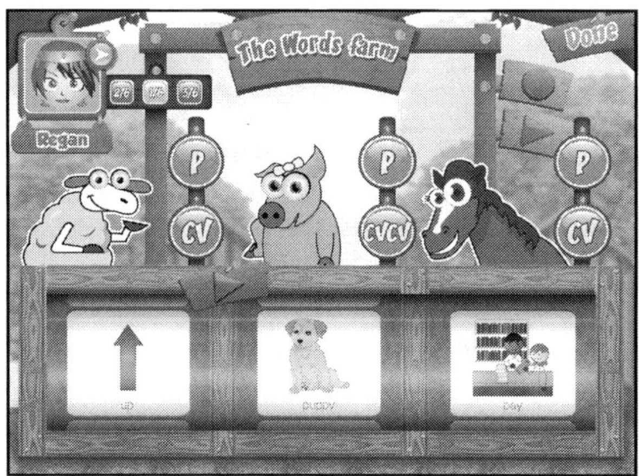

**FIGURE 2–36.** Smarty Ears Words Farm screenshot. Reproduced with permission of Smarty Ears, LLC. All rights reserved.

Step 5:  At the end of the session, review the session results and create a homework (carryover) worksheet by returning to the home screen and tapping on "Reports & Homework."

a.  Tap the client name/avatar to review results. The data include date of practice, target phoneme, syllable structure level, percent accuracy, and number of words attempted. This information can be printed for the client file or shared via email.

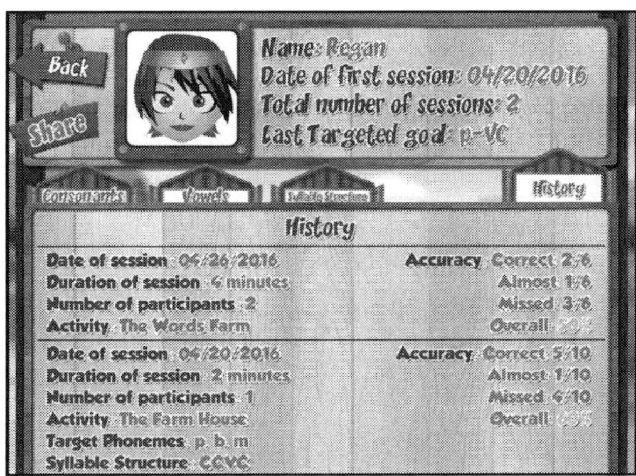

**FIGURE 2–37A.** Smarty Ears Results 1 screenshot. Reproduced with permission of Smarty Ears, LLC. All rights reserved.

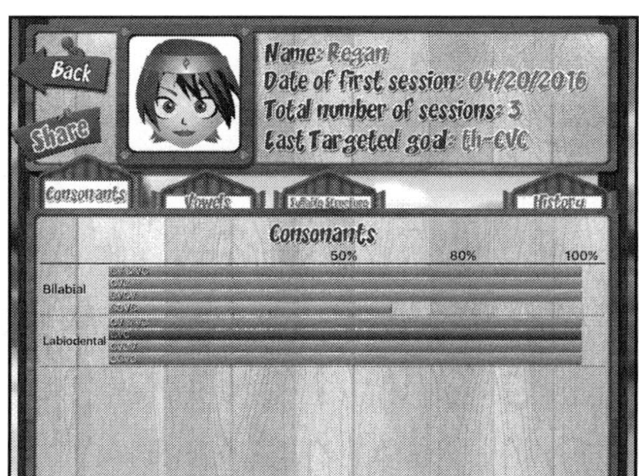

**FIGURE 2–37B.** Smarty Ears Results 2 screenshot. Reproduced with permission of Smarty Ears, LLC. All rights reserved.

b. Tap "Homework" and choose the "Homework File" by selecting the phoneme and syllable structure for the carryover. Tap "Open" to create the file. The file can be printed or shared via email.

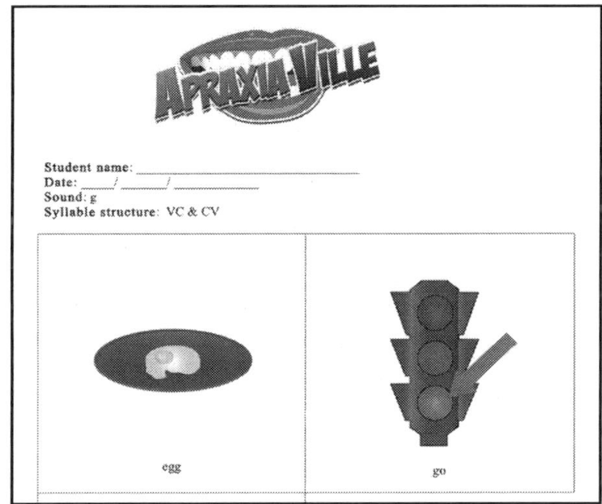

**FIGURE 2–38A.** Smarty Ears Homework example screenshot. Reproduced with permission of Smarty Ears, LLC. All rights reserved.

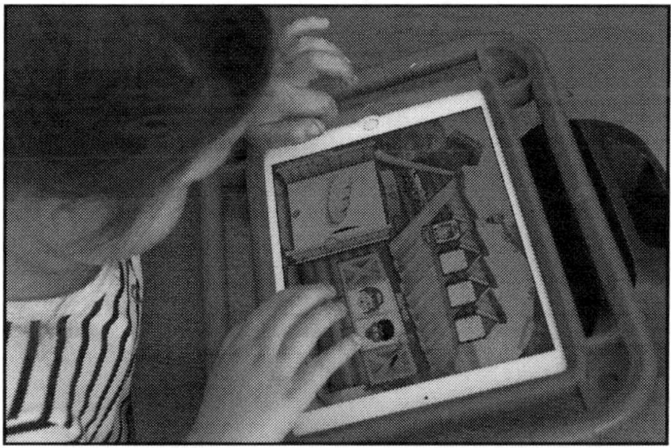

**FIGURE 2–38B.** Hannah Clark Apraxia Ville.

## Activity 3

Apraxia RainbowBee to elicit opportunities of utterances for clients who have an apraxic component that impacts their speech production.

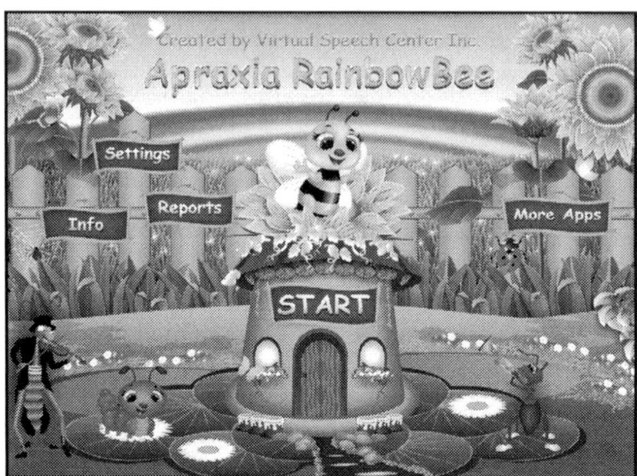

**FIGURE 2–39.** Virtual Speech Center apraxia rainbow main screenshot. Reproduced with permission of Virtual Speech Center.

Apraxia RainbowBee by Virtual Speech Center is a multistep, multimodality program with colorful graphics, photos, audio, and video target. The app includes two fun games: Flashcards and a board game. Apraxia RainbowBee features three levels of complexity with the ability to manipulate the prompting (cue) of visual, auditory, tactile, and lexical stimuli presented to the client. Adding customized images and recordings is a valuable feature and makes speech therapy more individualized.

To download Apraxia RainbowBee or to be able to view an in-depth tutorial, visit https://www .virtualspeechcenter.com

**FIGURE 2–40.** Virtual Speech Center QR code.

### *Task Setup*

Step 1:  Create client profiles and adjust settings. Add client targeted objectives as needed prior to the therapy session.

a.  Open the app and tap "Settings" to enable the built-in reward system, assign player turns (i.e., Alternate Count: up to five trials per client per turn), adjust the scoring sounds (i.e., three unique sound options), remove the text from the image/word, or add custom words and images to individualize the session. *NOTE:* Settings will remain constant for all clients during the session time. It's important to make sure the settings are appropriate for all clients within the session.

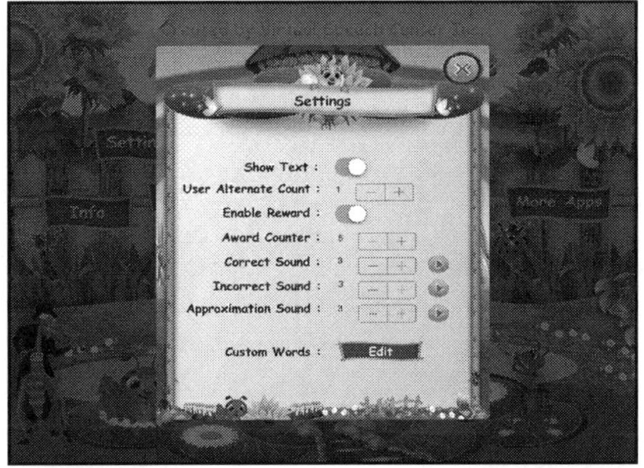

**FIGURE 2–41A.** Virtual Speech Center settings screenshot. Reproduced with permission of Virtual Speech Center.

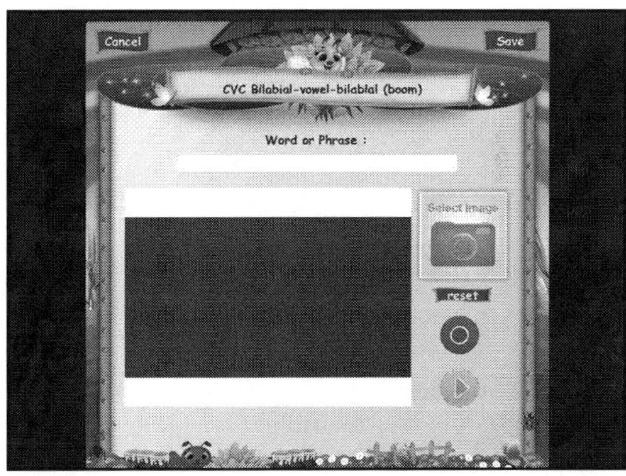

**FIGURE 2–41B.** Virtual Speech Center add image screenshot. Reproduced with permission of Virtual Speech Center.

b.  Tap "Start" to begin, "Add Student" to add client names, and "Save" when finished adding clients.

c.  Tap "Client Name(s)" to choose all clients participating in the session, choose either activity (Flashcards or Board Game), and tap "Next."

d.  Select the syllable structure (i.e., VC, CV, CVC, two-syllable words, three-syllable words, or phrases) and identify and select (i.e., EDIT) only the words to be targeted for each client.

> For a more efficient therapy session, always prepare lesson/task setup prior to therapy session. SLPAs should take initial direction from the supervising SLP as to the appropriate targets for each client.

### *Individual or Small Group Session*

Step 1:  With the client sitting aside or across from you, explain the intended therapy lesson (i.e., "today we will be practicing sounds, syllables, and words with the Apraxia RainbowBee app"). *NOTE:* SLPAs should take initial direction from the supervising SLP in regard to the client's ability and targeted objectives.

Step 2:  Tap on client names for all who are participating in the therapy session.

Step 3:  Choose an activity: Flashcards or Board Game. *NOTE:* The activity will remain the same for each client.

Step 4:  Confirm that the targeted objectives have been properly set for each client and modify if needed (i.e., CV, CVC, and phoneme). Tap "Next" to begin the session.

Step 5:  When the Flashcards activity is selected, the image or a "nonsense word" will appear.

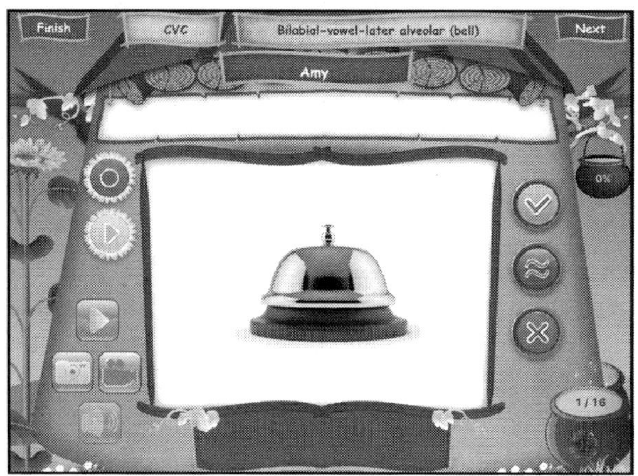


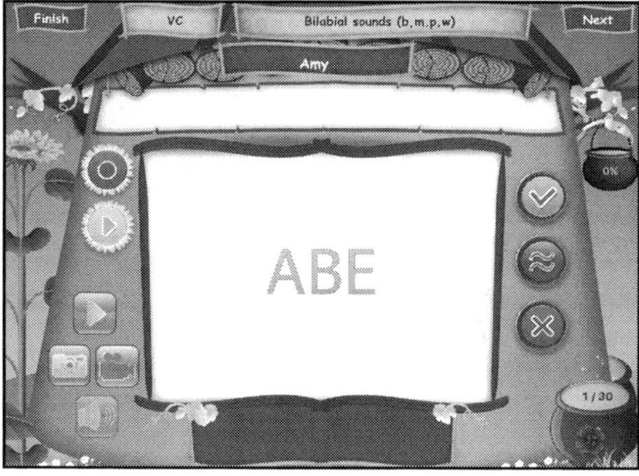


**FIGURE 2–42A.** Virtual Speech Center Flashcard Screenshot 1. Reproduced with permission of Virtual Speech Center.

**FIGURE 2–42B.** Virtual Speech Center Flashcard Screenshot 2. Reproduced with permission of Virtual Speech Center.

a.  Begin the session for the client's name that appears at the top of the screen. Set the cueing icons (i.e., tap the camera icon to display the image or word, tap the video camera icon to display a realistic voiced model, tap the speaker icon to turn off the audio for the voice model). *NOTE:* The visual cue displaying the text above the image can be turned off within the settings.

b.  Tap the "play arrow" icon to activate the cue that was selected.

c.  Use the record button to record a client's production. Use this opportunity for self-monitoring and correcting.

d.  Score as appropriate (correct, approximation, or incorrect), then tap "Next" to present the next flashcard. *NOTE:* Depending on the "Alternate Count" setting chosen prior to the therapy session, a new flashcard will be presented for the same client or a new flashcard will be presented for the next client. The clients' names will appear above the stimulus at the top of the screen.

e.  If the "Enable Reward" option and the "Award Counter" have been activated within the settings, "small bees" will appear on the stem of the flower on the left side of the screen as the client elicits correct responses. A variety of leveled puzzle games are offered upon completing the number of correct responses.

f.  Repeat the above steps for additional clients in the therapy session.

g.  Tap "Finish" to end the board game and view session results.

Step 6:  When the Board Game activity is selected:

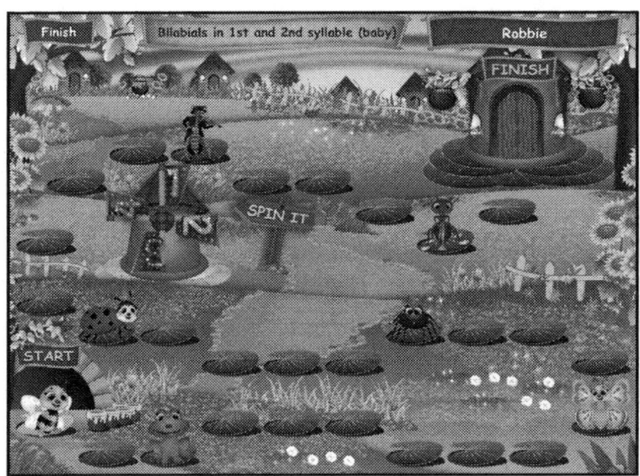


**FIGURE 2–43A.**  Virtual Speech Center board game screenshot. Reproduced with permission of Virtual Speech Center.

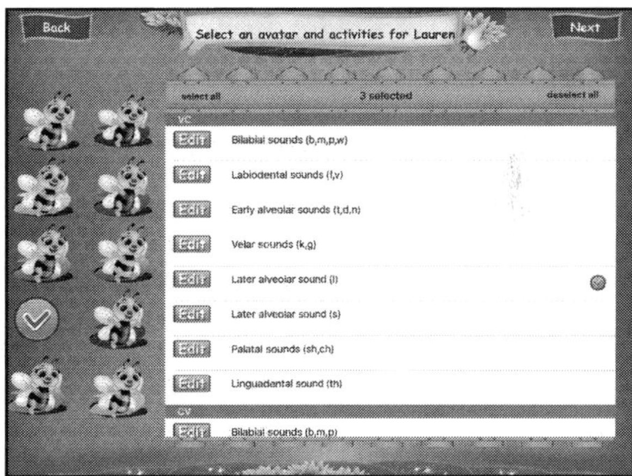


**FIGURE 2–43B.**  Virtual Speech Center avatar setup screenshot. Reproduced with permission of Virtual Speech Center.

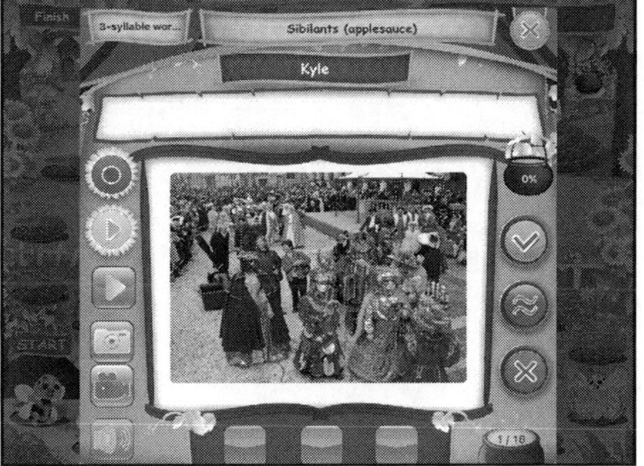


**FIGURE 2–43C.**  Virtual Speech Center board game stimuli screenshot. Reproduced with permission of Virtual Speech Center.

a.  Confirm that the targeted objectives have been set properly for the client and modify if needed (i.e., CV, CVC, and phoneme) and allow the client to choose a bee avatar as a playing piece. Tap "Next" to set up the avatar and confirm objectives for additional clients and to begin.

b.  The client's name and objective will appear at the top of the screen. Allow the client to spin the spinner to move his or her representative avatar and display the stimuli for practice.

c.  Set the "cueing" icons (i.e., tap the camera icon to display the image or word, tap the video camera icon to display a realistic voiced model, tap the speaker icon to turn off the audio for the voice model). *NOTE:* The visual cue displaying the text above the image can be turned off within the settings.

d.  Tap the "play arrow" icon to activate the cue that was selected. *NOTE:* The number of consecutive turns per player is dependent upon the "Alternate Count" setting chosen prior to the therapy session. It is suggested that the "Alternate Count" be set to "1" for board game play to alternate one turn between clients.

e.  Use the record button to record a client's production. Use this opportunity for self-monitoring and correcting.

f.  Score as appropriate: correct, approximation, or incorrect. Tap "X" to close the stimuli.

g.  Repeat for additional clients.

h.  Tap "Finish" to end the board game and view session results.

Step 7:  Review and document session results in the client file. Results may also be accessed from the main screen at any time by tapping "Reports."

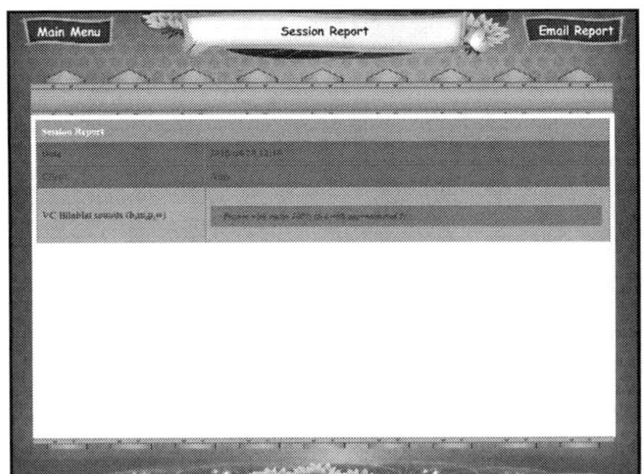

**FIGURE 2–44A.** Virtual Speech Center session results Screenshot 1. Reproduced with permission of Virtual Speech Center.

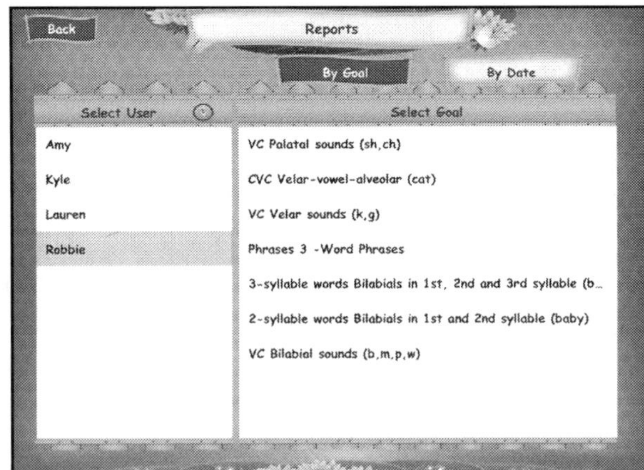

**FIGURE 2–44B.** Virtual Speech Center session results Screenshot 2. Reproduced with permission of Virtual Speech Center.

## Activity 4

Tackling Apraxia CV & CVC Early Sounds by Mia McDaniel for clients needing to improve intelligibility by working on early sounds. Versatility to use word/picture cards with your personal Cariboo game!

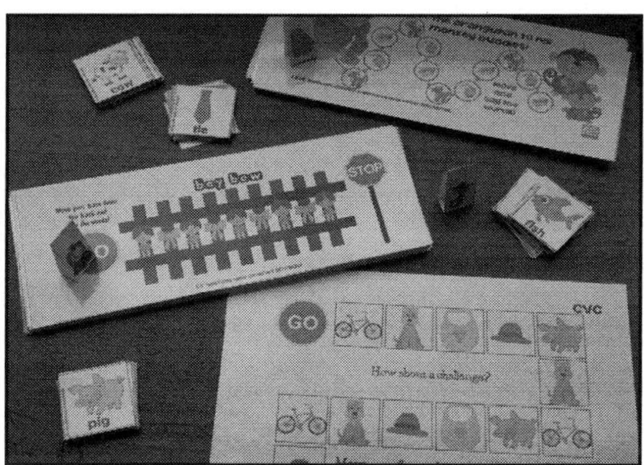

**FIGURE 2–45.** Tackling Apraxia product image.

Tackling Apraxia by Mia McDaniel, MA, CCC/SLP, is an activity that addresses early sounds, /b, j, p, t, d, k, g, m, n, w, h, f/. This activity contains CV and CVC word/picture cards, CV and CVC pacing cards, CVC challenge boards, and customizable open-ended boards.

To download Tackling Apraxia, visit https://www.teacherspayteachers.com/Product/Tackling-Apraxia-CV-CVC-Early-Sounds-Edition-bptdkgmn-jwhf-1106219

**FIGURE 2–46.** Putting Words in Your Mouth QR code.

For a more effective and efficient therapy session, this activity should be prepared and can be printed on cardstock and laminated for durability prior to the therapy session.

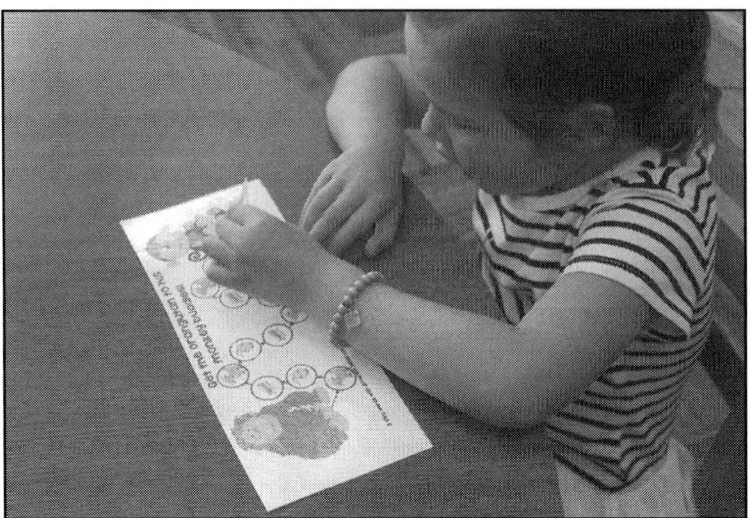

**FIGURE 2–47.** Hannah Clark apraxia card.

### *Individual or Small Group Session*

Step 1:  With the client sitting aside or across from you, explain the intended therapy lesson (i.e., "today we will be practicing sounds and words using these fun characters and cards"). *NOTE:* SLPAs should take initial direction from the supervising SLP in regard to the client's ability and targeted objectives.

Step 2:  Place the appropriate picture/word card, pacing card, challenge board, or open-ended board in front of the client to address specific client objectives:

   a.  CV or CVC picture/word card to teach words in isolation: bow, tie, cat, moon, etc. Practice until the client is proficient before moving to the pacing cards.

   b.  CV or CVC pacing cards to practice repetition of successfully learned words: pea/pow, key/car, bow/bee/tie, and so on. Practice until the client is proficient before moving to the challenge boards.

   c.  CV or CVC challenge boards to practice five alternating CVC words: toe, cow, bow, pie, key, and so on. Practice until the client is proficient before moving to the open-ended boards.

   d.  Open-ended boards that allow for writing in your own targets for specific customization for client.

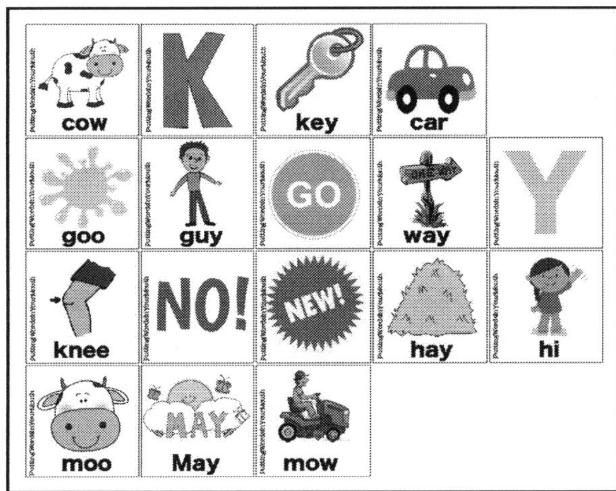

**FIGURE 2–48A.** Mia McDaniel Putting Words in Your Mouth picture word card screenshot. Reproduced with permission of Mia McDaniel, MA, CCC-SLP, http://www.puttingwordsin-yourmouth.com

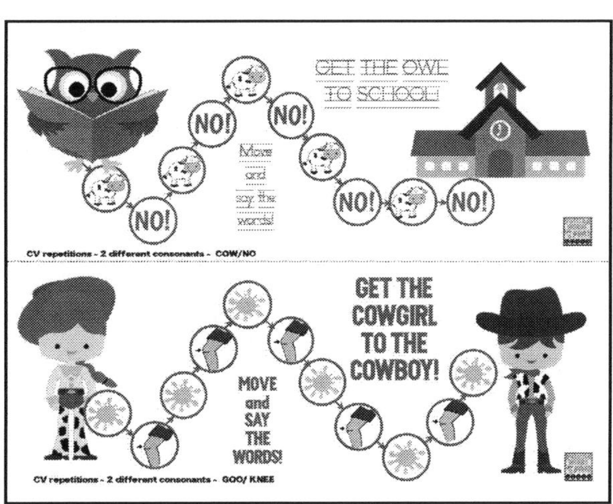



**FIGURE 2–48B.** Mia McDaniel Putting Words in Your Mouth pacing card screenshot. Reproduced with permission of Mia McDaniel, MA, CCC-SLP, http://www.puttingwordsinyour-mouth.com

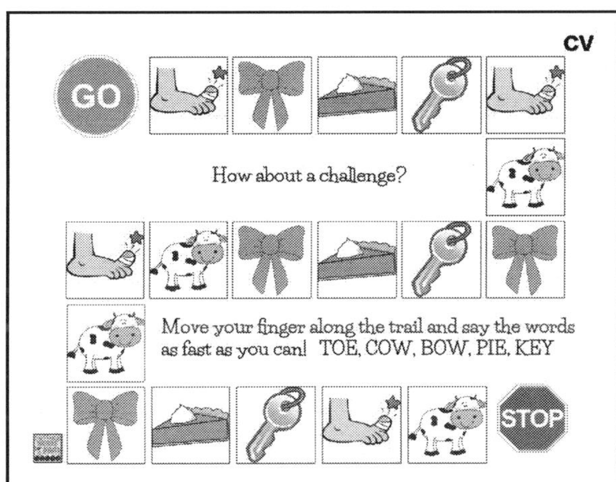



**FIGURE 2–48C.** Mia McDaniel Putting Words in Your Mouth challenge board screenshot. Reproduced with permission of Mia McDaniel, MA, CCC-SLP, http://www.puttingwordsin yourmouth.com

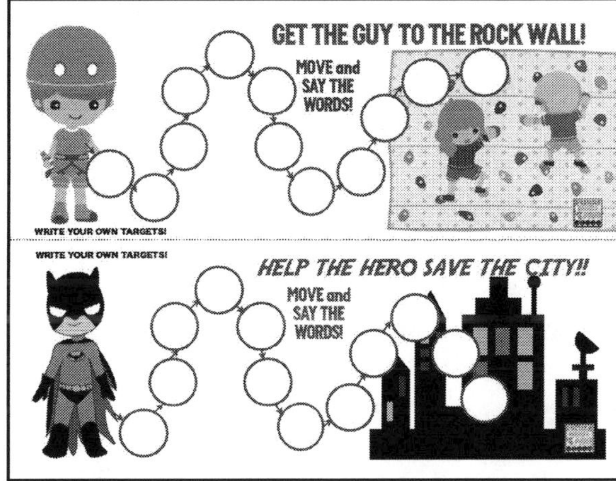



**FIGURE 2–48D.** Mia McDaniel Putting Words in Your Mouth open-ended board screenshot. Reproduced with permission of Mia McDaniel, MA, CCC-SLP, http://www.puttingwordsin yourmouth.com

Step 3:  If the client is working at the CV word/picture level, use the cards individually or a fun option is to place the individual cards in a Cariboo game to add an extra element of engagement.

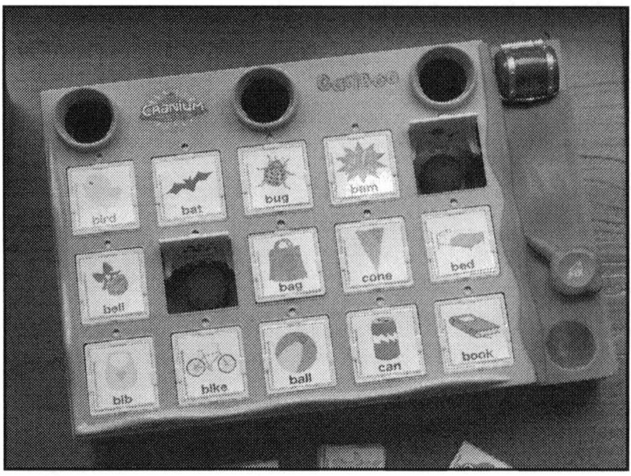

**FIGURE 2–49.** Cariboo example.

Step 4: If using one of the CV or CVC pacing cards, allow the client to choose his or her favorite hopper (board piece) or any other small object to move along the card.

Step 5: If needed, model word(s) for client. Have the client move the hoppers along the card while saying the sound/word or word sequence. Initially, encourage rhythm and slow rate, increasing speed as the client becomes more proficient. As the client becomes faster and more proficient, time the client and encourage him or her to beat his or her own time in each trial.

### Essential Resources

For more excellent ideas, freebies, and low-cost resources from Mia McDaniel, visit http://www.puttingwordsinyourmouth.com

**FIGURE 2–50.** Putting Words in Your Mouth QR code

## REFERENCE

Super Duper Publications. (2013). Word FLiPS for iPad (Version 1.0.2) [Mobile application software]. Retrieved from http://itunes.apple.com

# Communicative Intent



Communicative intent is the use of any type of behavior to deliver a message to a communication partner. Intentional communicative intent is the purposeful delivery of this message to convey information to another person. Nonintentional communicative intent is a spontaneous behavior that expresses a need but is not purposeful or directed toward a communication partner. Intentional communicative intent is an essential element to the development of a functional communication system. This is where children show a desire to communicate with another child or adult using a behavior that is widely understood and socially acceptable. Children with speech and language delays may struggle communicating secondary to their inability to understand the value of intentional communication. These children may display nonintentional communicative intent, also called behavioral communication. Behavioral communication is often expressed by crying, screaming, and using other more automatic types of communication. Once a child understands the relationship between intentional communicative intent and reinforcement, a world of possibilities opens up. The activities included in this chapter will help you address the communicative intent needs of children on your caseload. As you become familiar with these activities, you will begin to gain confidence working with children with communication intent needs and, under the guidance of your supervising speech-language pathologist (SLP), can develop your own therapy materials to fit the therapy goals established by the SLP.

## ACTIVITIES FOR COMMUNICATIVE INTENT

### Objectives

The following are some sample objectives for communicative intent within a therapy session:

1. Client will reach toward a desired item indicating a choice between items without prompting in 9 out of 10 opportunities across three sessions.

2. Client will use specific gestures such as knocking, signing "more," waving "bye-bye," or signing, "all done" to indicate a desire for a specific item, gain access to desired items, and request cessation of an activity in 8 out of 10 opportunities across three sessions.

3. Client will establish shared attention by making eye contact with the therapist, looking to the desired item and back to the therapist in 8 out of 10 opportunities across three sessions.

4. Client will point to a desired item with an isolated index finger to indicate desire for the item in 8 out of 10 opportunities across three sessions.

## Introduction to the Knock-Knock Box Program

The knock-knock box (KKB) program, created by speech-language therapists and behavior specialists Amy Prince and Amber Ladd, has the capacity to teach a wide variety of speech and language skills. For the purposes of this chapter, all communicative intent activities will use the knock-knock box. The focus will be on the beginning communicator and the process of teaching intentional communicative intent.

### *What It Is*

The knock-knock box is simply a clear box with a well-fitting lid that contains a variety of toys. You want to be able to keep the box shut when a client attempts to pull it open because many will attempt to bypass communication and access it independently. There is no one right way to build a knock-knock box. The beauty of this program is that the items within the box can be chosen to match each client's individualized interests and/or specific goals. As long as the guidelines are met, the box will be effective in teaching any skill that you choose.

While teaching the initial portions of the knock-knock box program, your language should match the level of the client or be slightly higher. While you are using physical prompting to ensure communicative intent, your language model should be single words. The only words you should say at this point are "knock-knock," "open," "more," "bye-bye," labeling the item that the client chooses with a single word, and your "play words." An occasional "yay!" or "good!" is okay to use but you really want to emphasize that the words or communicative acts are resulting in the really exciting items that they are accessing.

Creating a language-rich environment is important for clients to ensure that they are being exposed to a wide variety of vocabulary and language structures. While working with minimally verbal clients, it is important that EVERY WORD we use in a session has a very specific purpose. The words used at this point should consist of modeling the request words, verbally prompting the request words if you are able to fade out your model, and reinforcing the request words with the request words again. It may sound redundant, but by only utilizing these words, we are emphasizing that these are really important words. Using a limited vocabulary also results in our voice not being "tuned out" because we use more words than our clients are able to take in at one time.

Once the client is able to use the gestures independently to communicate his or her desires, it is time to start increasing the verbal attempts at these words. While modeling the single words, it is extremely effective to pair visual hand signals with your model. As your expectations increase, the visual prompt of the hand signal can be a less intrusive way of prompting a sound/word and is easier to fade out than continued verbal prompting.

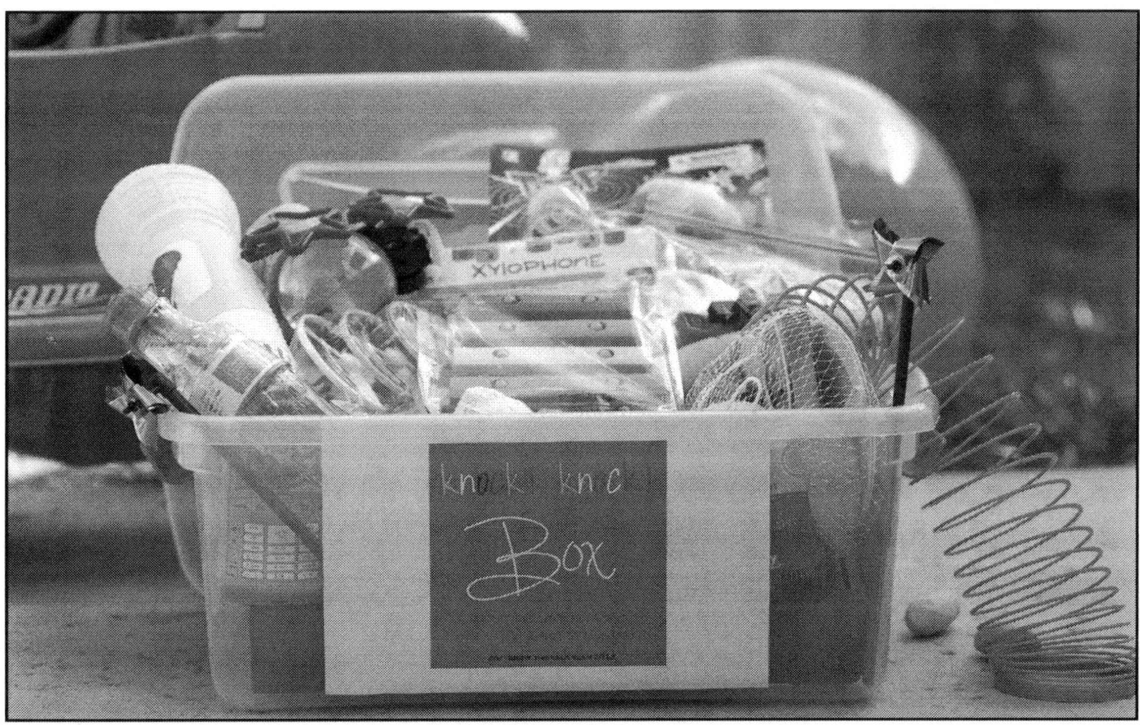


**FIGURE 3–1.** Knock-knock box pic. Reproduced with permission of The Talk Team.

When choosing the toys that your knock-knock box will contain, it is important to consider the following factors. Each toy should be clearly named with a noun and a verb. For example, a car becomes "car" and "drive" and helicopter becomes "copter" and "fly." The items should be small enough that you can have a wide selection in your box at all times. It should be relatively easy to manipulate by a small client. The only exception to this is a toy that requires a client to ask for your help to utilize. This can be a powerful motivator for a client as long as asking for help is not too difficult. "Asking" for help can be as simple as teaching the client to hand the object to you. If there are multiple people using the knock-knock box, it is important that each speech-language pathology assistant (SLPA) use the same words for each item. It can be helpful to put labels on each item to maintain fidelity between teachers.

### What It Is Not

The knock-knock box is not simply a box of toys. You provide the magic that makes the knock-knock box become an effective and motivating tool! If the box is simply left with the client, the interaction that creates communicative intent will be lost. If the box is available and played with at will at any point, it will lose its ability to create meaningful communicative exchanges.

### Before Beginning

Before you begin the activity as outlined below, it is important to establish rapport with your client. Forming a relationship and establishing yourself as a person that your client wants to spend time with is paramount. It can be scary and overwhelming for our clients to interact with someone new, especially if the time spent is demanding, hard, or unpleasant. When a fun, interactive relationship is established, trust is developed and our clients are more willing to interact and learn new skills. The more fun you have, the more skills you will be able to teach. If your clients view you as someone who is engaging, silly, and the deliverer of everything they want, you have reached a point to begin teaching.

Additionally, you need to have a plan to arrange your environment to keep the client physically present with you. Face to face is the best scenario, but if you must start with a young client on your lap, that can work as well. Sitting is more effective, but this can be used while standing. It is rarely, if ever, effective to chase a client around while carrying your knock-knock box!

### In the Beginning

Initially, you want to "show" the clients how fun the box is while teaching them how to appropriately access the toys. When a client has significant speech and language delays, there is often an accompanying delay in functional play skills. Clients may not play with toys appropriately or show any interest in toys at all. It may be necessary to watch the client interact with available items and play with them in a variety of ways to see how the client is motivated. If necessary, you may need to show how each toy works so that the client understands that they are fun. We often assume that our clients "know" how fun a toy is or that they have even seen it before! It is important to follow the clients' lead and observe what they do with a toy and determine what makes it reinforcing to them. While we may have an idea of what makes a toy fun, your client may have a completely different idea. It is important to eventually teach clients how to play appropriately, but when teaching communicative intent, clients should be allowed to play "their way" so that motivation is maintained. If a client is forced to play your way, the toys may lose their reinforcing components and the desire to play can be lost. If your client has intact play skills, it can be helpful to allow the client to look into the box briefly before you initiate a trial. If you decide to use this step, be careful that you keep this portion very brief so that the client doesn't get too many "freebies." Once you have visually gained the client's attention and he or she has demonstrated interest in the box, it is time to teach!

### Teaching Beginning Gestures

Initially, the client must demonstrate a reach toward a desired item. Visual and physical prompting may be necessitated to initiate this reach. Often clients can be distracted by the environment or themselves and need extra engagement to realize that fun items/activities are present and available. Gaining attention can typically be prompted by holding items close to the client's visual field, using a sensory strategy such as driving a vehicle on the client's arms, tickling (when appropriate), or modeling playing with the item. With beginning communicators, visual prompting is preferred over verbal cues. Clients with expressive delays often display receptive delays as well. These clients may not always respond to their name being called or follow simple directions, so verbal prompting can be ineffective and may be ignored or not understood.

### *Playing*

While the client is playing with the toy, model appropriate phrasing (one to two words) that you would want to hear the client say at some point in the future. A good standard rule is "MLU plus 1 or 2." Mean length of utterance, or MLU, is the average number of morphemes in a client's utterance. If your client is not saying words, your utterances should never be more than two words. If your client uses single words, your sentences should never exceed three words. This standard should be adhered to throughout your speech and language session. All directions, cues, prompts, and models should fall into this "MLU plus 1 or 2" guideline. If the client is playing with a car, you might state, "You are driving car!" "That is a car," "You are playing with the car," or "vroom" repeatedly while the client is playing with it, regardless if he or she is playing with it appropriately or attending to your voice. Your goal is to become the voice in

**TABLE 3–1.** The KKB Program at a Glance

| Skill | Example |
| --- | --- |
| Request to open the box | Various target responses: <br> Knocking (use hand-over-hand guidance if necessary) <br> "Open" |
| Anticipatory eye contact | With items that require activation, use phrases like "Ready . . . Set . . . " and wait for intentional eye contact before stating "go" and providing activation |
| Requesting recurrence | Target response: signing "more" or stating "more" verbally |
| Requesting the items inside by name | Target response: "truck" |
| Requesting the items with a verb + noun combination | Target response: "drive truck" |
| Receptive identification of objects and/or pictures | "Find truck" |
| Receptive identification of functions | "Show me the one that flies" |
| Asking/answering questions | Put object in brown lunch bag <br> Child: "What's in the bag?" |
| Requesting items with functions | "Can I verb the noun?" <br> Child: "Can I drive the truck?" |
| Specific vocabulary | Use the list below for a variety of ways to use each toy and elicit specific vocabulary targets |
| Turn-taking | Target response: "My turn," "Your turn" |

*Source:* Reproduced with permission of The Talk Team.

his or her head so that someday down the road, the words that you continuously model are the words that come to mind and ultimately out of his or her mouth. It is also appropriate to use the same words as your "request" when you take the item back from the client. If you repeatedly request the car with the phrase, "Can I drive car?" you are demonstrating an acceptable way to verbally request. There are a variety of effective ways to play with the car when you take it from the client, before you place it back in the box. These techniques include modeling appropriate play (i.e., driving the car), playing with a tactile component (i.e., driving the car up the client's arm), or using anticipatory play. Inserting this play scheme between turns will keep your client engaged and wanting to continue to play with you. Remember that YOU are what IS fun, not the car, so don't be afraid to be silly and try different things. You never know what will gain each client's attention.

### Filling Your Box

These are just a few of the items you might put in a KKB, but it is a constantly growing and changing kit. Discount stores and dollar bins are great places to find content, and there is no limit to what you can use!

**TABLE 3–2.** KK Box Builder

| Object (What Toy) | Targets (What I Say) |
| --- | --- |
| Car | Verbs:  drive, push, crash<br>Concepts:  fast/slow, prepositions, drive on body parts, stop/go, color identification |
| Tube | Verbs:  pull, push ("Pull tube"), I see you<br>Concepts:  long/short, color identification, push/pull |
| Book | Verbs:  read book, turn page, open the _______ (if flap book)<br>Concepts:  picture identification, WH?'s, prediction |
| Bubbles | Verbs:  blow, pop, open bubbles<br>Concepts:  up high/down low, a little/a lot, small/big |
| Phone | Verbs:  talk on phone, push buttons<br>Concepts:  hello/goodbye, open/close, who?'s |
| Top | Verbs:  spin top, stop/go<br>Concepts:  prepositions  (in, on, next to, between) |
| Ball | Verbs:  throw, roll, bounce, kick, catch<br>Concepts:  Where?'s, fast/slow, high/low, big/small, prepositions |
| Play dough | Verbs:  squeeze/roll play dough, push/pull<br>Concepts:  a little/a lot, long/short, big/small, color ID |
| Kazoo | Verbs:  play music, start/stop, blow<br>Concepts:  loud/quiet, dance |

| Object (What Toy) | Targets (What I Say) |
|---|---|
| Slinky | Verbs:  bounce, "boing"<br>Concepts:  up/down, I see you, long/short, sneeze game (on head) |
| Balloon | Verbs:  blow balloon, let go<br>Concepts:  where is it?, fast/slow, big/bigger, long/short, "help me" |
| Microphone | Verbs:  talk/sing microphone<br>Concepts:  loud/quiet, long/short |
| Dice | Verbs:  roll dice<br>Concepts:  big/small, number ID, counting, prepositions, more/less, how many? |
| Pull toy—snakes/lizards | Verbs:  pull<br>Concepts:  long/short, prepositions, stop/go |
| Flashlight | Verbs:  shine ______, turn on/off<br>Concepts:  up/down, high/low, prepositions |
| Pinwheel | Verbs:  blow, spin, go<br>Concepts:  fast/slow, soft/hard, around, spinning |
| Pop-up toy (bird) | Verbs:  push, pop, jump, ready-set-go!<br>Concepts:  up/down, big/little, wait, go |
| Maracas | Verbs:  shake, stop, go<br>Concepts:  fast/slow, dance, loud/quiet |
| Mirrors | Verbs:  look, "see me"<br>Concepts:  Receptive facial feature identification |

*Source:*  Reproduced with permission of The Talk Team.

## Activity 1

Teaching "knock-knock" as a form of intentional communicative intent for approximate ages 12 months to 12 years.

### *Materials Needed*

1. Knock-knock box

> Teaching communicative intent is best done in a one-to-one setting. While we understand that setting and caseload may often cause a need for group therapy, if a client on the caseload is at this level, it is highly recommended to set up an individual session.

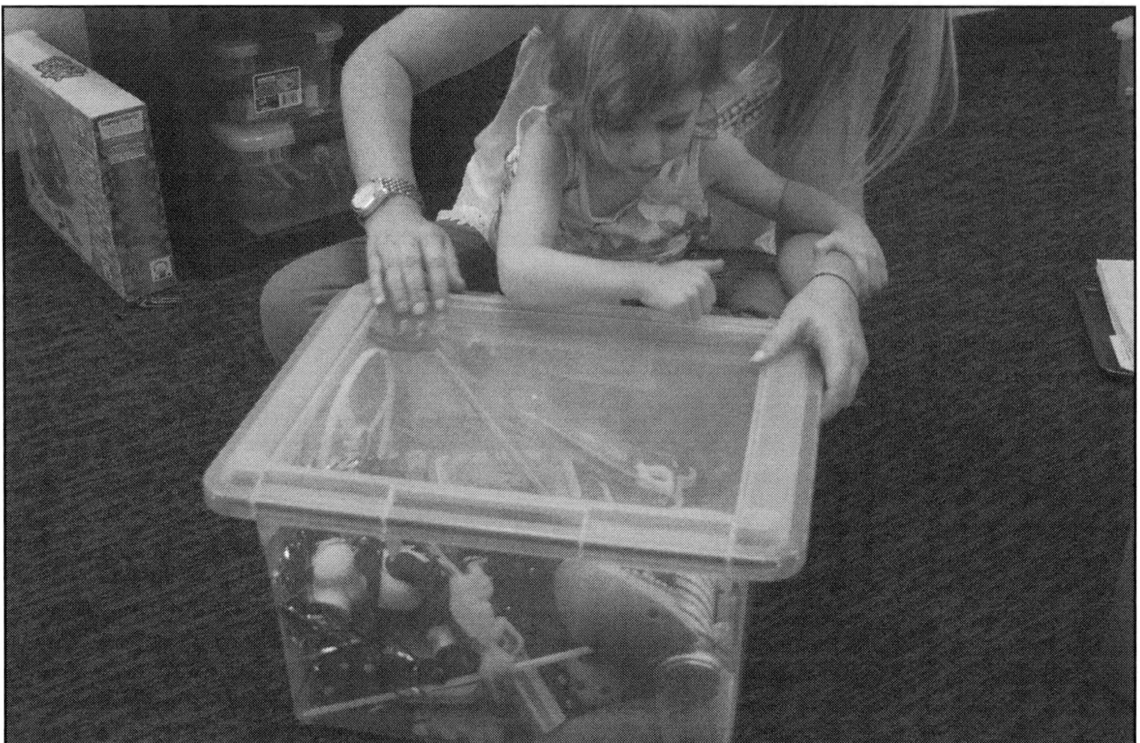

**FIGURE 3–2.** Calista Folsom knock-knock box.

### *Individual or Small Group Session*

Step 1:  Teaching the "knock"

    a.  Present the box to the client while modeling knocking on the lid and at the same time stating, "Knock-knock!"

    b.  Wait for 1 to 2 seconds to give the client an opportunity to imitate your action. If the client does not imitate the knock, initiate hand-over-hand prompting so that the client is successful with knocking on the box.

    c.  Once the client has imitated knocking or you have hand over hand prompted the response, state "Open!" while opening the box and allowing the client to choose a toy. Make sure that the box is opened for him within 1 to 2 seconds of the target behavior (knocking). It is important that the selected reinforcers, in this case the opening of the box, are delivered in this very brief time frame so the connection between the "request" and the delivery of the reinforcer is recognized.

    d.  Once the client has picked a toy, place the lid back on and remove the box. The removal of the box is important initially to ensure that it doesn't serve as a visual cue to knock again. Once the client understands how the knock-knock box works, leaving the box or using it is a table is acceptable.

    e.  Allow the client to play with the toy for approximately 10 to 20 seconds and then take the toy back and place it back in the box.

    f.  Immediately present the box again and proceed with the same sequence.

## Activity 2

Teaching anticipatory eye contact and shared attention as a form of intentional communicative intent for approximate ages of 6 months to 10 years.

Anticipatory responding is an amazing tool to gain engagement and ultimately shared attention from your client. This technique is used to gain clients' attention and teach them that our presence equals "great things"—much like intentional communicative intent. Anticipatory responding is the act of gaining eye contact (or other voluntary behaviors that can be shaped) that results in the activation of a toy or activity. For example, when playing with the car, you can state, "I'm . . . going . . . to . . . (insert anticipatory look and pause) . . . DRIVE!!" and then drive the car up to the client, resulting in tickles, the car driving under the shirt, or anything silly and fun that makes the client laugh or smile. The goal is to use your tone of voice and BIG anticipation so that the client begins to predict at what point you will deliver the "fun." Once this occurs, you wait expectantly for eye contact or a glance toward your face and consider that the "communication" intent of the client.

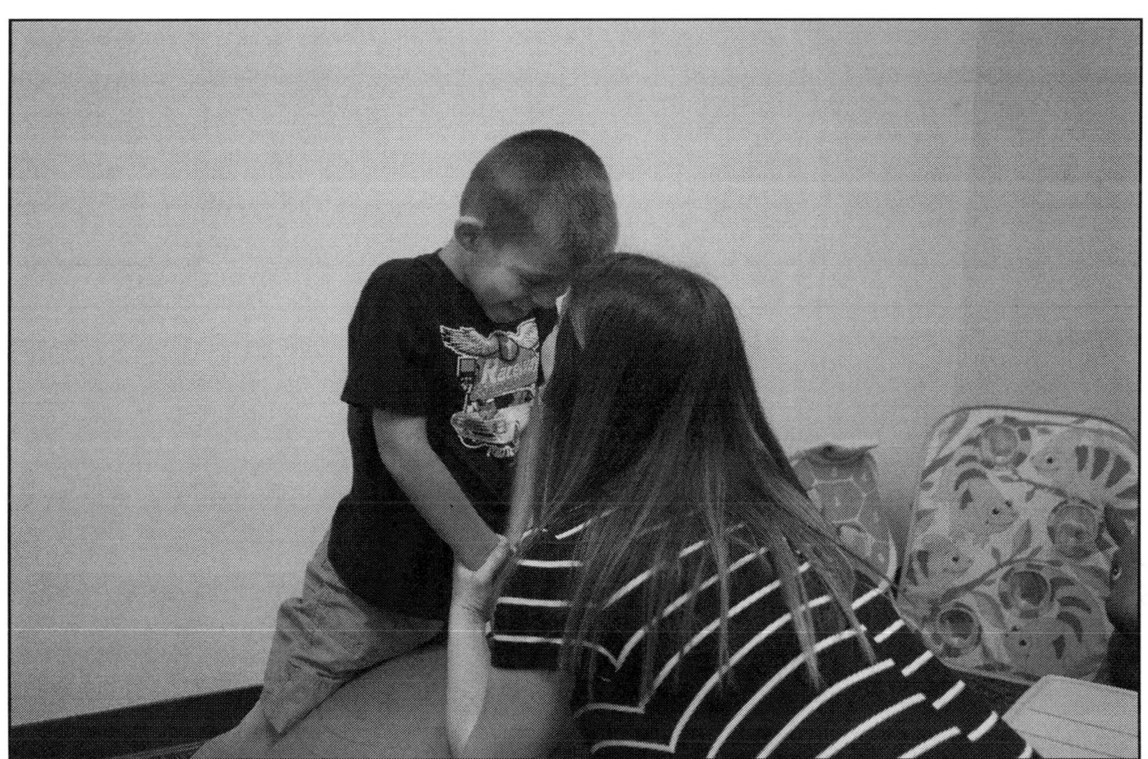

**FIGURE 3–3.** Koen Withrow eye contact.

If your client is not responding to your anticipatory activities with intention eye contact, you can choose another voluntary behavior to shape. At the point of your anticipatory look and pause, if you see a brief glance toward you or the item, you can accept that as the communication you are looking for and provide the reinforcement. Once you have reinforced this behavior and delivered the activation of the fun activity, you can start waiting for a little bigger glance in your direction and eventually shape this into eye contact. This process should be slow and you should wait for a small shift in the client's behavior that signals intent you'd like to reinforce.

### Materials Needed

1. Knock-knock box

2. Any reinforcers that the client exhibits interests in

3. Optional: any other toy or activity that captures the client's interests

> Teaching communicative intent is best done in a one-on-one setting. While we understand that setting and size of caseload may require group therapy, if a client on the caseload is at this level, it is highly recommended to set up an individual session.

### Individual or Small Group Session

Step 1: Teaching anticipatory responding

    a. Introduce a play routine that includes an anticipation step. The activity should be selected based on what the client is showing interest in at the time. For example, "I'm . . . going . . . to . . . TICKLE YOU!!" Make sure that you include a pause between each word so that the anticipation is exaggerated.

    b. Practice the routine two to three times so that the client understands what the result of the routine will be (the tickle).

    c. Once the routine has been practiced, introduce the beginning of the routine, including expectant pauses between each word.

    d. At the end of the routine, use an expectant pause and an expectant look and wait for purposeful eye contact. Once eye contact is achieved, deliver the end of the routine (i.e., the tickle).

    e. If eye contact is not achieved, look for a different behavior that can be shaped into intentional eye contact. If a client moves his or her face toward you, looks in your direction, or reaches his or her hand toward you, recognize that these are all behaviors that can be comprehended as intentional communication.

f.  If you begin to shape an alternative behavior, gradually expect the behavior that is exhibited to become closer to intentional eye contact. This procedure should be done extremely slowly so that the client does not become discouraged and continues to participate in these play routines.

## Activity 3

Teaching the sign for "more" to request recurrence of a play routine or item.

Once the client has learned the "knock" or is not demonstrating frustration with the learning process, you can introduce "more."

### *Materials Needed*

1.  Knock-knock box

2.  Any other toy or activity that captures the client's interests

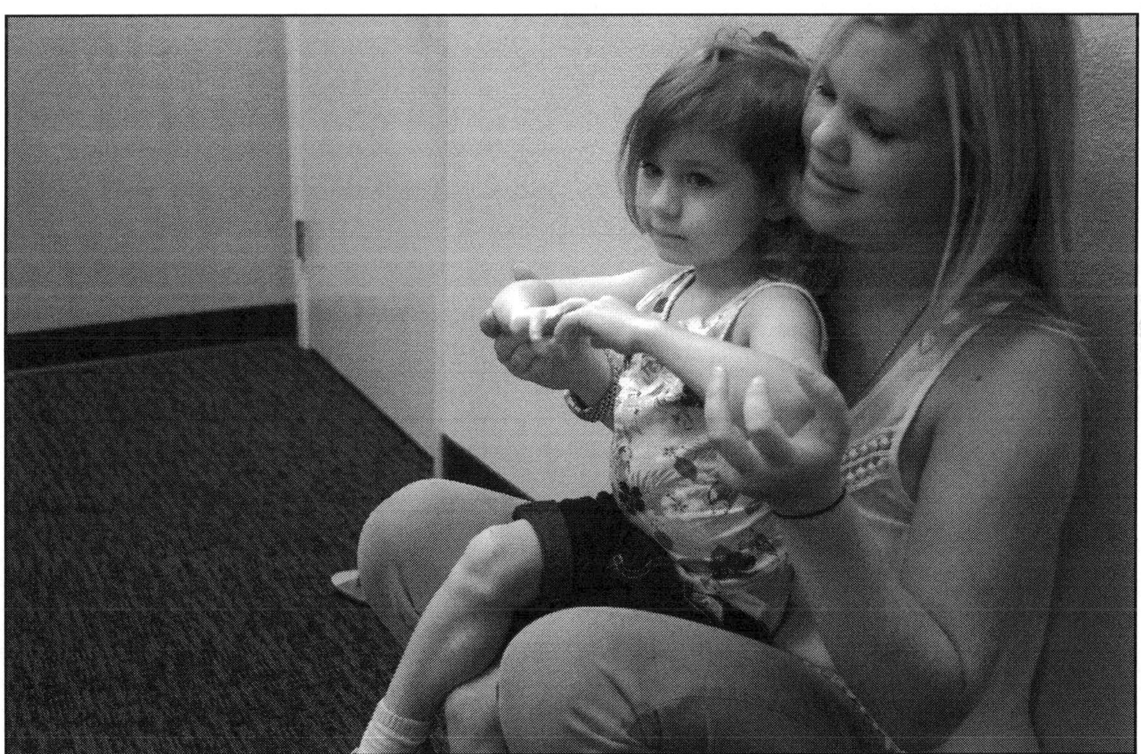

**FIGURE 3–4.** Calista Folsom "more" with Cara Lambert (therapist).

> Teaching communicative intent is best done in a one-to-one setting. While we understand that setting and caseload may often cause a need for group therapy, if a client on the caseload is at this level, it is highly recommended to set up an individual session.

### Individual or Small Group Session

Step 1:  Introducing more

    a.  After a client has knocked on the box and gained access to the toys, place the box to the side. After 10 to 20 seconds of play, state "more" while signing more and take the toy from the client.

    b.  Immediately initiate hand-over-hand prompting and shape the client's hands to sign, "more." Repeat, "more" and hand the toy back to the client within 1 to 2 seconds.

    c.  Continue with this sequence and give the client the opportunity to imitate your model of the sign for more.

    d.  If the client continues to require tactile prompting to sign "more," fade your prompting out as quickly as possible until the client is able to sign independently.

> As the SLPA and the language model, it is important to request the item exactly how you want the client to request it. When we use the language that we are expecting to hear, the client learns that this is the way that everyone makes a request. As we teach more involved language skills, we use this strategy to really ensure that the clients make the connection between the "words" that they use and the reinforcement that they receive.

## Activity 4

Teaching isolated finger pointing as a form of intentional communicative intent to gain access to desired items/toys using "The Dot" (a simple written dot that provides a concrete visual cue).

Many beginning communicators have not learned how to point with an isolated index finger to indicate that they want something. This skill is generally developed in typically developing children by 12 months of age. Pointing is universally understood and develops joint attention with others in the client's environment. Pointing is one of the most important gestures that a client can learn to communicate effectively with others. Teaching a point can be difficult because trying to use hand-over-hand guidance can be cumbersome and frustrating to the client and difficult to fade.

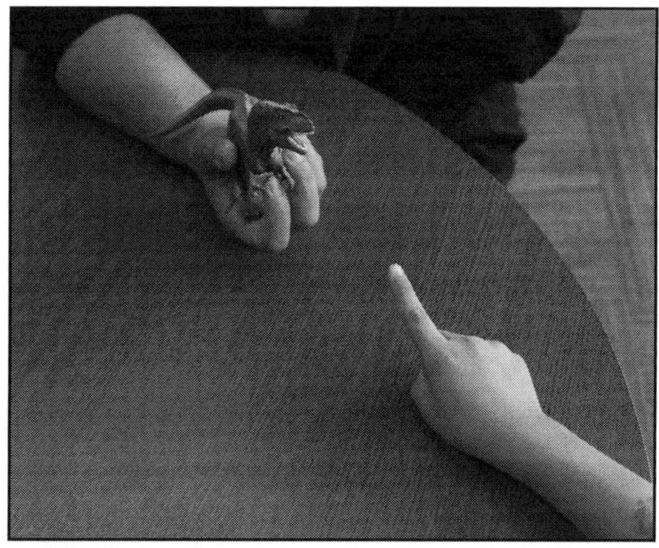

**FIGURE 3–5A.** Point dinosaur.

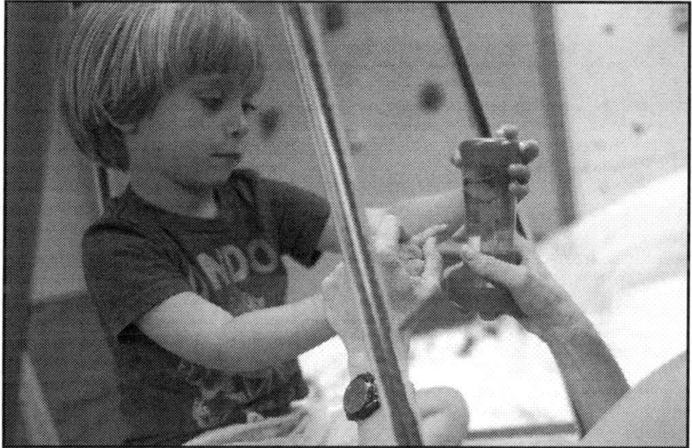

**FIGURE 3–5B.** Parker Kelly hand-over-hand point.

### Materials Needed

1. Knock-knock box

2. Sticky note or small piece of paper with a dot written on it

3. Any toy or item that the client exhibits interest in

### Individual or Small Group Session

Step 1:  Introducing the point

      a.  First, draw a dot on a sticky note or other small piece of paper and place the paper or note on the item that the client wants. The dot can be placed on the knock-knock box itself, and the knocking can be incorporated once the box has been pointed at or you can utilize the toys from the knock-knock box.

b. Model the point by placing your extended index finger on the dot and encourage the client to imitate you.

c. If the action is not imitated, use hand-over-hand prompting to guide the client's finger to the dot.

d. Once the client has touched the dot with an extended index finger, state the label for the item and deliver the item to the client within 2 seconds (remember the importance is FAST reinforcement!).

e. This sequence should be repeated while fading the visual prompt. The dot can be faded by drawing smaller dots as less prompting is required or by removing sections of the sticky note itself, as prompting is decreased. Continue fading in either manner until a dot is no longer needed to facilitate an isolated finger point.

f. Once an independent isolated finger point is established, the desired materials should be placed in different locations in reference to the client to ensure that generalization is occurring.

## Activity 5

Teaching a client to wave "bye-bye" to indicate that he or she is finished with the item.

When you see any behaviors that indicate that the client is no longer interested in a chosen toy (e.g., turning away, no longer interacting with the item, throwing, or dropping the item), it is appropriate to teach the client an acceptable way to communicate that he or she no longer wants it.

It is imperative that you read the client's behavior so that you can prompt the appropriate response. It is only valid to ask a client, "Do you want more?" or "Do you want more or are you done?" if you are expecting a response to the question. If the client does not have the ability to answer a question or choose between two options, it is your job to provide the words for what his or her actions indicate is desired. If a client is engaged with an item, looking at it, or reaching for it, it is indicative of desire and prompting a way to request it is appropriate. If the client is looking away, appearing uninterested, or pushing an item away, you can prompt a wave to say goodbye to the item.

### *Materials Needed*

1. The item that the client is engaged with

2. Items that the client does not want

> Teaching communicative intent is best done in a one-to-one setting. While we understand that setting and caseload may often cause a need for group therapy, if a client on the caseload is at this level, it is highly recommended to set up an individual session.

### *Individual or Small Group Session*

Step 1:  Introduce the wave

    a.  As soon as you observe lack of interest or any behaviors that indicate that the client is not engaged any longer, model waving your hand while stating "bye-bye!"

    b.  Give the client a chance to imitate the wave.

    c.  If the client does not imitate the wave, initiate hand-over-hand prompting to ensure that the client waves before the toy disappears.

    d.  As soon as the client waves, either independently or with hand-over-hand prompting, make sure that the item is taken away within 1 to 2 seconds. When the reinforcement of the item "going away" occurs quickly, clients will begin make the correlation that when they wave, unwanted items are removed.

# 4

# Language Disorders

Language disorders are often categorized as being receptive, expressive, or mixed in nature. The majority of the activities can be easily adapted to fit the child's area of need, regardless of category. As you may recall from your coursework on language development and language disorders, receptive abilities include following directions and listening comprehension. Children with receptive language disorders typically struggle understanding what is said to them. In terms of expressive language abilities, they include verbal and nonverbal skills as well as "how" a child uses language. Children with expressive language disorders typically struggle using words to express themselves. They may use incorrect grammar, use short phrases, or have a limited vocabulary. The activities included in this chapter will help you address the specific needs of children with language disorders. As you become familiar with these activities, you will begin to gain confidence working with children with language disorders and thus, under the guidance of your supervising speech-language pathologist (SLP), can develop your own therapy materials to fit the therapy goals established by the SLP.

## ACTIVITIES FOR LANGUAGE

## Objectives

The following are some sample objectives targeting language needs:

1. Client will increase the use of verbs for specific actions in 8 out of 10 opportunities across three consecutive data collection points.

2. Client will categorize common objects/pictures of objects in 8 out of 10 opportunities across three consecutive data collection points.

3. Client will be able to increase sentence complexity (use of prepositional phrases) in 8 out of 10 opportunities across three consecutive data collection points.

## Activity 1

Language skills, functions, categories, irregular verbs, antonyms, comparatives, and superlatives using Candy Town Language cards by Jenna Rayburn for ages pre-K through fifth grade.

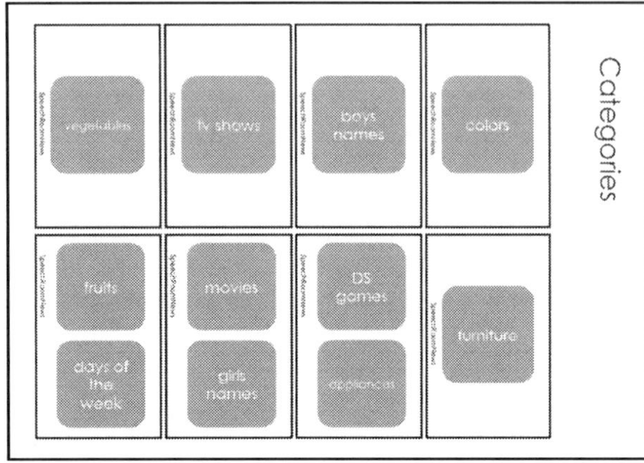

**FIGURE 4–1A.** Jenna Rayburn Speech Room News Candy Cards screenshot. Reproduced with permission of Jenna Rayburn, MA, CCC-SLP, http://www.TheSpeechRoomNews.com

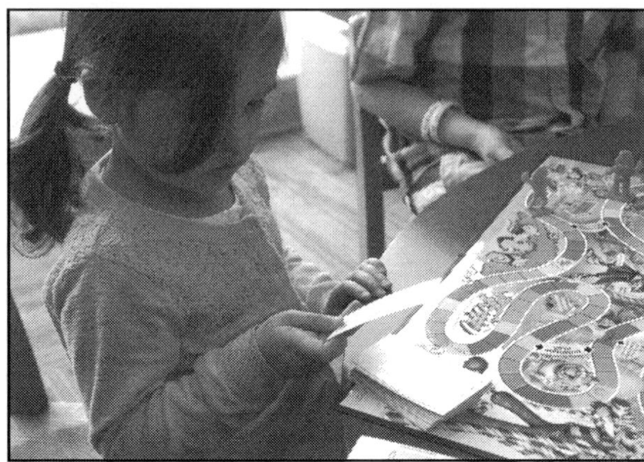

**FIGURE 4–1B.** Hannah Clark Candy Town.

The Candy Town cards can be used in accompaniment with the trademarked Candy Land game to target language skills. These cards are look-alike cards that are used with the board game. Option: If a game board is not available, create a block chart for stamping or coloring during the activity time. Have the clients color or stamp a block each time they provide an answer to a drawn card. Five sets of cards are included: irregular verbs, categories, antonyms, comparatives and superlatives, and functions. For purposes of this activity, the category and functions cards will be used.

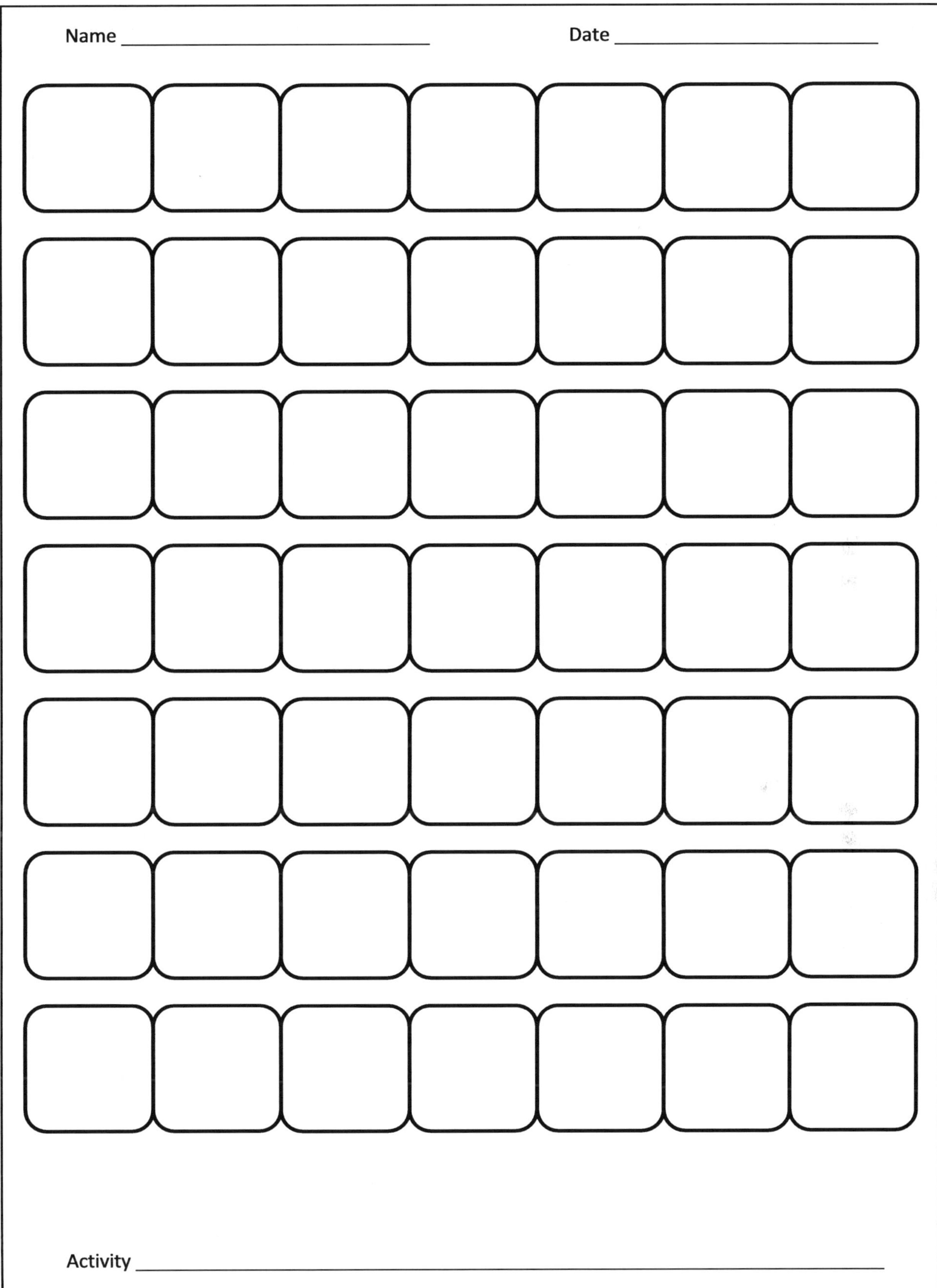


**FIGURE 4–2.** Image of color block.

To download the Candy Town Language cards, visit https://www.teacherspayteachers.com/Product/Candy-Town-Language-Cards-274010

**FIGURE 4–3.** Candy Card QR code.

This activity can be printed on cardstock and laminated for durability.

### *Individual or Small Group Session*

Step 1:  If using the Candy Land board game, set up the game and select appropriate Candy Town card decks that target each client's goals. The Candy Town language card decks replace the Candy Land color block cards. If using a block chart, provide each client with a copy and some coloring markers or pencils. *NOTE:* The SLPA should take initial direction from the supervising SLP in regard to the client's language ability and goals and objectives.

Step 2:  Explain both the object of the game and from which pile of Candy Town cards each client will be choosing from (i.e., "Mary will be playing with this deck (function words) and Johnny you will be playing from this deck (categories)").

Step 3:  The client will choose his or her playing piece for moving along the board game.

Step 4:  The first client will draw one card from his or her assigned decks and respond to stimuli on the card. The SLPA will model as needed (i.e., "Name three items that belong in the silverware category or what is the function (reason) of a toaster?").

Step 5:  After the client responds, he or she will move the playing piece to the corresponding color(s) on the card or color or stamp in one or two spaces on the block chart. The SLPA then collects data on client responses and notes prompting when needed.

Step 6:  The next client will draw a card from his or her pile and respond to stimuli on the card. The SLPA will model as needed.

Step 7:  Have the client repeat Steps 5 and 6 until session/activity time is completed.

Step 8:  Record data in clients' files as needed.

### *Essential Resources*

Jenna Rayburn of Speech Room News (http://thespeechroomnews.com/) also offers a variety of speech and language activities both free and paid. Visit at https://www.teacherspayteachers.com/Store/Jenna-Rayburn-26

**FIGURE 4–4.** Jenna Rayburn TPT store QR code.

## Activity 2

Following and giving directions with emphasis on positional concepts and using manipulatives for a variety of ages. Optional reinforcement/generalization with companion Sago Sago mini apps.

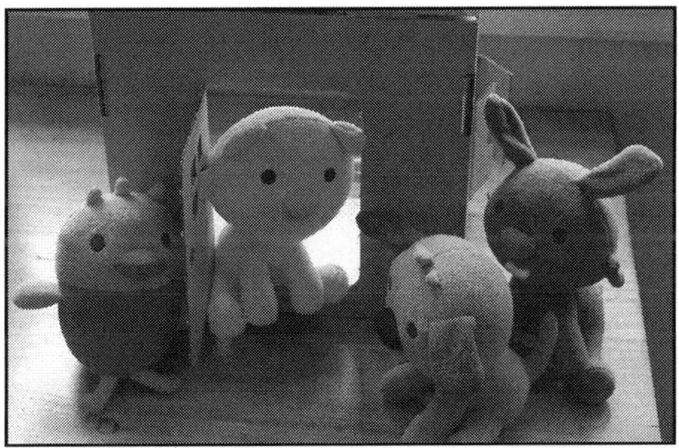

**FIGURE 4–5A.** Sago plushies.

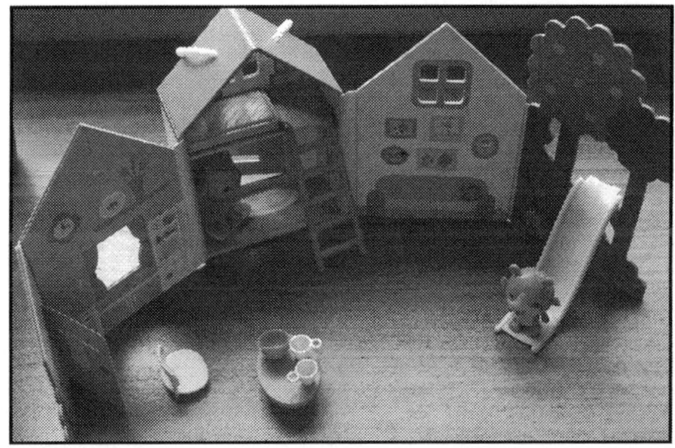

**FIGURE 4–5B.** Sago toyhouse.

Using manipulatives, this activity can target both expressive and receptive language skills. We recommend using verbing for following directions, positional concepts, and more. For purposes of this lesson, use positional concepts such as next to, under, behind, in front of, in, out, on, or under while providing simple directions to the client or when having the client give instructions to another (i.e., put the rabbit next to the house). Manipulatives (Sago Sago mini plush toys and Sago mini toyhouse) will be shown for illustrative purposes. Any engaging manipulative (favorite animals, superheroes, objects) can be used for this lesson. Companion Sago Sago mini apps will be illustrated to complement this activity.

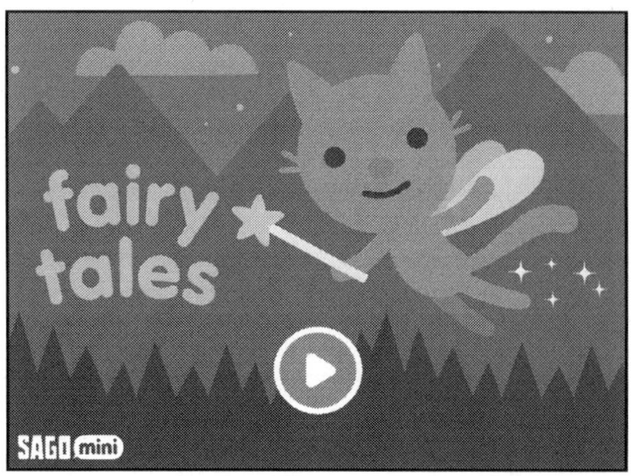


**FIGURE 4–6A.** Sago Sago fairytale main screenshot. Reproduced with permission of Sago Sago.

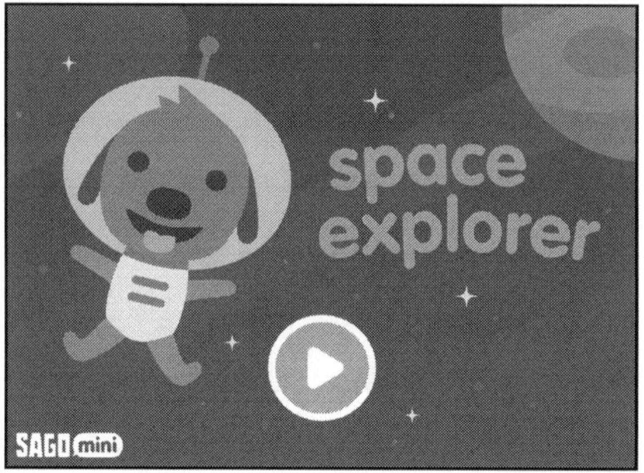


**FIGURE 4–6B.** Sago Sago space explorer main screenshot. Reproduced with permission of Sago Sago.

To download the Sago Sago mini apps or purchase Sago mini toys, visit http://www.sagomini.com

**FIGURE 4–7.** Sago Sago QR code.

### *Individual or Small Group Session*

Step 1:   With the client sitting next to or beside you, explain that you will be using manipulatives to learn about position words (i.e., "We will be playing with this toy house and animals to practice words like next to, behind, above").

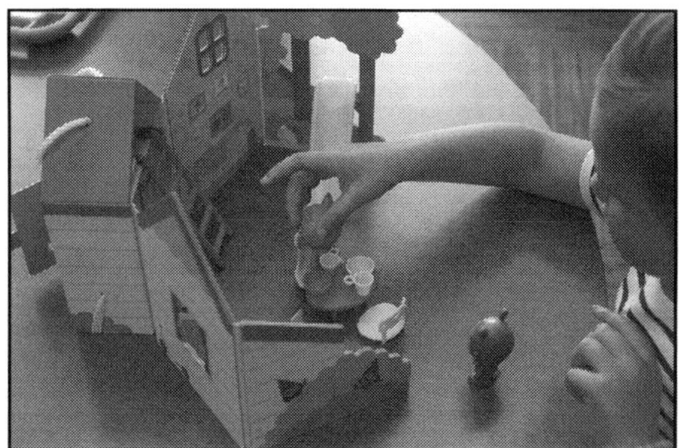

**FIGURE 4–8A.** Hannah Clark toyhouse.

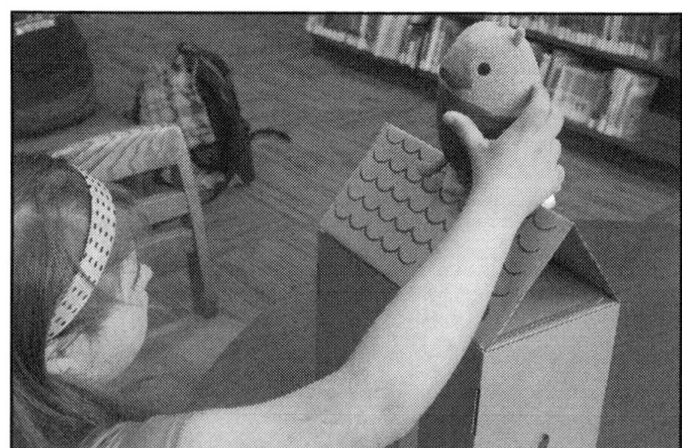

**FIGURE 4–8B.** Elizabeth Giese plushie.

Step 2: To target receptive language skills, provide positional concept instructions to the client to "put the cat behind the house or on the bed," "put the squirrel between the trees," "put one of the animals on the top floor," or "make the squirrel go down the slide." Additional positional words that might be used are on, off, next to, beside, in, out, under, near, through, over, left, right, bottom, above, and front.

Step 3: To target expressive language skills, have the client explain using specific positional words where the toy is or what he or she wants a peer (or the SLPA) to do with the toy (i.e., the squirrel is climbing "up" the ladder or going "down" the slide, the cat is "behind" the door, the hose is "around" or "on" the hanger). Asking WHERE questions also provides opportunities for clients to practice their expressive language skills (i.e., Where is the window? The window is "above" the pictures. Where are the pillows? The pillows are "on" the sofa.). *NOTE:* Modify this lesson as needed for client skill level. You may need to model the sentence or provide a framework before the client explains (i.e., the squirrel is going ______ the slide).

Step 4: Creating positional word cards or using sticky notes is another option to provide needed cues and prompts for the client.

Step 5: Continue practicing expressive and receptive positional concepts by using highly engaging Sago Sago mini apps. Sago mini fairytales All the Sago apps are capitalized as they were based on the website and Sago mini space explorer will be used for illustrative purposes.

   a. Open the Sago mini fairytales or the Sago mini space explorer or any other app that provides opportunities for positional concept practice. *NOTE:* To turn off "Sago News or Parent Info" on the home screen, visit the settings within the device and slide the "Sago News and/or Parent Info" buttons to off.

   b. Demonstrate for the client how the character (princess cat or space dog) moves through the app by using finger motions and allow him or her to explore.

   c. As the client moves the character through the fairytale forest or space, use this opportunity to ask WHERE questions, have the client tell where the character is, or model a grammatically correct sentence for the client.

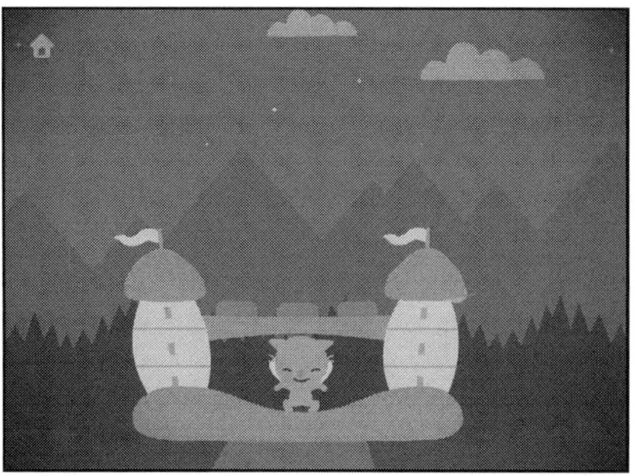

**FIGURE 4–9A.** Sago Sago bounce castle screenshot. Reproduced with permission of Sago Sago.

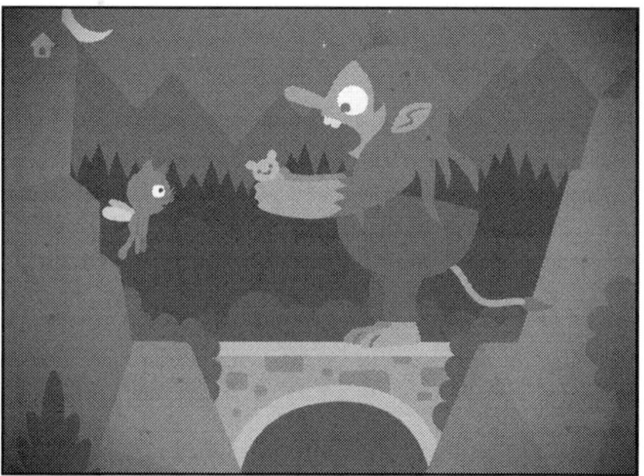

**FIGURE 4–9B.** Sago Sago monster bridge screenshot. Reproduced with permission of Sago Sago.

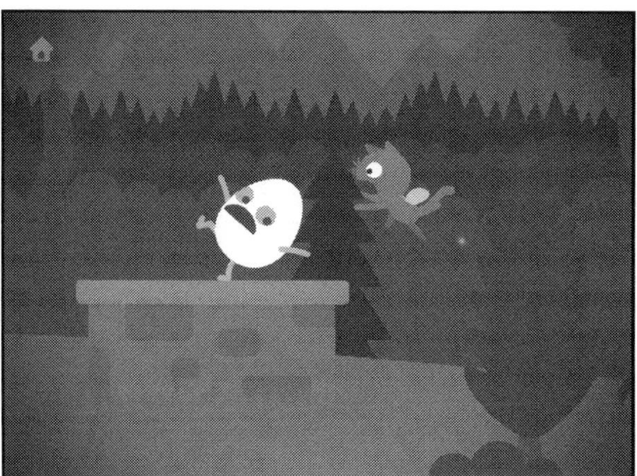

**FIGURE 4–9C.** Sago Sago monster bridge falling off screenshot. Reproduced with permission of Sago Sago.

d. Sample scripted language for the fairytale app: "Look, the egg is falling 'off' the wall!" "What happened to the egg?" "The green dinosaur is 'in' the nest." "The monster is 'on' the bridge." "The cat is above the house." "The purple squirrel is in the doorway." "The cat is jumping 'inside' the bounce castle." "Should we move the cat to the 'left' or the 'right'?" "Or should we go 'up' or 'down'?"

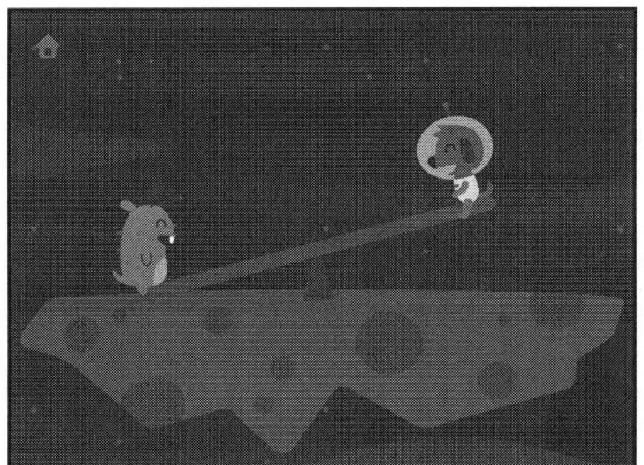

**FIGURE 4–10A.** Sago Sago space teeter-totter screenshot. Reproduced with permission of Sago Sago.

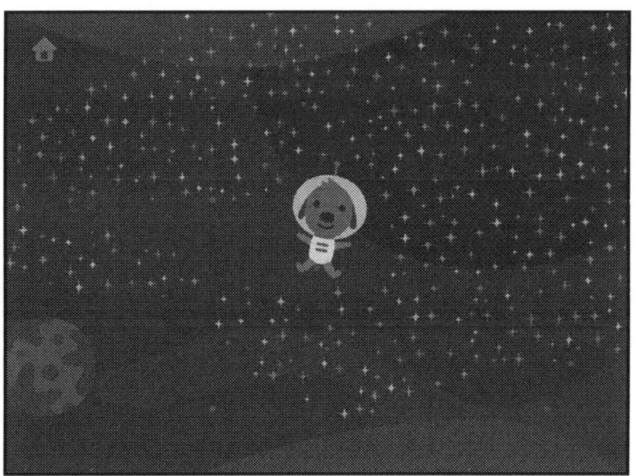

**FIGURE 4–10B.** Sago Sago stars screenshot. Reproduced with permission of Sago Sago.

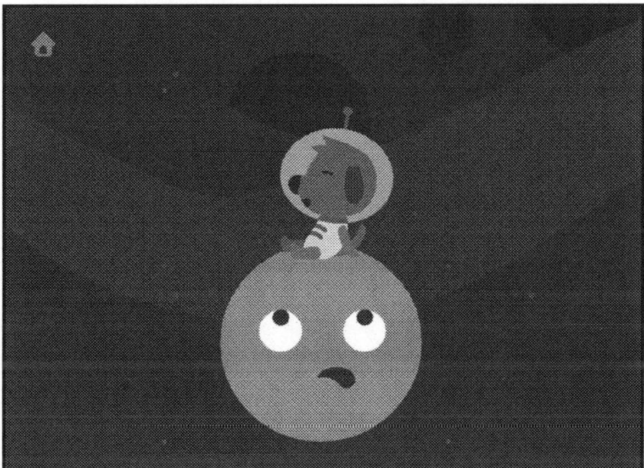

**FIGURE 4–10C.** Sago Sago on top of planet. Reproduced with permission of Sago Sago.

e. Sample scripted language for the space explorer app: "The green alien is under the blanket or on the bed." "The light is above his head." "The toys are on the floor." "The dog is on the teeter-totter and it is going up and down." "The space dog is flying through the stars!" "Should we make space dog fly to the right or to the left?" "Space dog is next to or on top of the planet."

## Activity 3

Increasing functional and everyday receptive vocabulary with StoryToys Jr. Touch, Look, Listen interactive book apps for a variety of ages and second language learners.

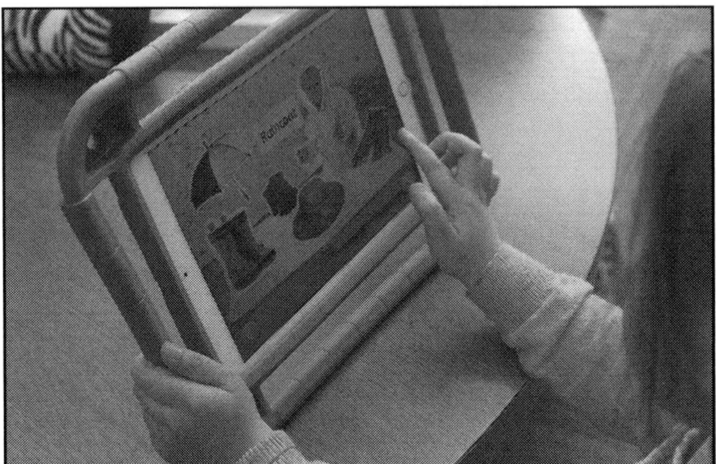

**FIGURE 4–11.** Hannah Clark StoryToys.

This activity will target categories, simple comprehension of new words learned, and key concepts such as colors and numbers. *NOTE:* Print books can also make for appropriate vocabulary activities. The Touch, Look, Listen series by StoryToys Jr. are interactive book apps that provide a wonderfully rich pop-up 3D visual experience. Built-in questions provide comprehension reinforcement as well as a setting for multiple languages, including English, French, German, Spanish, and Chinese.

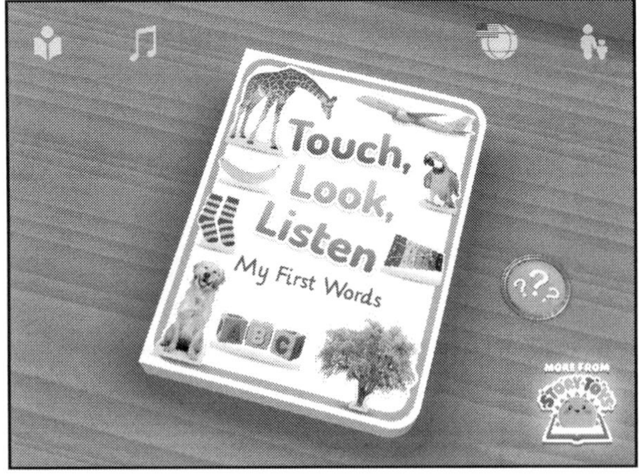


**FIGURE 4–12A.** StoryToys Entertainment Limited TLL first words screenshot. Reproduced with permission of StoryToys Limited.

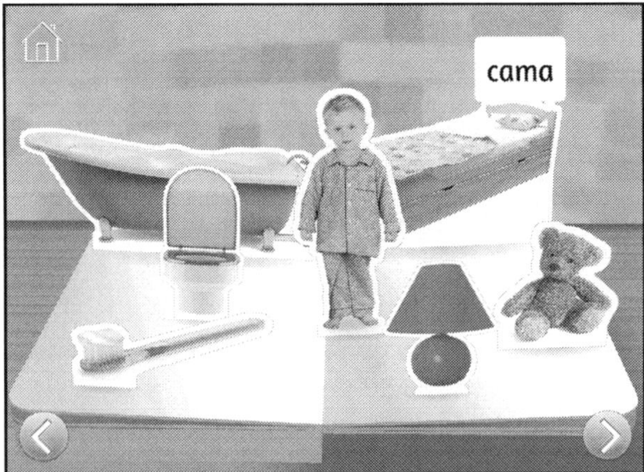


**FIGURE 4–12B.** StoryToys Entertainment Limited TLL Spanish first words screenshot. Reproduced with permission of StoryToys Limited.

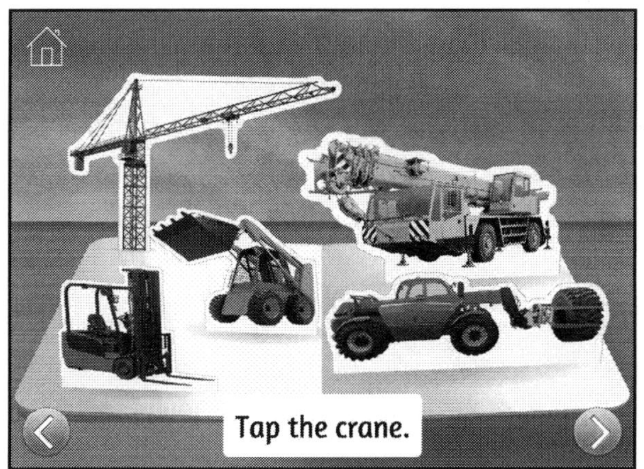


**FIGURE 4–12C.** StoryToys Entertainment Limited TLL comprehension vehicles screenshot. Reproduced with permission of StoryToys Limited.

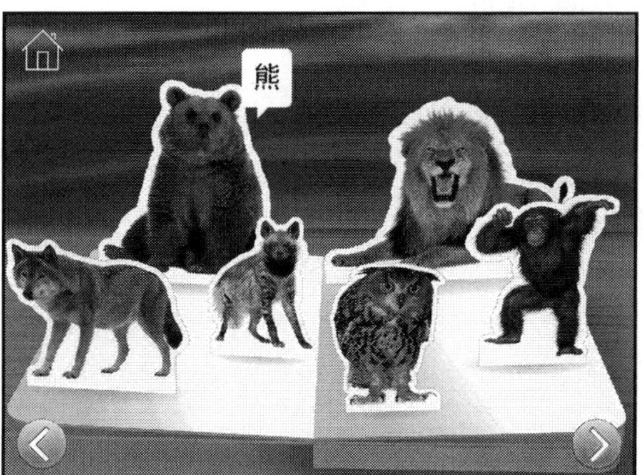


**FIGURE 4–12D.** StoryToys Entertainment Limited TLL Chinese zoo animals screenshot. Reproduced with permission of StoryToys Limited.

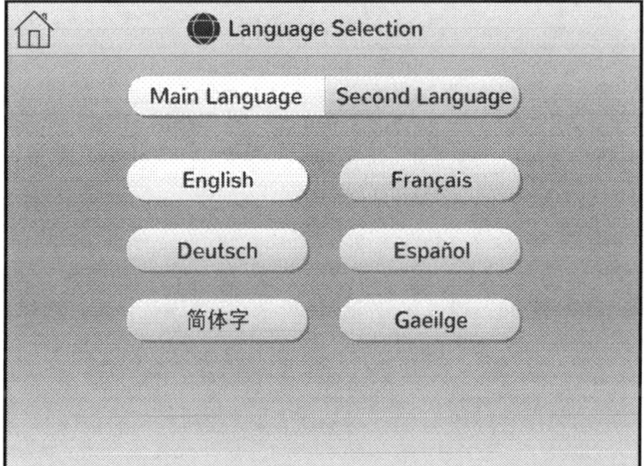


**FIGURE 4–12E.** StoryToys Entertainment Limited language screenshot. Reproduced with permission of StoryToys Limited.

To download the Touch, Look, Listen apps (Zoo Animals, My First Words, What Do I Wear? Things That Go) or to become familiar with other highly engaging, interactive, and useful StoryToys apps, visit http://storytoys.com

**FIGURE 4–13.** StoryToys QR code.

### Individual or Small Group Session

Step 1:  With the client sitting next to or beside you, explain that you will be using an interactive book app to target learning new vocabulary during the speech/language session.

Step 2:  Open the StoryToys Jr. Touch, Look, Listen app. Depending on your client objectives, choose one of the four apps:

- Touch, Look, Listen—My First Words (animals, body parts, family members, household items, clothing, food, vehicles, numbers)

- Touch, Look, Listen—Things That Go (trucks, cars, buses, motorbikes, boats, and more)

- Touch Look, Listen—Zoo Animals (all types of zoo animals)

- Touch Look, Listen—What Do I Wear? (clothing for all seasons)

Step 3:  As appropriate for client objectives, tap the globe icon at the top of the screen to set the main language to English, Spanish, Chinese, German, or French and the second language to None, English, Spanish, Chinese, German, or French.

Step 4:  Allow the client to explore the book app and become familiar with how to turn pages and tap images appropriately. *NOTE:* It is important that you become familiar with this app prior to the therapy session.

Step 5:  Once the client is familiar with the app you have chosen, use this opportunity to ask the client to tap a "specific item" to check receptive skills and vocabulary knowledge. For early learners, tap each image so they can see the printed word and hear the narration (in the language you have chosen for main language). *NOTE:* An option is to turn the volume down/off on the tablet and narrate the word for the client. If client is a reader, you can choose to have him or her read the word after the image is tapped.

Step 6:  Ask your client to create a verbal or written sentence using the vocabulary. If needed, model an appropriate sentence for the client (i.e., "I wear mittens in the winter to keep my hands warm," "A sailboat needs wind to move across the water," "I brush my teeth with a toothbrush," "A bird can fly").

Step 7:  Asking your clients questions that allow them to answer using their new knowledge will support their understanding and generalization skills (i.e., "Which animals fly or have fur?" "What type of transportation flies or is used on water?" "When do you wear mittens or a raincoat?").

## Activity 4

Asking and answering questions using the Question Therapy app by Tactus Therapy for a variety of ages and skill levels.

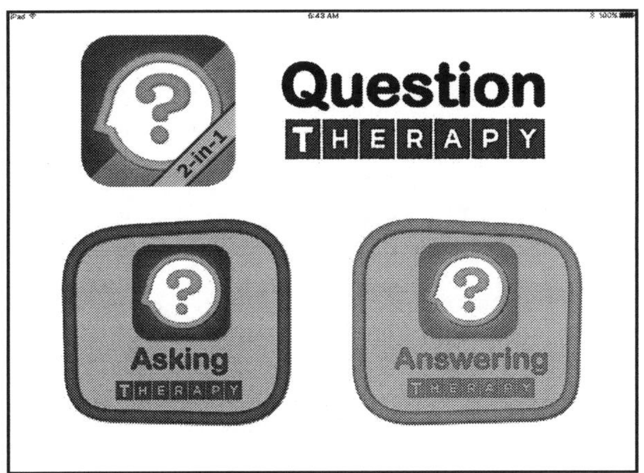

**FIGURE 4–14A.** Tactus Therapy question main screenshot. Reproduced with permission of Tactus Therapy Solutions, Ltd.

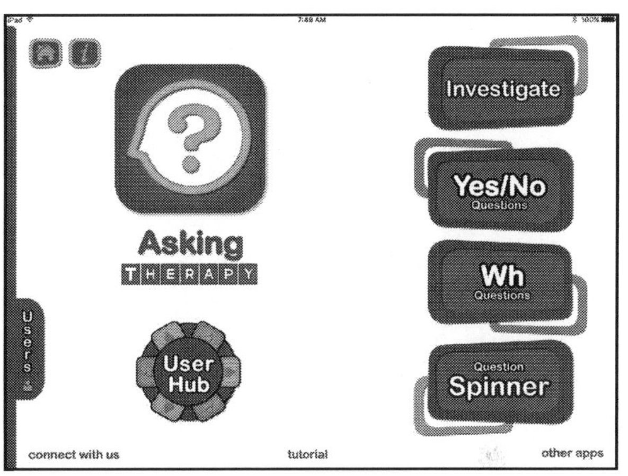

**FIGURE 4–14B.** Tactus Therapy asking screenshot. Reproduced with permission of Tactus Therapy Solutions, Ltd.

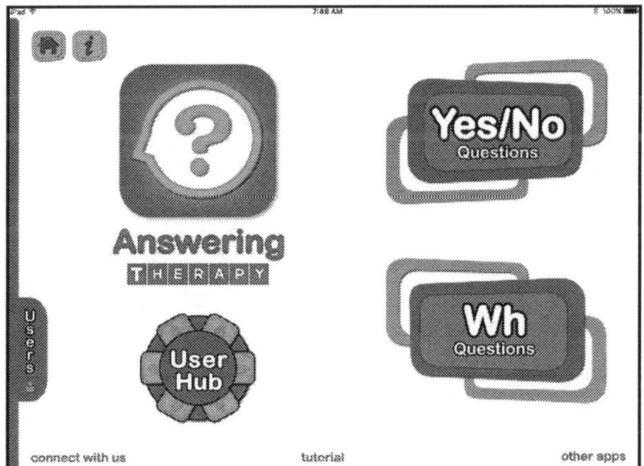

**FIGURE 4–14C.** Tactus Therapy answering screenshot. Reproduced with permission of Tactus Therapy Solutions, Ltd.

Question Therapy by Tactus Therapy consists of two features within one app. Answering Questions allows the user to work on yes/no and wh-questions, questions geared toward personal orientation and ability for unlimited customized questions. Asking Questions gives the user the opportunity to learn to ask yes/no and wh-questions, as well as work on clarifying and requesting. This comprehensive language app has the ability to

- Work with multiple clients

- Customize stimulus with audio, text, or both

- Set levels (question types)

- Customize questions

- Show visual images and give hints

- Work in receptive or expressive mode

- Record user response

- Adjust the number of answer choices

- Provide data results

To download Question Therapy by Tactus Therapy, the free version of Question Therapy Lite, or additional apps and therapy resources, visit http://tactustherapy.com

**FIGURE 4–15.** Tactus Therapy QR code.

For a more efficient and effective therapy session, take time to enter the optional user information on the personal survey, customize questions, and become familiar with the app prior to the therapy session.

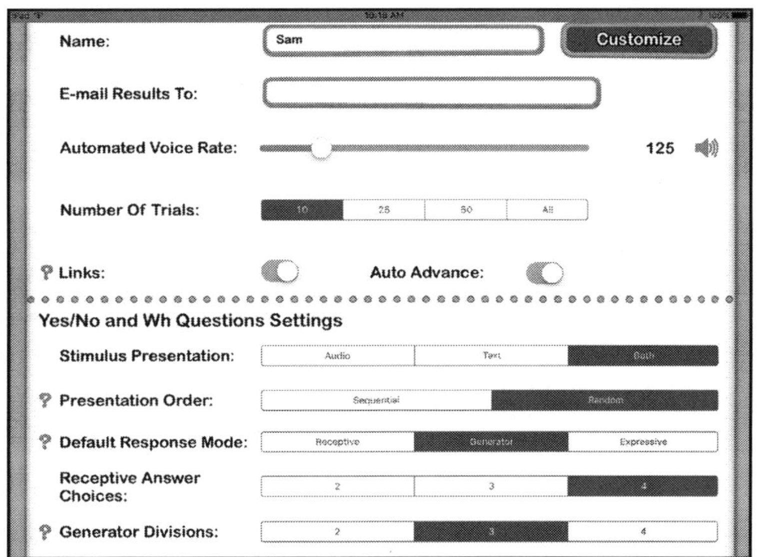

**FIGURE 4–16.** Tactus Therapy QT settings screenshot. Reproduced with permission of Tactus Therapy Solutions, Ltd.

### *Individual or Small Group Session*

Step 1:  With the client sitting next to or across from you, explain that you will be using an app to help target asking and answering questions based on targeted objectives.

Step 2:  Open Question Therapy.

Step 3:  Depending on the clients' objectives, tap Asking Therapy or Answering Therapy

    a.  Asking Therapy is intended for all ages and focuses on asking yes/no and wh-questions. Answering Therapy gives users the opportunity to practice understanding and answering questions for all ages with seven levels of yes/no questions and nine categories of wh-questions.

    b.  Tap USERS and choose the client to work with. *NOTE:* Each client's profile information and settings should be entered prior to the therapy session to maximize therapy session time.

c.  If selecting Asking Therapy, choose the type of activity to work on: Investigate, Yes/No Questions, Wh-Questions, or Question Spinner.

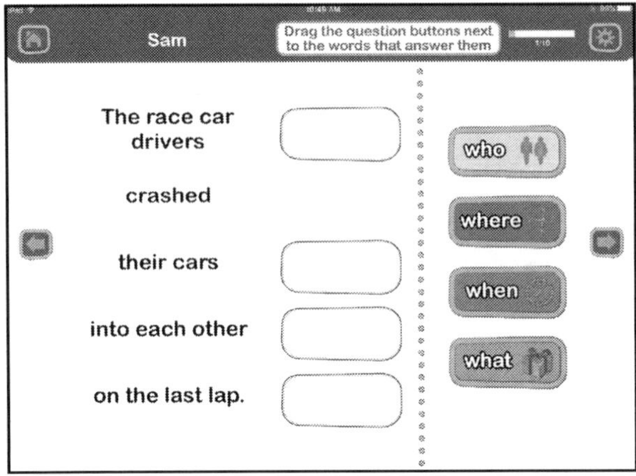

**FIGURE 4–17A.** Tactus Therapy investigate screenshot. Reproduced with permission of Tactus Therapy Solutions, Ltd.

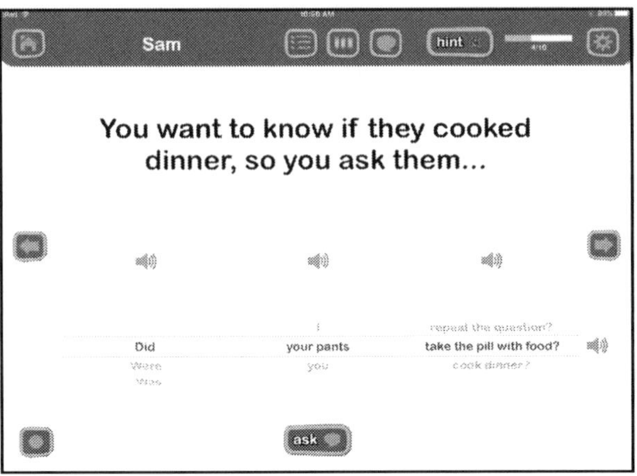

**FIGURE 4–17B.** Tactus Therapy ask yes/no screenshot. Reproduced with permission of Tactus Therapy Solutions, Ltd.

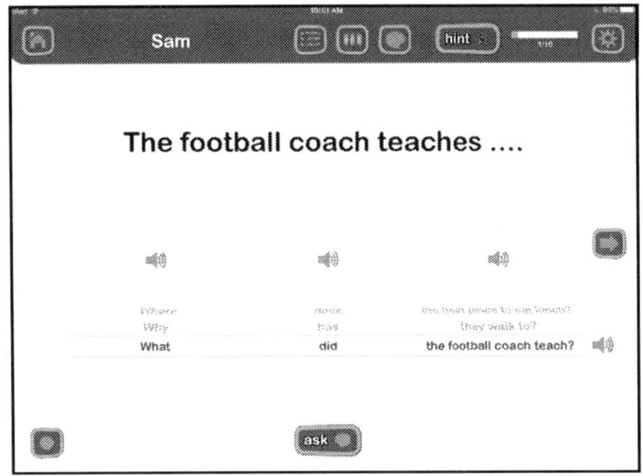

**FIGURE 4–17C.** Tactus Therapy ask WH screenshot. Reproduced with permission of Tactus Therapy Solutions, Ltd.

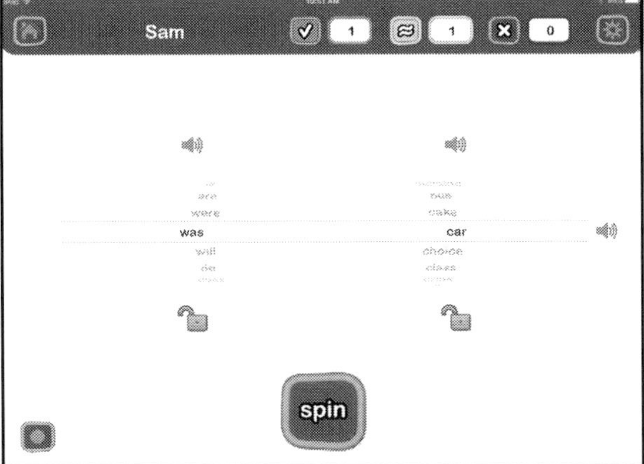

**FIGURE 4–17D.** Tactus Therapy ask spinner screenshot. Reproduced with permission of Tactus Therapy Solutions, Ltd.

d. If selecting Answering Therapy, choose the type of activity to work on: Yes/No Questions or Wh-Questions.

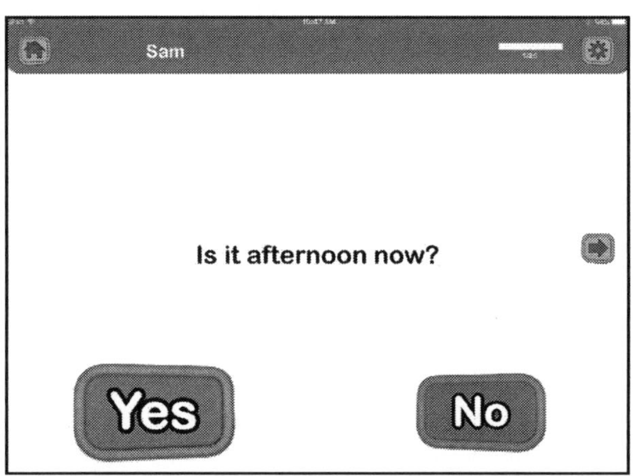


**FIGURE 4–18A.** Tactus Therapy answer yes/no A screenshot. Reproduced with permission of Tactus Therapy Solutions, Ltd.

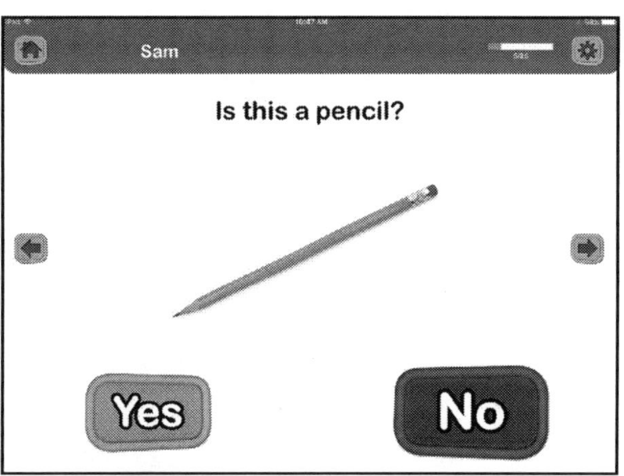


**FIGURE 4–18B.** Tactus Therapy answer yes/no B screenshot. Reproduced with permission of Tactus Therapy Solutions, Ltd.

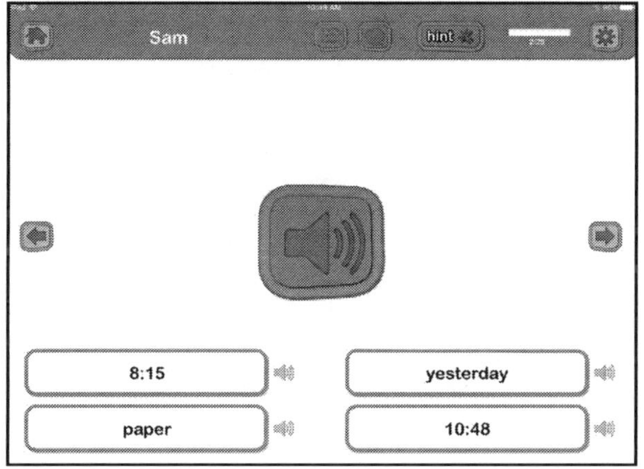


**FIGURE 4–18C.** Tactus Therapy answer WH A screenshot. Reproduced with permission of Tactus Therapy Solutions, Ltd.

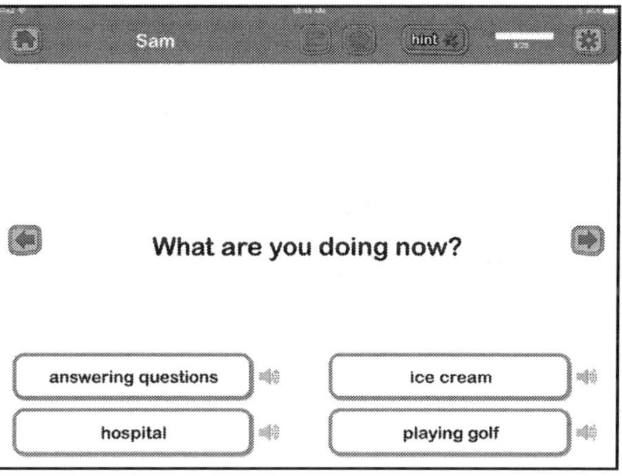


**FIGURE 4–18D.** Tactus Therapy answer WH B screenshot. Reproduced with permission of Tactus Therapy Solutions, Ltd.

Step 4: Work directly with the client on selected questions for the number of trials that have been set within the settings.

Step 5: When working in small group sessions, reselect USERS and choose the next client to work with and proceed with Step 3c.

Step 6: Record data in the client file as required.

## Activity 5

Addressing receptive and expressive language skills using the MyPlayHome App series by Shimon Young.

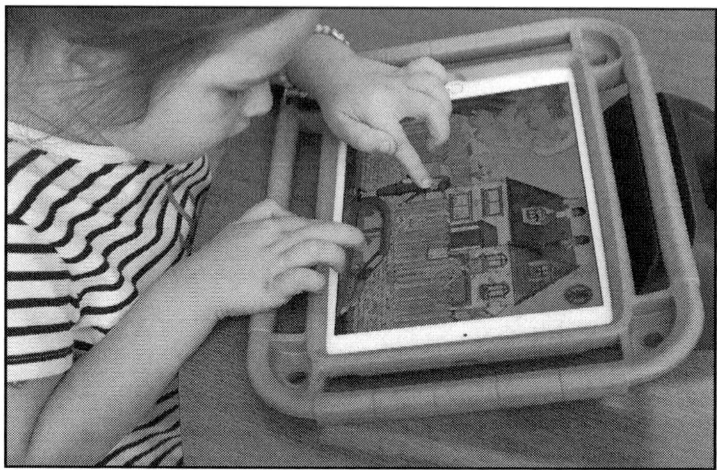

**FIGURE 4–19.** Hannah Clark MyPlayHome.

MyPlayHome, MyPlayHome School, MyPlayHome Stores, and MyPlayHome Hospital are appropriate for a variety of ages. Work on following directions, building vocabulary and pronouns, asking and answering questions, retelling sequences, storytelling, and much more in functional home and community settings with culturally diverse characters. It is not necessary to have all of the apps for this activity; however, moving from one environment to another adds extra engagement and many more learning opportunities.

The MyPlayHome Apps are a series of highly interactive individual apps that allow users to role-play within the home, school, store, and hospital environments. The apps are interactive with each other, and users can travel from home to school, store, hospital, and back again and even take items along with them.

MyPlayHome is a virtual home containing a kitchen, living room, bathroom, two bedrooms, and a backyard. There are many diverse family members to choose from by dragging and dropping them into the room. View the assortment of people by tapping the people icon in the upper right corner. Move from room to room by tapping the arrows. People can be dragged and dropped from area to area. To move to the front yard/street level, tap the "down area" in the living room so that you may go to one of the other environments (you must have the MyPlayHome Stores, MyPlayHome School, or MyPlayHome Hospital to move to another environment). Use the arrow, put a person in the car, or have him or her walk to the next environment (school, hospital, or stores).

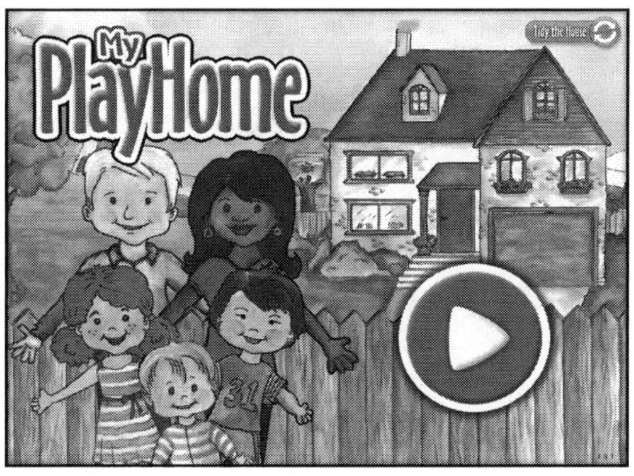

**FIGURE 4–20A.** MyPlayHome main screenshot. Reproduced with permission of Shimon Young.

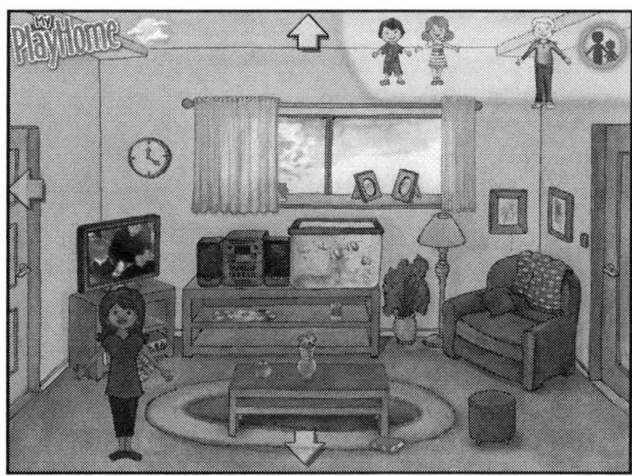

**FIGURE 4–20B.** MyPlayHome LR screenshot. Reproduced with permission of Shimon Young.

To download MyPlayHome, visit http://www.myplayhomeapp.com

**FIGURE 4–21.**
MyPlayHome QR code.

MyPlayHome Stores is a virtual community with access to four stores: a fruit smoothie shop, a clothing store, an ice cream shop, and a grocery store. As in MyPlayHome, there are many diverse people to choose from and that can interact within the different stores. Move from store to store using the arrows or drag and drop the people from store to store. Scan your grocery items, pack your groceries, buy an outfit in the clothing store, and take them back to MyPlayHome by using the arrow at the bottom of the ice cream store or visit one of the other environments (school or hospital).

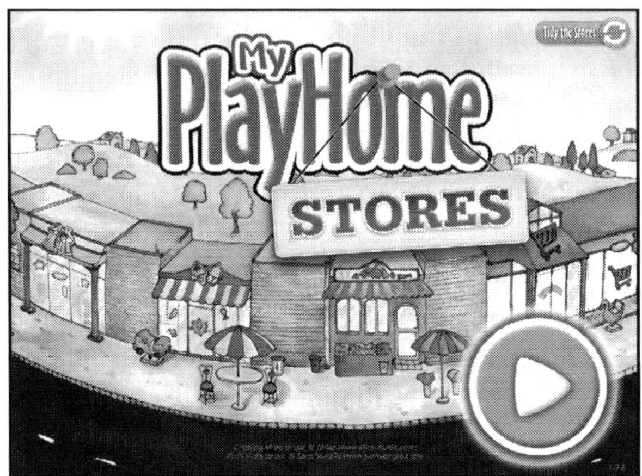

**FIGURE 4–22A.** MyPlayHome Store main screenshot. Reproduced with permission of Shimon Young.

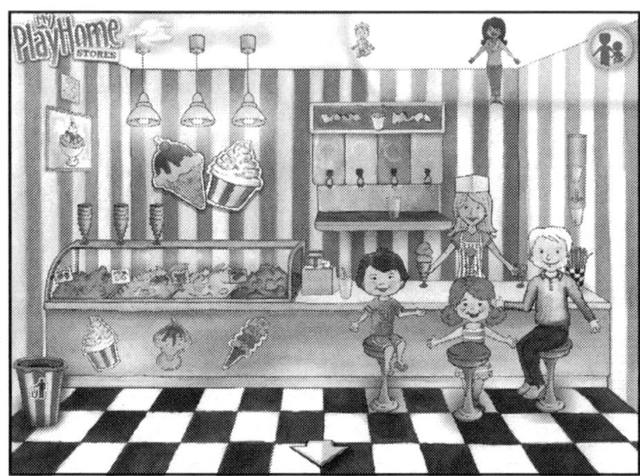

**FIGURE 4–22B.** MyPlayHome Store ice cream shop screenshot. Reproduced with permission of Shimon Young.

To download MyPlayHome Stores, visit https://itunes.apple.com/us/app/my-playhome-stores/id683942610?mt=8.

**FIGURE 4–23.**
MyPlayHome Store
QR code.

MyPlayHome School is a virtual school with two floors that can be accessed by stairs or elevator, a theater, a playground, a cafeteria, restrooms, lockers, a classroom, a janitor closet, a school office, and more. Interactivity within each area is abundant. Move from area to area using the arrows or drag and drop the people where you'd like them. Walk back to MyPlayHome (or one of the other environments) by using the down arrow in the school office. You can also access the playground by using the arrow at the front of the school building.

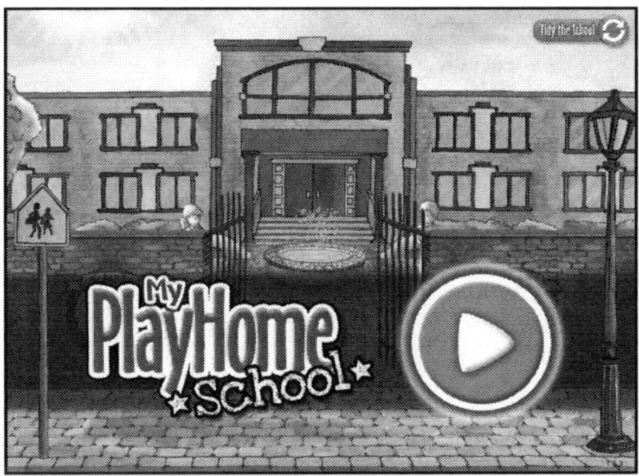

**FIGURE 4–24A.** MyPlayHome School main screenshot. Reproduced with permission of Shimon Young.

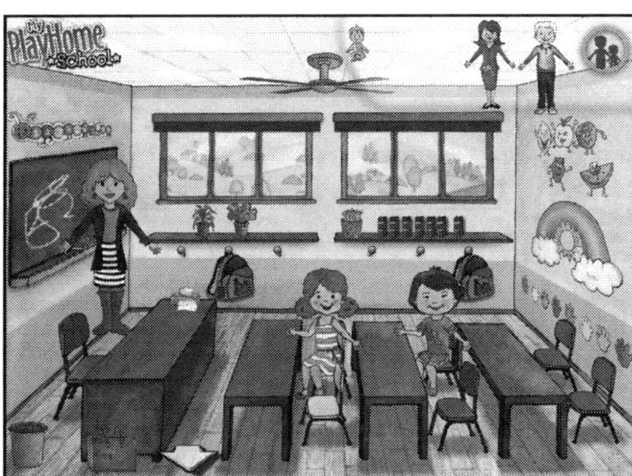

**FIGURE 4–24B.** MyPlayHome School classroom screenshot. Reproduced with permission of Shimon Young.

To download MyPlayHome School, visit https://itunes.apple.com/us/app/my-playhome-school/id922188121?mt=8

**FIGURE 4–25.**
MyPlayHome School
QR code.

MyPlayHome Hospital is a virtual hospital for when the family needs a doctor, wants to visit a sick friend, or mom is a nurse or doctor and the hospital is where she works. Just as in the sister PlayHome apps, you can access areas by dragging and dropping the people to the desired location or using the arrows. Visit the gift store and bring a balloon to a sick friend, let family members wait in the waiting room, use a stethoscope and hear a heartbeat, get an x-ray, and so much more. Learn hospital- and doctor-related vocabulary.

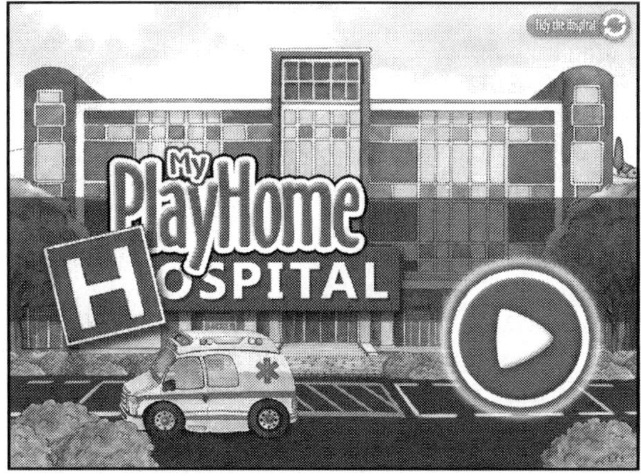

**FIGURE 4–26A.** MyPlayHome Hospital main screenshot. Reproduced with permission of Shimon Young.

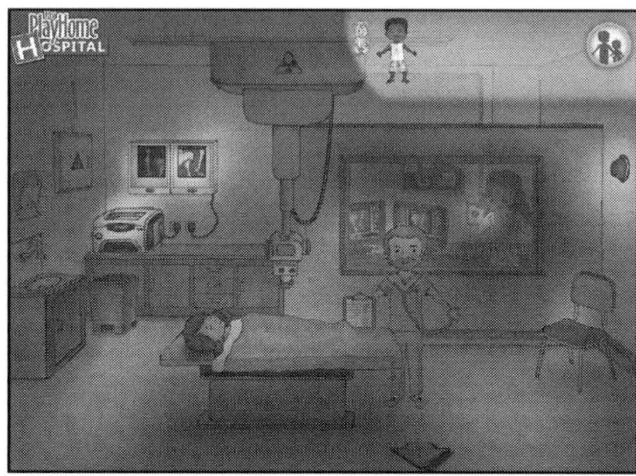

**FIGURE 4–26B.** MyPlayHome Hospital x-ray screenshot. Reproduced with permission of Shimon Young.

To download MyPlayHome Hospital, visit https://itunes.apple.com/us/app/my-playhome-hospital/id1095280287?mt=8

**FIGURE 4–27.**
MyPlayHome Hospital
QR code.

> For a more effective and efficient therapy session, become familiar with the apps prior to the therapy session.

### Individual or Small Group Session

Step 1:  With the client sitting next to you or across from you, explain that you will be working speech and language goals using the MyPlayHome apps.

Step 2:  Open any of the MyPlayHome apps to begin the therapy session.

Step 3:  Demonstrate and allow your client to become familiar with how to interact within each screen and move people to and from rooms and the other environments (school, store, hospital).

Step 4:  With client objectives and goals in mind (i.e., pronouns, verbs, vocabulary, categories, following directions, etc.), begin targeting language goals. Below are examples that might be used; modify as needed.

Expressive

- What is the boy/girl/mom/dad/baby doing? Require the client to use correct grammar and pronouns (i.e., "She is eating").
- Move through the people at the top of the screen and ask the client to identify male and female by using "he" and "she."
- Put an object (i.e., book) in the hand of a character and ask the client what he or she is doing.
- Go to the store and make a smoothie. Require the client to give directions to a peer or SLPA (i.e., first put in a banana, then an apple, and last a carrot).
- Allow the client to tell the story and then role-play with the character within the environment.

Receptive

- Point or touch the _____.
- Put the boy in the chair and turn on the TV.
- Turn off the TV, turn on the light, and play some music.
- Go to the kitchen and give the girl a popsicle.
- Put a man and boy in the car and drive to the store to get smoothie.

Step 5:  When working in small group settings, give clients opportunities to take turns.

Step 6:  Record session data within client files as needed and required.

### Essential Resources for This Activity

Teach Speech 365 from Teachers Pay Teachers offers therapy companion packets for the MyPlay-Home series. Visit https://www.teacherspayteachers.com/Store/Teach-Speech-365

**FIGURE 4–28.** Teach Speech 365 QR code.

## Activity 6

Listening, sequencing, and recalling information using Auditory Memory Club by Smarty Ears.

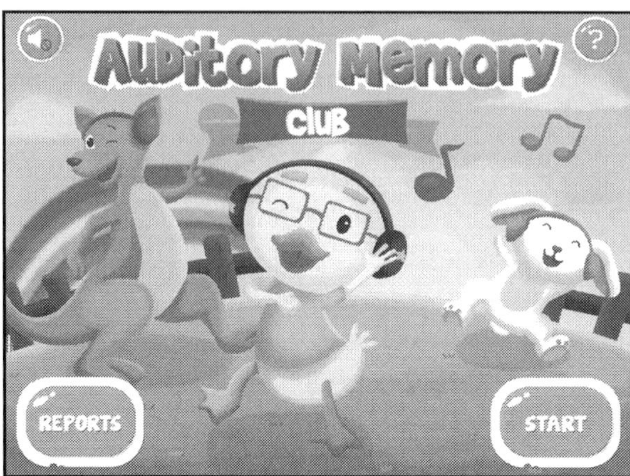

**FIGURE 4–29.** Smarty Ears Auditory Memory Club main screenshot. Reproduced with permission of Smarty Ears, LLC. All rights reserved.

Auditory Memory Club by Smarty Ears is a single- or multiclient (up to four) app that encourages individuals to develop better active listening skills, which in turn help develop language processing and memory skills.

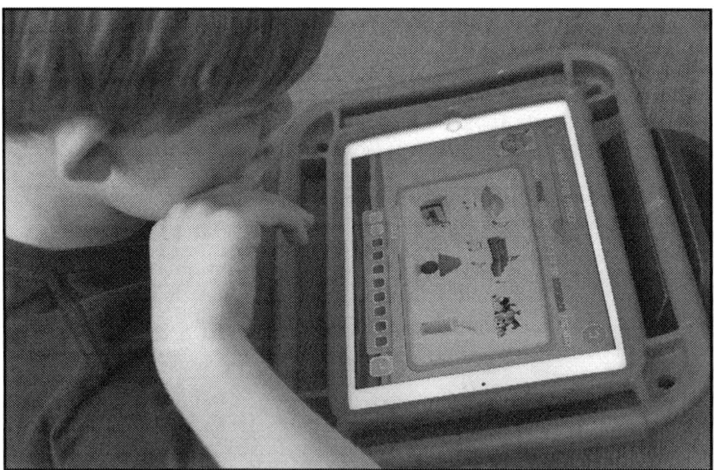

**FIGURE 4–30.** Riley Clark auditory memory.

To download Auditory Memory Club, visit http://smartyearsapps.com

**FIGURE 4–31.** Smarty Ears QR code.

For a more efficient and effective therapy session, take time to enter the client profile information, adjust activity settings as needed, and become familiar with the app prior to the therapy session.

### Individual or Small Group Session

Step 1:  With the client sitting next to or across from you, explain that you will be using an app to help target language processing skills based on targeted objectives.

Step 2:  Open Auditory Memory Club and select the client(s) participating in the therapy session. You may choose up to four clients to participate within the session.

Step 3:  Choose the appropriate activity (i.e., I Say You Do, What Was That?, Remember for Amber, Let's Put Some Order) for the individual or small group session. *NOTE:* If you are working in small groups, clients will all work on the same activity.

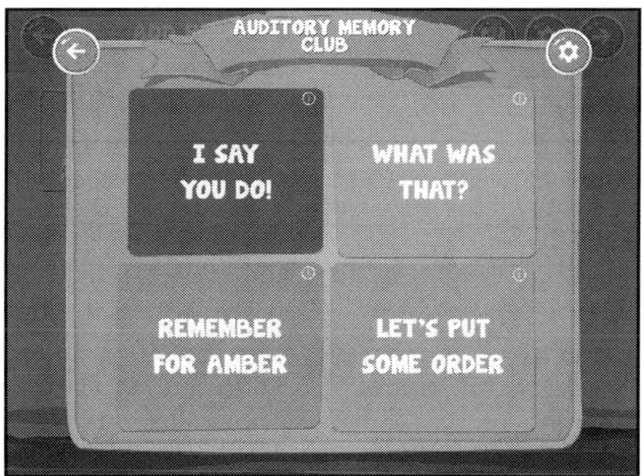


**FIGURE 4–32.** Smarty Ears auditory memory activity screenshot. Reproduced with permission of Smarty Ears, LLC. All rights reserved.

Four activity areas include:

    a. I Say You Do—one-step to multiple-step commands with a delay (pause) for up to 100 seconds

    b. What Was That?—listen to an audio clip and then identify what made the sound

    c. Remember for Amber—listen to a series of words and then identify the items mentioned

    d. Let's Put Some Order—listen to a series of words and then put the images in correct order

Step 4: Proceed with the activity chosen. *NOTE:* Activities What Was That?, Remember for Amber, and Let's Put Some Order are automatically scored based on the client's response (i.e., tap/touch). Score is based on observation for the I Say You Do activity.

Step 5: Print or record data for the client file as needed.

## Activity 7

Positional concept cards and cutouts by Mia McDaniel for preschool through second-grade clients.

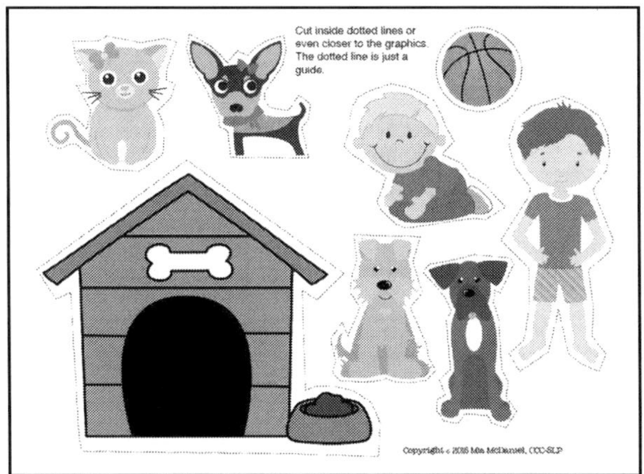


**FIGURE 4–33A.** Mia McDaniel Putting Words in Your Mouth positional concepts Screenshot 1. Reproduced with permission of Mia McDaniel, MA, CCC-SLP, http://www.puttingwordsinyourmouth.com

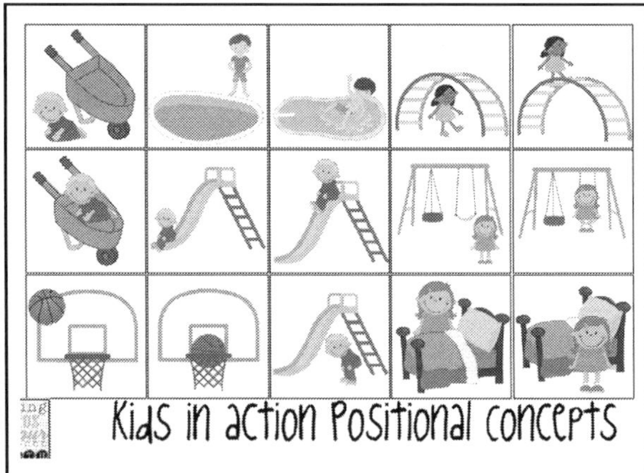


**FIGURE 4–33B.** Mia McDaniel Putting Words in Your Mouth positional concepts Screenshot 2. Reproduced with permission of Mia McDaniel, MA, CCC-SLP, http://www.puttingwordsinyourmouth.com

This activity can be use with or without a Cariboo game to target positional concepts. The Cariboo Cards for Positional Concepts activity by Mia McDaniel is designed to be used with a personal Cariboo game. The cards can also be used as a stand-alone card game.

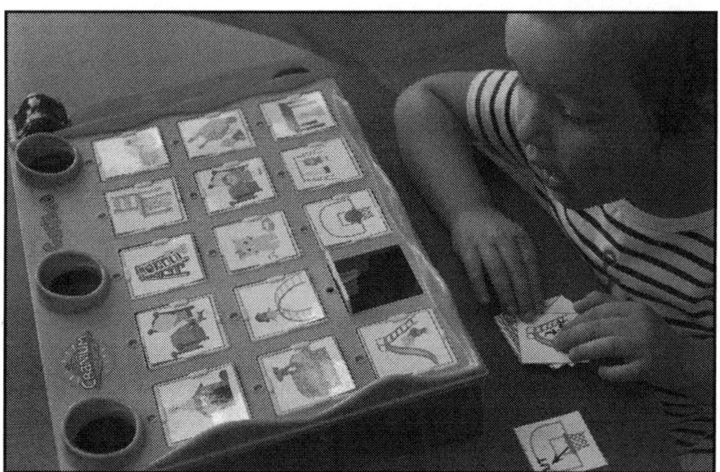

**FIGURE 4–34.** Hannah Clark positional concepts.

To download Cariboo Cards for Positional Concepts, visit https://www.teacherspayteachers .com/Product/Cariboo-Cards-for-Positional-Concepts-2-sets-teaching-materials-1784813

**FIGURE 4–35.** Cariboo cards QR code.

For a more effective and efficient therapy session, this activity can be printed on cardstock and laminated for durability and set up prior to the therapy session.

### *Individual or Small Group Session*

Using Cariboo game with activity

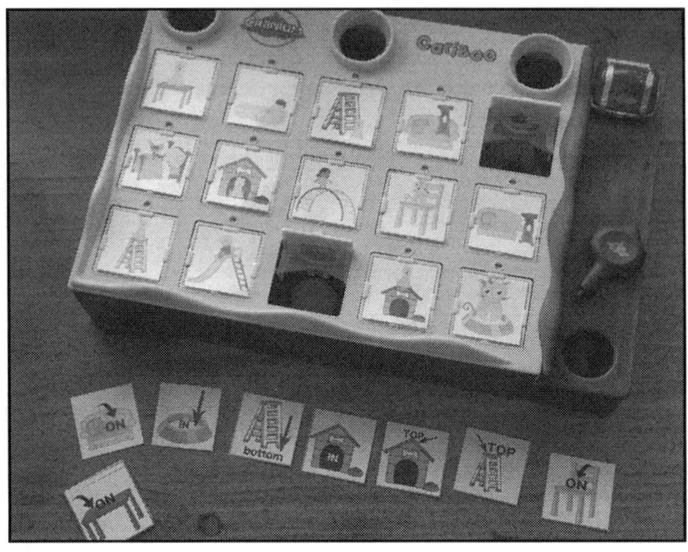

**FIGURE 4–36.** Cariboo.

Step 1:  With the client sitting aside or across from you, give an explanation of what the intended therapy lesson will be (i.e., "Today we will be practicing language concept with this fun activity and using the Cariboo game"). *NOTE:* The SLPA should take initial direction from the supervising SLP in regard to the client's ability and targeted objectives.

Step 2:  Place the stack of corresponding cards (the name/picture representation cards) in close proximity to the client. *NOTE:* Pets, kids in action images, or a combination of the pets/kids cards should be already placed on the game doors of Cariboo prior to the therapy session.

Step 3:  Allow the client to choose a card from the deck and then scan the images on the game doors to find the one that portrays the card chosen from the deck. If the client is successful in identifying the match, the game door will open. *NOTE:* If the client is unable to relate to the concepts chosen, you can simply provide a command related to the object that he or she should open (i.e., "open the dog under the table," "the dog is under" or just "under").

Step 4:  As with typical Cariboo play, if the client finds a ball, he or she gets to deposit it toward opening the treasure chest.

Step 5:  If the client requires additional support, use the image cutouts (i.e., character, animal, pool, slide, etc.) to model "the dog on the bed."

Step 6:  Record data as needed and required in the client file.

Using activity without the Cariboo game

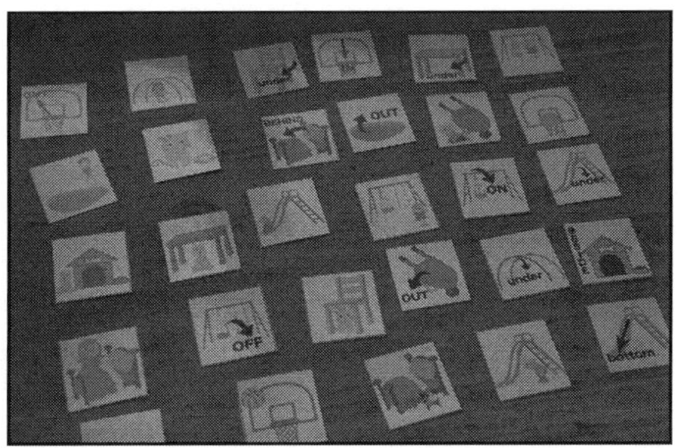

**FIGURE 4–37A.** Positional cards Cutout 1.

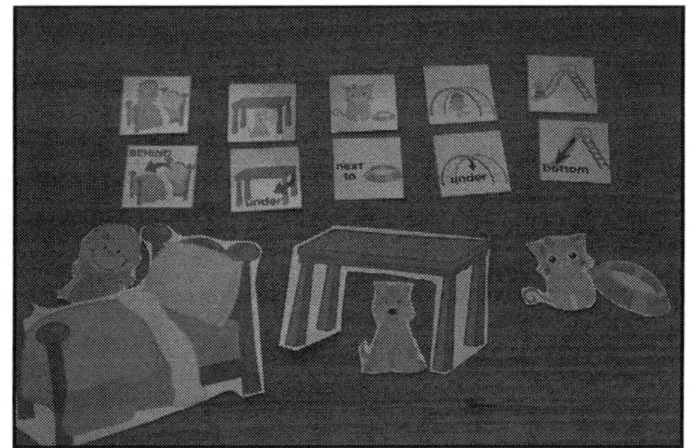

**FIGURE 4–37B.** Positional cards Cutout 2.

Step 1: With the client sitting aside or across from you, give an explanation of what the intended therapy lesson will be (i.e., "Today we are going to learn new words"). *NOTE:* The SLPA should take initial direction from the supervising SLP in regard to the client's ability and targeted objectives.

Step 2: Put the entire pet and kids in action image cards face down in a deck.

Step 3: Have the client choose a card and describe the picture including the positions (i.e., "the dog is in the doghouse").

    a. Option: You can place all cards (action image cards and position word cards) face up on a table and have the client choose a position word card and find the matching concept image card.

Step 4: If the client needs additional support, use the image cutouts (i.e., character, animal, pool, slide, etc.) to model "the dog on the bed."

Step 5: Record data as required and needed in the client file.

## Activity 8

Targeting grammar using the Syntax Workout app created by a certified speech and language pathologist and developed by the Virtual Speech Center.

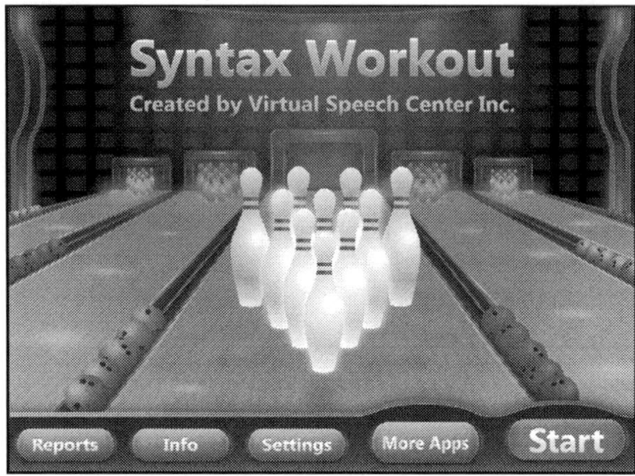


**FIGURE 4–38A.** Virtual Speech Center Syntax Workout main screenshot. Reproduced with permission of Virtual Speech Center.

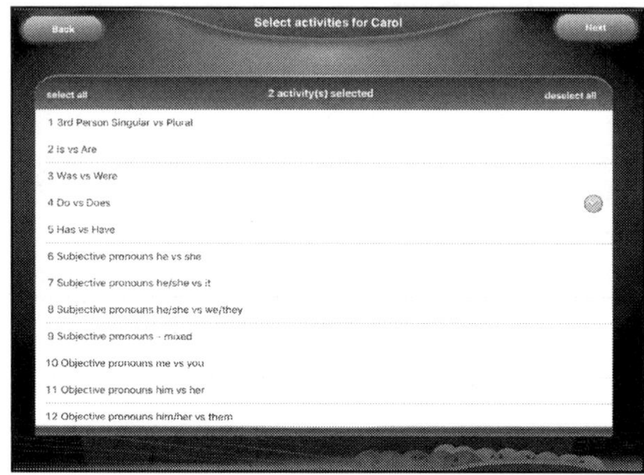


**FIGURE 4–38B.** Virtual Speech Center Syntax Grammar activities screenshot. Reproduced with permission of Virtual Speech Center.

Syntax Workout includes 1,500 stimuli in the following activities: third-person singular, do vs. does, has vs. had, is vs. are, was vs. were, subjective pronouns (I, you, he she, etc.), objective pronouns (me, you, him, her, etc.), possessive pronouns (my, your, his her, etc.), and demonstrative pronouns (this, that, those, these). Syntax Workout has an option to play a built-in reward bowling game after a selected number of correct trials are completed by the client.

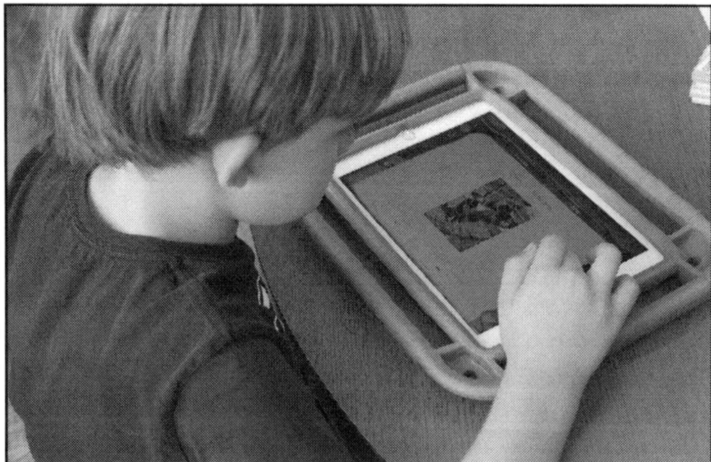

**FIGURE 4–39.** Riley Clark syntax app.

To download Syntax Workout and to access many other speech and language resources, visit https://www.virtualspeechcenter.com

**FIGURE 4–40.** Virtual Speech Center QR code.

For a more efficient and effective therapy session, take time to enter the client profile information into the app and adjust activity settings as needed. We also suggest you become familiar with the app prior to the therapy session.

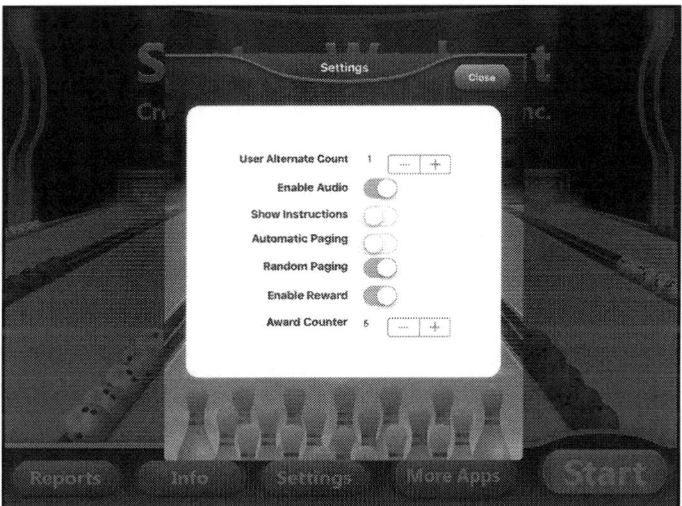


**FIGURE 4–41.** Virtual Speech Center Syntax settings screenshot. Reproduced with permission of Virtual Speech Center.

- User Alternate Count—use this setting to select the number of trials before switching to the next client (i.e., three trials per client).

- Enable Audio—use this setting to provide a narration.

- Show Instructions—use this setting to display text on the image screens.

- Automatic Paging—use this setting to automatically have the app move to the next page of stimuli. If off, the user will press next to advance the page.

- Random Paging—use this setting if you have more than one activity chosen for a client and want the stimuli to be randomly presented during session.

- Enable Reward—use this setting to automatically display a bowling game reward.

- Award Counter—set this to the number of correct trials when Enable Reward is on (i.e., five correct trials and then the reward game will be displayed).

### *Individual or Small Group Session*

Step 1: With the client sitting aside or across from you, give an explanation of what the intended therapy lesson will be (i.e., "Today we will be practicing grammar using an app"). *NOTE:* The SLPA should take initial direction from the supervising SLP in regard to the client's ability and targeted objectives.

Step 2: Open Syntax Workout and tap "Start."

Step 3: Select the client(s) participating in the therapy session and tap "Next." *NOTE:* The client's profile information should be set up prior to the therapy session.

Step 4: Based on objectives and goals, select the syntax activities for client. The client's name will be displayed at the top of the screen. Tap "Next." If more than one client was selected to participate in the therapy session, select activities for each client and tap "Next."

Step 4: The selected stimuli will be displayed on the screen. *NOTE:* It is important to have all the proper settings selected prior to the therapy session (i.e., number of trials per client before switching to the next client, audio option, text option, enable built-in reward, etc.).

Step 5: Have the client tap the selection that he or she believes is correct or respond according to visual stimuli (i.e., if the direction option is on, text prompts will be displayed and the app will autoscore based on the client's answer selection. If the enable audio option is off, the SLPA will score, correct or incorrect, based on the client's chosen response.). *NOTE:* If appropriate, use the recording feature by selecting the record button on the top left of the screen. Clients can repeat the grammatically correct sentence and play back for self-monitoring.

Step 6: If more than one client was selected for the therapy session, the next client will be displayed along with the targeted stimuli. Repeat Step 5 for each additional client.

Step 7: Tap "Finish" to end the session.

Step 8: Tap "Reports" to view client results by activity or by date. Reports may be printed for the client file or emailed to an appropriate supervising SLP.

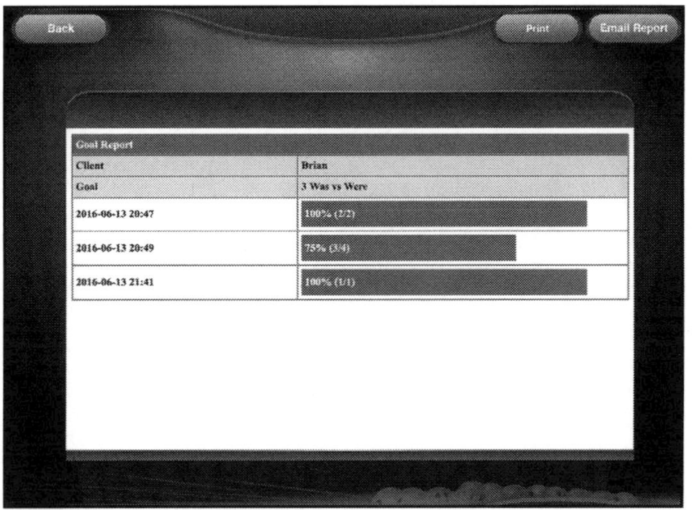

**FIGURE 4–42.** Virtual Speech Center Syntax results screenshot. Reproduced with permission of Virtual Speech Center.

# 5

# Social Language and Pragmatics

Social language, or as it is commonly referred to as pragmatics, is the ability to appropriately "use" language based on the context of the communication exchange. Although this skill continues to develop (mature) throughout childhood, typically developing children are able to vary their language use to match the need of the listener(s). It should be noted that social language rules vary across cultures; therefore, knowledge of culture is imperative to social language acquisition. A social communicative disorder is defined by the American Psychiatric Association (2013) as a deficit using communication for social purposes, such as greetings, appropriately considering the social context.

As such, clients with social communicative disorders struggle following rules such as turn taking, reading verbal and nonverbal cues, making inferences, and figurative language. This chapter includes activities for topic maintenance, perspective-taking, figurative language, identifying and using idioms, and reasoning and will help you address the specific needs of children with social communicative disorders. As you become familiar with these activities, you will begin to gain with confidence working with children with these needs and, under the guidance of your supervising speech-language pathologist (SLP), begin to develop your own lessons based on these activities.

## ACTIVITIES FOR SOCIAL LANGUAGE AND PRAGMATIC NEEDS

### Objectives

The following are some sample objectives for social language and pragmatic needs within a therapy session:

1. Client will interrupt appropriately (i.e., "excuse me, . . . ") in 9 out of 10 opportunities across three data points.

2. Client will change the topic appropriately in 9 out of 10 opportunities across three data points.

95

3. Client will avoid topics that are inappropriate for the setting in 9 out of 10 opportunities across three data points.

4. Client will notice when his or her conversation partner is bored in 9 out of 10 opportunities across three data points.

## Activity 1

This activity targets social language (such as turn-taking, interrupting appropriately, asking about others, changing topics, and noticing when others are bored) using the Talking Together app for two to four clients within a small group.

Talking Together, developed by Virtual Speech Center and authored by Jennifer Rogers, MA, CCC-SLP, is a comprehensive app that encourages clients in groups of two to four to hold and maintain conversation. Clients use a tablet as a board-type game by placing it in the center of the table and competing to participate in conversation. Talking Together contains 25 pragmatic goals divided into categories (basic conversation, tone and body language, turn-taking, and topic maintenance) with over 100 topics that are assigned to client profiles prior to play.

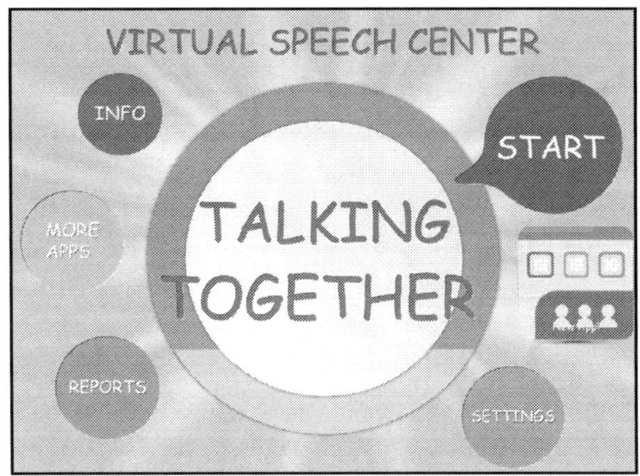


**FIGURE 5–1.** Virtual Speech Center talking together main screenshot. Reproduced with permission of Virtual Speech Center.

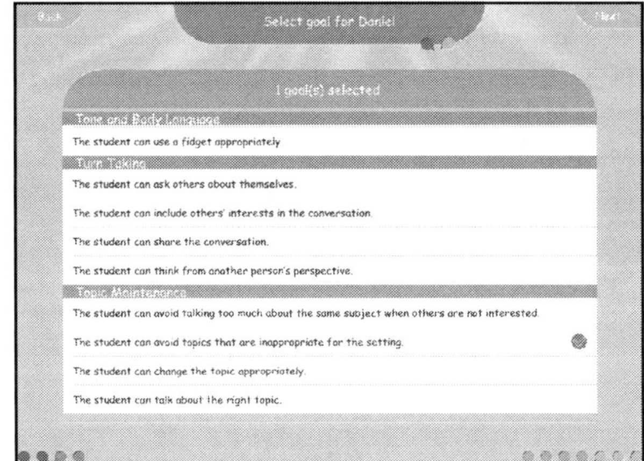


**FIGURE 5–2.** Virtual Speech Center goals screenshot. Reproduced with permission of Virtual Speech Center.

To download Talking Together, visit https://www.virtualspeechcenter.com

**FIGURE 5–3.** Virtual Speech Center QR code.

> To make for a more effective and efficient therapy session, enter specific client data (i.e., names and target objective/goals) into the app prior to the therapy session.

### *Task Setup*

Step 1:  Add client names.

Step 2:  Tap client names that will be participating in the therapy session and tap "Next."

Step 3:  Select goal(s) for the client and press "Next." *NOTE:* The speech-language pathology assistant (SLPA) should take guidance from supervising SLP for appropriate goals.

Step 4:  Repeat Step 3 for all clients participating in the therapy session.

Step 5:  Tap the content to be used during session and tap "Next." There are five choices: About Me, Favorites, Hypothetical Questions, Recreation, and School. To edit the content, tap "edit" and tap the specific content to be selected or deselected.

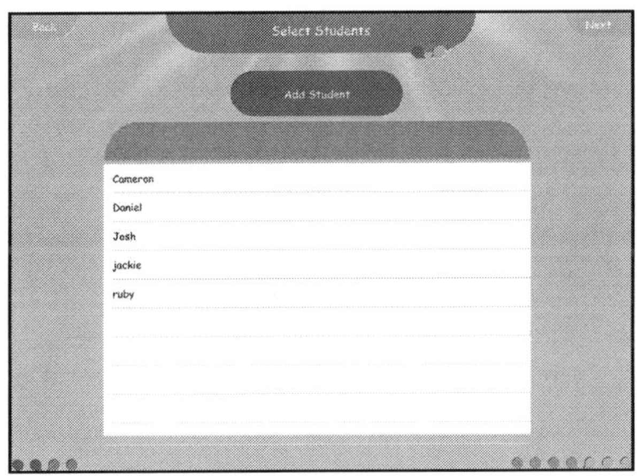

**FIGURE 5–4A.** Virtual Speech Center add student screenshot. Reproduced with permission of Virtual Speech Center.

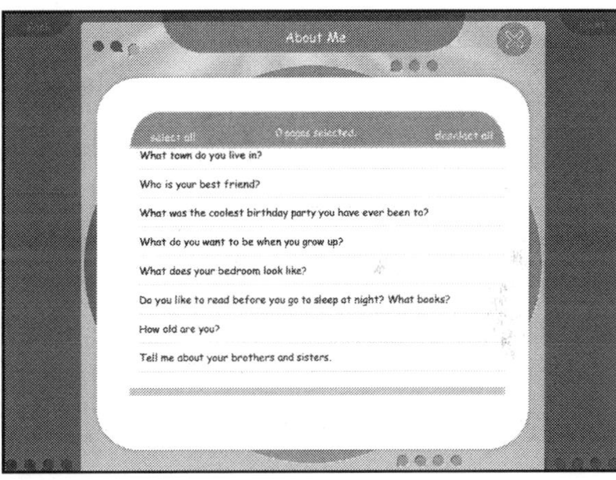

**FIGURE 5–4B.** Virtual Speech Center content screenshot. Reproduced with permission of Virtual Speech Center.

Step 6: Access the "Settings" to adjust the audio and customize the scoring sounds if needed.

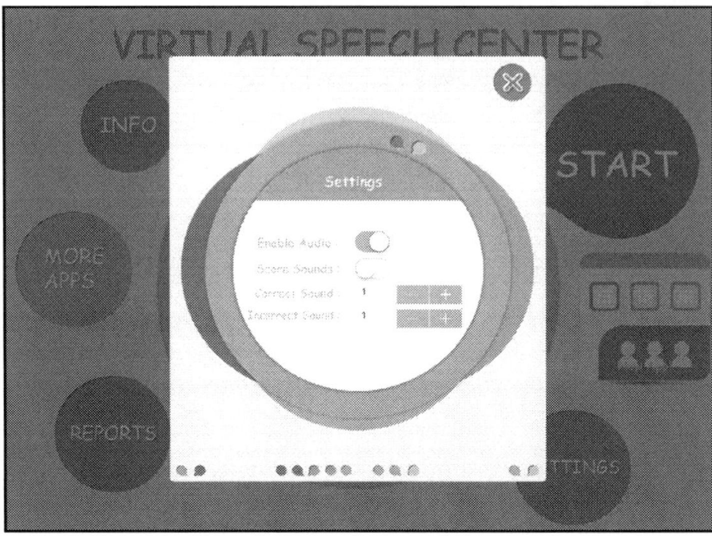


**FIGURE 5–5.** Virtual Speech Center settings screenshot. Reproduced with permission of Virtual Speech Center.

### Small Group Session

Step 1: Open the Talking Together App and place the tablet on the table or workspace so that all clients participating can easily reach it.

Step 2: Explain to the clients that they will be working on their individual communication skills using the Talking Together app.

Step 3: Model and explain to the clients that they will compete to practice their conversation skills by tapping the "GO" button that corresponds to their name as it rotates. The first one to tap "GO" will have a turn. An option is to have the clients sit around the table or workspace so that they are sitting on the same side where the tablet displays their name and allow them to take turns by moving in a clockwise direction. This will avoid a quicker client taking all the turns.

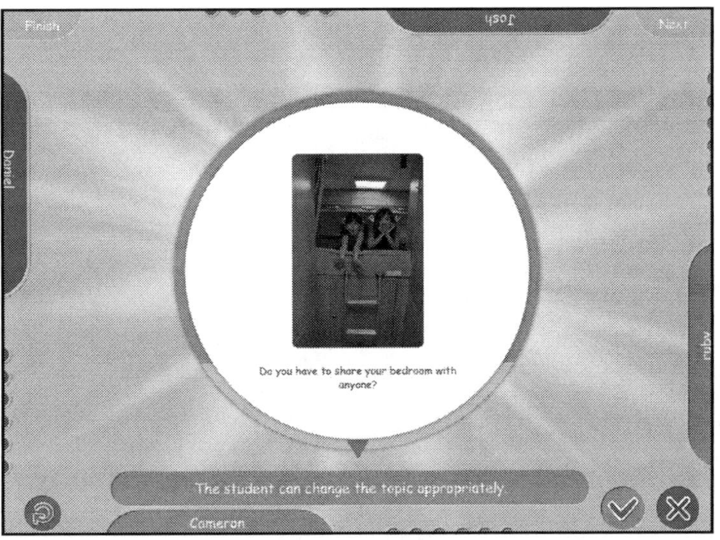


**FIGURE 5–6.** Virtual Speech Center game play 4 screenshot. Reproduced with permission of Virtual Speech Center.

Step 4:  The conversation spinner will point to the client that tapped "GO" while narrating the question (i.e., "Do you play any sports? If so, which one?"). Their individual goal will display above their name. Allow the clients to ask one of their conversation partners the question (i.e., "Josh, do you play sports?"). Press the "play arrow" to repeat the question if needed. *NOTE:* The audio can be disabled within the settings and, if appropriate, clients can read/ask the questions.

Step 5:  Tap "Next" to display another content question and continue the conversation opportunities.

Step 5:  Track progress by scoring correct (yes, the clients looked at their conversation partner when asking) by tapping the "check" or incorrect by tapping the "x." The data will be stored and can be emailed or printed at the end of the session by accessing the "REPORTS" area on the main home screen. Record needed data in the client file.

## Activity 2

Targets choosing (receptive) or responding with (expressive) correct social responses in a variety of social contexts using the Social Quest app for middle school clients. Depending on client abilities, this app may be used for younger or older clients.

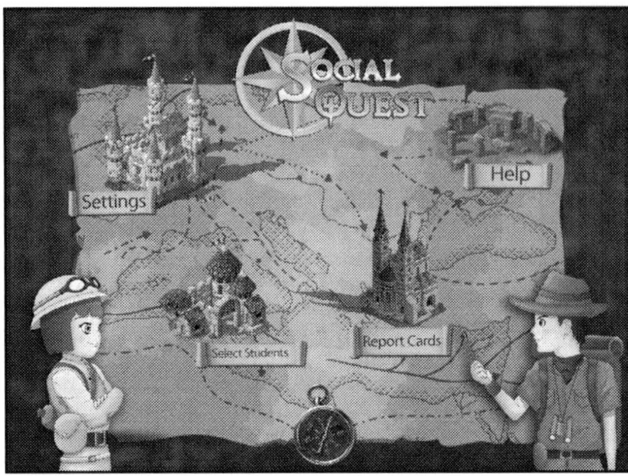

**FIGURE 5–7A.** Smarty Ears Social Quest main screenshot. Reproduced with permission of Smarty Ears, LLC. All rights reserved.

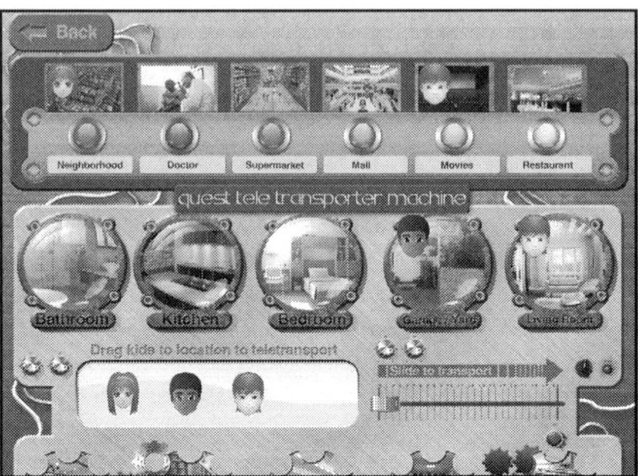

**FIGURE 5–7B.** Smarty Ears Social Quest scenario screenshot. Reproduced with permission of Smarty Ears, LLC. All rights reserved.

Social Quest, developed by Smarty Ears and authored by SLP Rosie Sims, is designed to help clients improve social language comprehension and expression. This app uses a variety of social settings (i.e., neighborhood, doctor, restaurant, specific areas inside the home) and photographs as visuals to help clients navigate real-world situations. A built-in motivational system allows clients to collect rewards along the way.

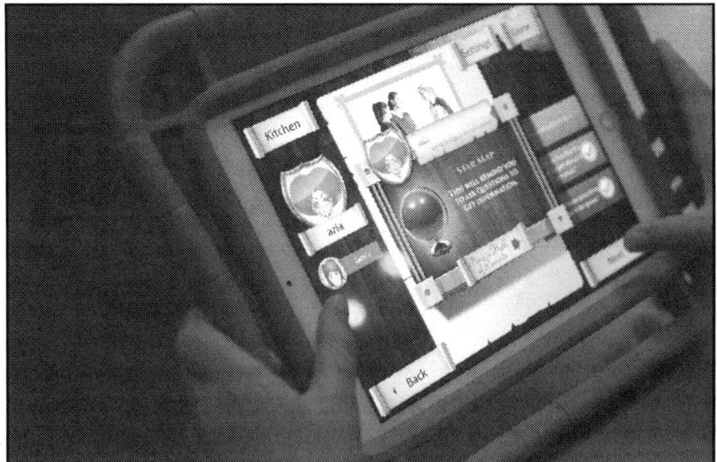

**FIGURE 5–8.** Reward screenshot.

To download or find out more about Social Quest, visit http://smartyearsapps.com

**FIGURE 5–9.** Smarty Ears QR code.

> To make for more effective and efficient therapy sessions, enter a specific client date (i.e., names) as needed into the app prior to the therapy session.

### *Task Setup*

Step 1:  Enter client names into "Select Students."

Step 2:  Select an avatar or photo to represent the client. An option is to allow the client to choose an avatar.

Step 3:  Select expressive or receptive as appropriate for the individual client. These settings also can be adjusted during the therapy session by tapping the "gear" icon at the top of the page. *NOTE:* If choosing a receptive activity, there is an option to require two correct answers versus one correct answer for any social situation by sliding the button to yes. This helps with teaching that often there is more than one correct answer for a particular social situation.

Step 4:  Within the "Settings" on the main screen, there is an option to remove the background image from the screen and allow for a cleaner and less distracting screen. Tap "Clean UI" to remove the background or "Default UI" to keep the background image. This setting can also be adjusted during the therapy session by tapping the "gear" icon at the top of the page. In addition, audio cues can be turned on or off.

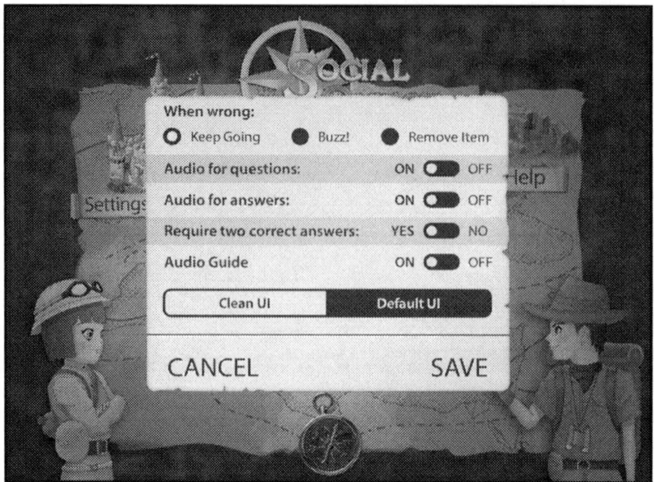


**FIGURE 5–10.** Smarty Ears settings screenshot. Reproduced with permission of Smarty Ears, LLC. All rights reserved.

### *Individual or Small Group Session*

Step 1:  With clients sitting aside or across from, explain that they will be using an app to help work on social language situations. *NOTE:* The SLPA should take initial direction from the supervising SLP in regard to the client's objectives and goals.

Step 2:  Tap the student name to select client(s) participating in therapy session and tap "Next."

Step 3:  Drag and drop the representative photograph or avatar to the social context that addresses each client's specific objective and goals and slide the lever to begin. A client may be dragged and dropped into multiple social contexts (i.e., neighborhood and kitchen).

Step 4:  For clients for whom you have chosen receptive activities, read the scenario to your clients, allow them to listen to the audio narration, or read aloud the social scenario. Clients participating in the session will appear on the left side of the screen with the first player at the top. Clients will tap one or two answer choices depending on the setup (i.e., two correct responses yes/no). The app will automatically keep data on correct and incorrect responses.

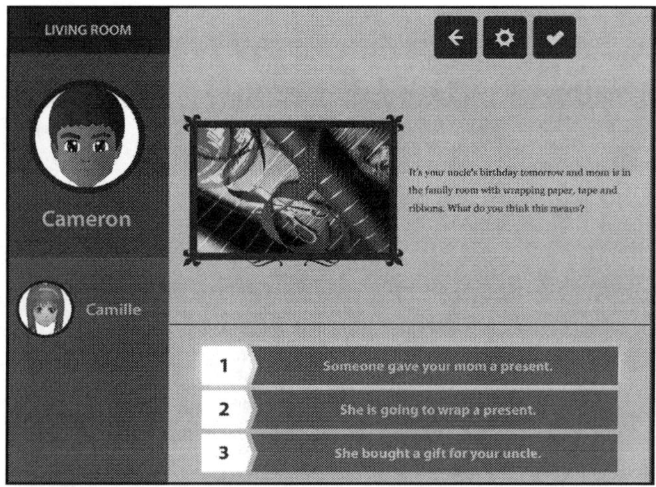



**FIGURE 5–11.** Smarty Ears receptive screenshot. Reproduced with permission of Smarty Ears, LLC. All rights reserved.

Step 5: For clients for whom you have chosen expressive activities, allow them to listen to the social scenario and then respond. You will score correct (got it) or almost or incorrect (missed). Tap "Next" to display a new scenario for the next client.

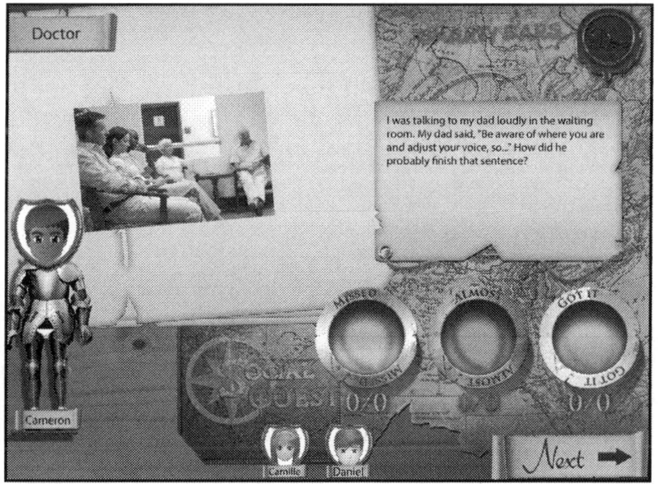



**FIGURE 5–12.** Smarty Ears expressive screenshot. Reproduced with permission of Smarty Ears, LLC. All rights reserved.

Step 6: Record data as needed in the client file. View saved data by tapping "Report Cards." Data can be shared via email, printed, or saved to an outside source such as Dropbox.

## Activity 3

Targeting pragmatic objectives such as perspective-taking, body language, facial expression, common expressions, auditory processing, and interpreting vocal intonation using Between the Lines app for elementary age through adolescent clients.

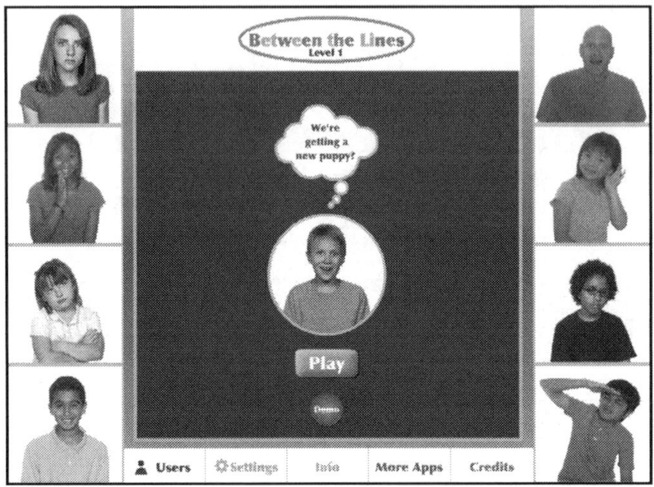


**FIGURE 5–13.** Hamaguchi Between the Lines 1 main screenshot. Reproduced with permission of Hamaguchi Apps.

Hamaguchi Apps has a series of Between the Lines apps: Level 1, Level 2, and Advanced. There are more than 60 available tasks/questions within three activities (Who Is Talking, What Is He/ She Thinking, and What Does That Mean?) and three built-in reward games that can be set to on or off. For purposes of this activity, Between the Lines Level 1 will be illustrated.

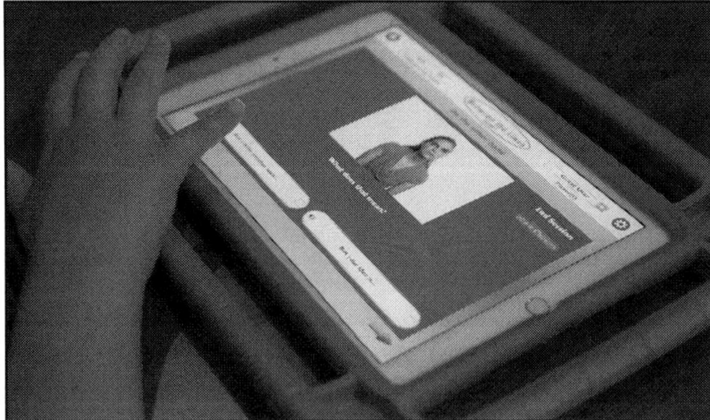

**FIGURE 5–14.** Between the lines.

To download Between the Lines Level 1, find out more about additional light versions of the Between the Lines series, or view demos of Hamaguchi Apps, visit http://www.hamaguchi apps.com

**FIGURE 5–15.**
Hamaguchi QR code.

To make for more effective and efficient therapy sessions, enter the specific client data into the User section, set up therapy groups, and customize settings as needed prior to the therapy session.

### Task Setup

Step 1:  Tap "Users" to enter client names or set up groups.

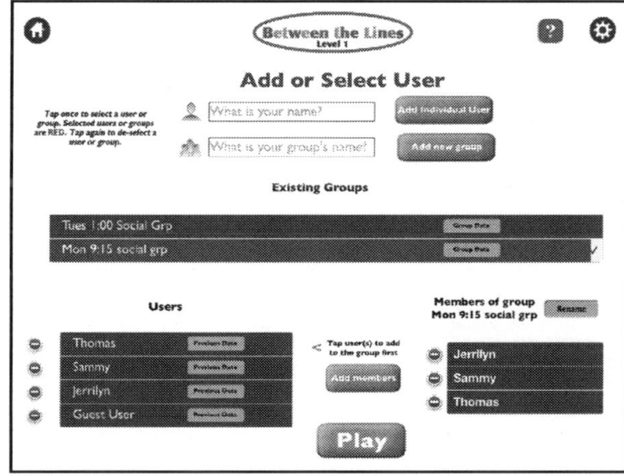

**FIGURE 5–16.** Hamaguchi user screenshot. Reproduced with permission of Hamaguchi Apps.

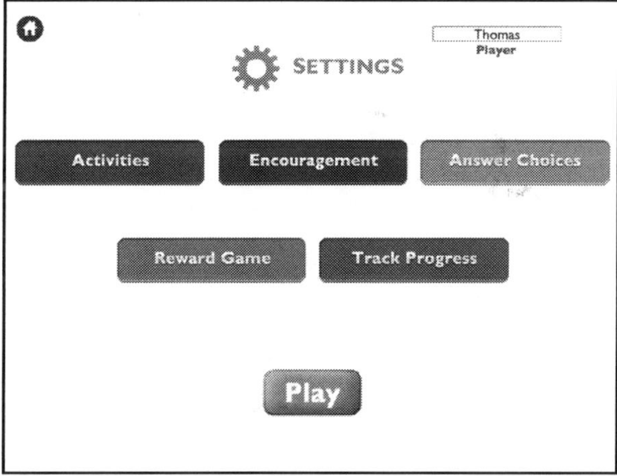

**FIGURE 5–17.** Hamaguchi setting screenshot. Reproduced with permission of Hamaguchi Apps.

Step 2:  Tap "Settings" to customize the following areas:

- Activities—choose one to three activities that address listening and facial expressions, body language and perspective taking, or expressions, idioms, and slang. If more than one activity is selected, there is an option to rotate one task within each activity or randomly have the activities display.

- Encouragement—choose to allow praise phrases after a selected number of correct answers and adjust the bell sound as needed.

- Answer Choices—select the number of manually shown or automatically shown answers to choose from.

- Reward Game—select to allow one of three games (Dunk Tank, Bull's Eye, or Knock 'Em Down) to play after a selected number of questions.

- Track Progress—select to allow progress to be tracked and scores to be displayed. *NOTE:* Progress is only tracked when clients are set up in the "User" area. The guest selection will not track data.

### Individual or Small Group Session

Step 1:  Confirm that the correct client or group is selected by tapping the individual client or group name. Questions and tasks will rotate between users when groups have been set up.

Step 2:  With the client across or aside from you, explain that he or she will be using an app to work on social language activities (i.e., "Johnny, today we will practice listening and figuring out who said it").

Step 3:  Open Between the Lines Level 1 and tap "Play" on the home screen. *NOTE:* Clients will receive the same stimuli when they are set up within a user group. When clients are set up as individual users, the activities/tasks can be customized for each client.

   a.  If the Who Is Talking? activity has been selected in the settings, the client will listen to a comment, view the visual choices of who said it, and select one of the choices.

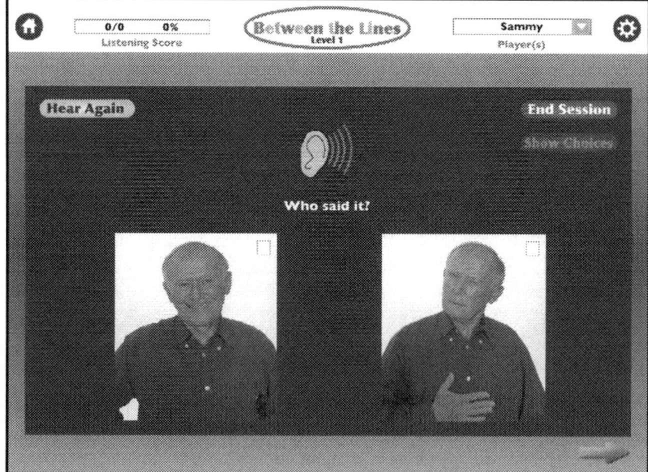


**FIGURE 5–18.** Hamaguchi Who Said That? screenshot. Reproduced with permission of Hamaguchi Apps.

b. If the What Is He/She Thinking? activity has been selected in the settings, the client will view a short video clip displaying a variety of facial expressions and body language, view text answer choices, and then select an answer.

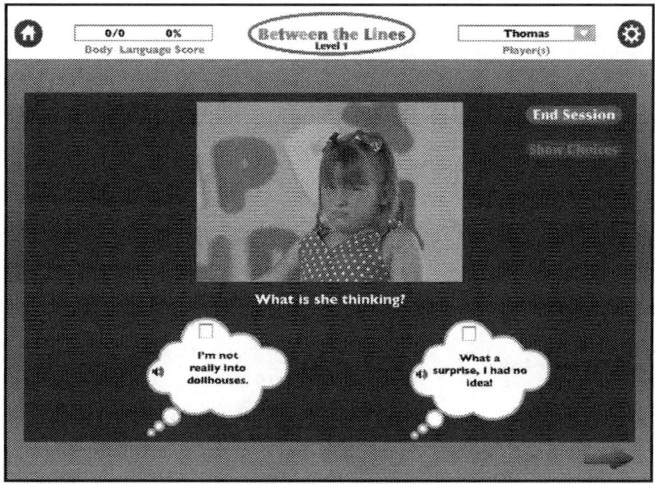



**FIGURE 5–19.** Hamaguchi What Is He/She Thinking? screenshot. Reproduced with permission of Hamaguchi Apps.

c. If the What Does That Mean? activity has been selected in the settings, the client will view a short video clip of common expressions, idioms, or slang; view text answer choices; and select an answer.

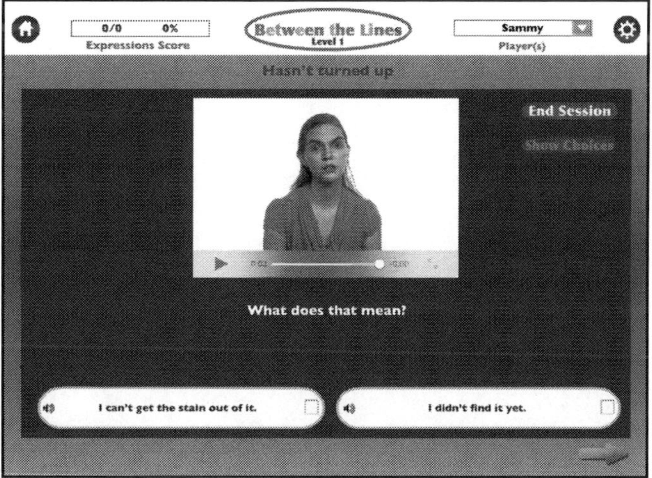



**FIGURE 5–20.** Hamaguchi What Does That Mean? screenshot. Reproduced with permission of Hamaguchi Apps.

Step 4:  Record data as needed in the client file. If the progress tracker was selected in settings, data may be viewed by accessing the user screen and tapping "previous data" for individual users or "group data" for clients who have been set up in groups.

## Activity 4

Targeting a variety of emotions for elementary age clients using a comprehensive social skills curriculum by Miss V's Speech World.

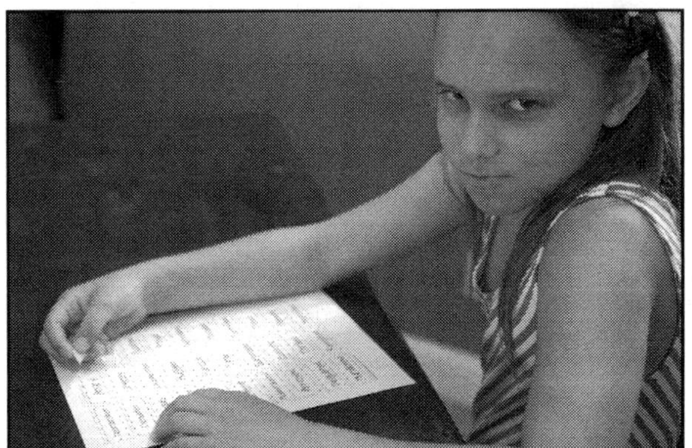

**FIGURE 5–21A.** Aria Derryberry angry.

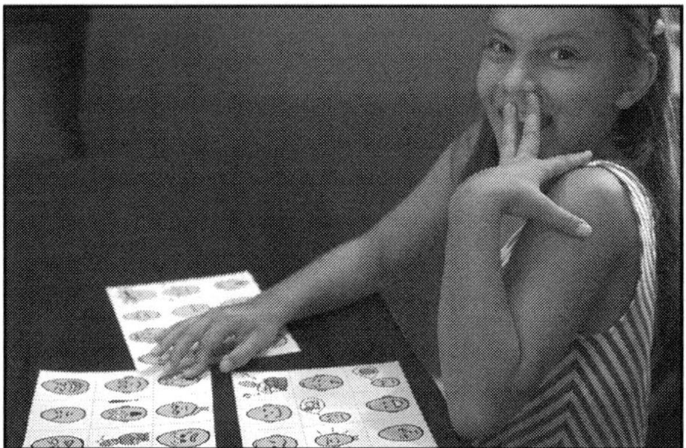

**FIGURE 5–21B.** Aria Derryberry surprised.

SLP Viola Dean of Miss V's Speech World has created a social skills group curriculum that contains 40 lessons and 252 activities that are appropriate to use with ages 6 through 17. For purposes of this activity, Part III (Feelings) of the curriculum will be illustrated.

To download Part III of the Social Skills Group Curriculum or the curriculum in its entirety, visit https://www.teacherspayteachers.com/Store/Miss-Vs-Speech-World

**FIGURE 5–22.** Miss V's Speech World QR code.

> For a more effective and efficient therapy session, the supplement materials can be printed on cardstock and laminated for durability prior to the therapy session.

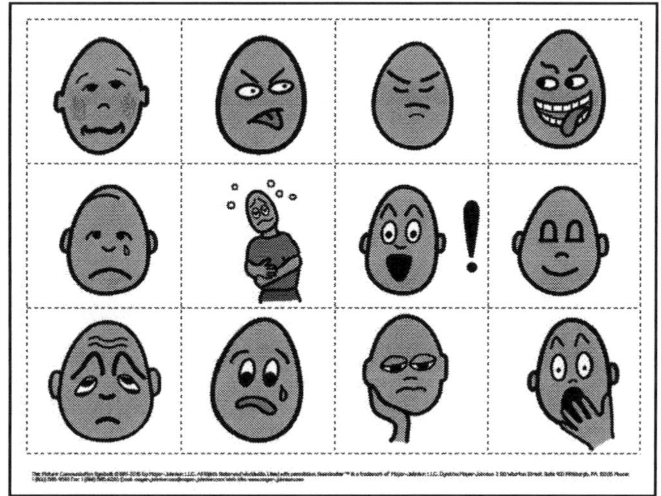

**FIGURE 5–23.** Miss V's Speech World emotion screenshot. Reproduced with permission of Miss V's Speech World.

### Task Setup

Step 1:  Print, cut, and laminate (optional) the emotion cards.

### Individual or Small Group Session

Step 1:  With the client(s) sitting aside or across from you, explain the purpose of the therapy lesson (i.e., "Today we will practice distinguishing positive from negative emotions"). *NOTE:* The SLPA should take initial direction from the supervising SLP in regard to the client's ability and targeted objectives.

Step 2:  Show each emotion card to the group and have the client(s) decide whether the depicted emotion is positive, negative, or neutral. Use a container to categorize them or create separate piles for positive or negative or neutral emotion cards. For a variation, instead of showing the emotion cards to the group, have the clients come up one at a time and imitate the facial expression of a card. Have the clients use a real-life model to determine whether the emotion is positive or negative.

Step 3:  Ask clients which clues they used to determine whether the emotion was positive or negative (i.e., eyebrows furrowed, mouth turned down).

Step 4:  Have clients take a guess as to what the emotion may be called or discuss which of these emotions they have felt recently and why.

Step 5:  Record data as needed in the client file for each client's progress.

For an additional or follow-up activity that addresses complex emotions using the same emotion cards and that can work for older clients, follow the steps below:

Step 1:  With the clients sitting aside or across from you, explain the purpose of the therapy lesson ("Today we will learn about more emotions, embarrassed, proud, nervous, guilty, and jealous"). *NOTE:* The SLPA should take initial direction from the supervising SLP in regard to clients' ability and targeted objectives.

Step 2:  Ask the clients which types of emotions they know or have learned about and create a list on paper or white board.

Step 3:  Ask the clients to name some other emotions that they might know. A few might be confused, embarrassed, proud, nervous or anxious, worried, disappointed, guilty, lonely, hopeful, ashamed, jealous, exhausted, shy, and so on.

Step 4:  Choose a few new emotions to work on (i.e., embarrassed, proud, jealous, etc.) and ask them for some synonyms for one of the emotions (i.e., embarrassed = mortified, self-conscious, humiliated; proud = fulfilled, rewarded).

Step 5:  Discuss whether or not feeling embarrassed or any other emotion you have chosen is a good feeling or a not so good feeling.

Step 6:  Ask your clients about some situations that might cause them to feel embarrassed (i.e., people are laughing at you, making a mistake in front of someone, everyone is looking at you) or any other emotion you have chosen.

## Activity 5

Targeting self-control for a variety of ages using a comprehensive social skills curriculum by Miss V's Speech World.

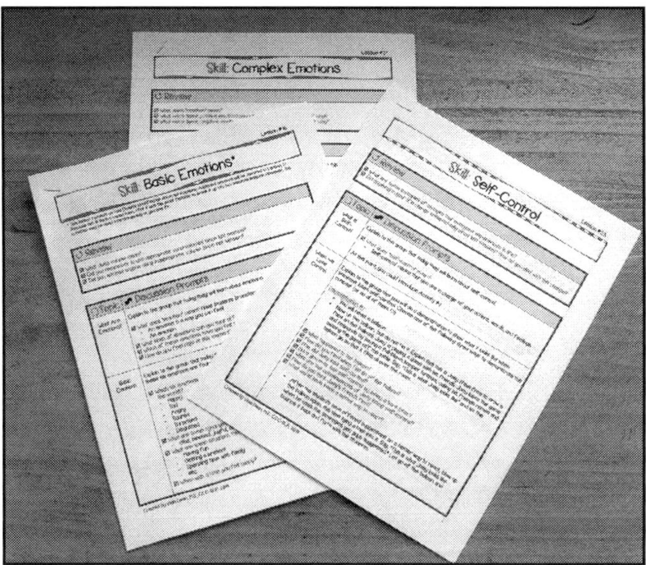

**FIGURE 5–24.**  Packet example.

SLP Viola Dean of Miss V's Speech World has created a social skills group curriculum that contains 40 lessons and 252 activities that are appropriate to use for ages 6 through 17. For purposes of this activity, Part III (Anger Management) of the curriculum will be used.

To download Part III of the Social Skills Group Curriculum or the curriculum in its entirety, visit https://www.teacherspayteachers.com/Store/Miss-Vs-Speech-World

**FIGURE 5–25.** Miss V's Speech World QR code.

For a more effective and efficient therapy session, the supplement materials can be printed on cardstock and laminated for durability prior to the therapy session.

*Task Setup*

Step 1: Print, cut, and laminate (optional) the situation cards.

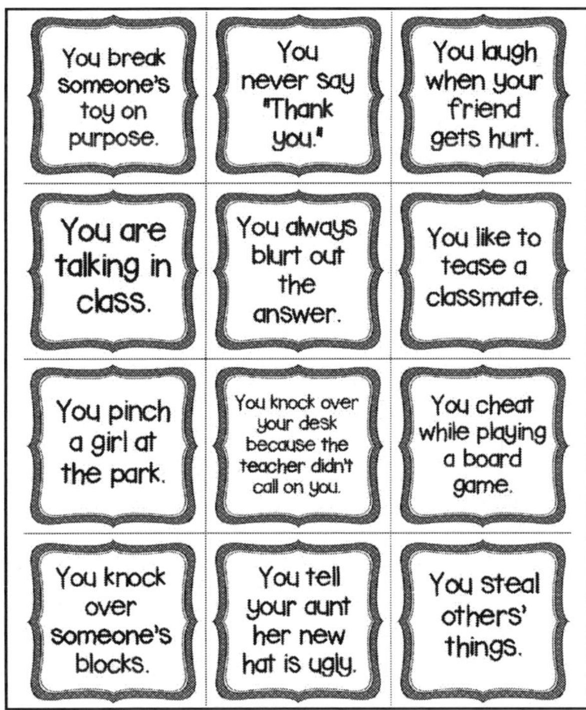


**FIGURE 5–26A.** Miss V's Speech World self-control scenarios Screenshot 1. Reproduced with permission of Miss V's Speech World.

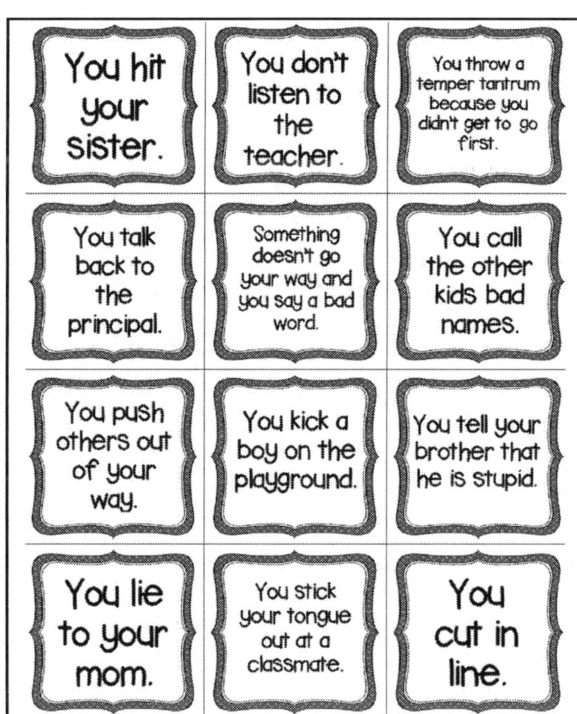


**FIGURE 5–26B.** Miss V's Speech World self-control scenarios Screenshot 2. Reproduced with permission of Miss V's Speech World.

### Other Materials Needed

- Balloon

- Tube of toothpaste or shaving cream

- Paper plate

### Individual or Small Group Session

Step 1:  With the clients sitting aside or across from you, explain the purpose of the therapy lesson (i.e., "Today we will be learning about self-control"). *NOTE:* The SLPA should take initial direction from the supervising SLP in regard to clients' ability and targeted objectives.

Step 2:  Ask the clients if they know what self-control means (i.e., self-control means that you are in charge of your actions, words, and feelings).

Step 3:  Give a demonstration to show what it looks like when someone loses self-control. A fun demonstration is to use a balloon.

  a.  Blow up the balloon but do not tie it.

  b.  Give the balloon a name (i.e., Joey) and give a potential scenario.

  Sample script:

  This is Joey (draw a face on the balloon if you would like). Joey is playing a game with his friends. Joey lost the game and responds by having a full-blown temper tantrum, calling his friends names and swiping the game off the table.

Step 4:  While holding the balloon, tell the clients, "This is what Joey looks like" and let the balloon go so that it flies all over the room.

Step 5:  Discuss with the client(s):

  a.  What happened to the balloon?

  b.  How did you feel when I let go of the balloon?

  c.  How did Joey lose self-control?

  d.  Have you ever lost self-control by being a sore loser?

  e.  What are the consequences of Joey losing self-control?

  f.  How do you think Joey's friends feel?

  g.  What would have been a better way to react?

Step 6: Allow the clients to offer suggestions on a better way to react. Blow up the balloon again, this time tying a knot in it. Tell the clients, "This is what Joey looks like when he uses the strategies you guys suggested." Release the balloon and bounce back and forth with the clients.

Step 7: Discuss with clients:

a.   Would you rather play with a balloon that has the knot tied or untied? Why?

b.   How do you feel around people who lose self-control?

For a follow-up activity (using the printed self-control scenarios) that demonstrates that our actions cannot always be undone, follow the steps below:

Step 1: With the clients sitting aside or across from you, give them an explanation of what the intended therapy lesson will be (i.e., "Let's learn more about self-control."). *NOTE:* The SLPA should take initial direction from the supervising SLP in regard to clients' ability and targeted objectives.

Step 2: Have the clients sit around a table or workspace with a paper plate in the middle.

Step 3: Allow clients to take turns choosing a self-control scenario card and read it aloud. While cards are being read, point out how the actions will affect others and how the characters are losing self-control.

Step 4: Each time a card is read, a client gets to squeeze a glob of toothpaste or shaving cream onto the paper plate.

Step 5: When all the cards are read, discuss that by losing self-control, a lot of feelings can get hurt. Now, ask, "How can we fix it once we have lost self-control and hurt others' feelings?"

Step 6: Allow clients to come up with suggestions and create a list. For each suggestion, tell them, "Okay, so put the toothpaste or shaving cream back in the tube." The clients will see that is impossible and begin to understand how actions cannot always be undone.

Step 7: For a less messy variation, have the clients pop bubbles on bubble wrap. They also will not be able to fix the popped bubble wrap.

## Activity 6

Using social stories to help clients understand proper social behavior within the Social Norms app or creating social stories with customized photos and text.

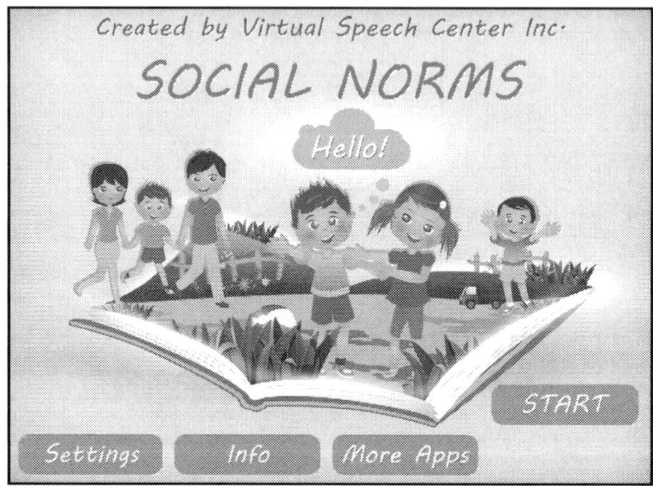


**FIGURE 5–27.** Virtual Speech Centers social norms main screenshot. Reproduced with permission of Virtual Speech Center.

The Social Norms app by Virtual Speech Center helps clients learn about social rules and behaviors through stories. It includes over 50 stories with visuals for a variety of categories: Manners (i.e., thank you, excuse me, waiting), Hygiene/Health (i.e., washing hands, runny nose, using toilet), Safety (i.e., crossing street, seat belts), Home (i.e., doing homework, cleaning up), School (i.e., answering questions in class, asking someone to play, fire drill), Community (i.e., shopping, restaurant, dentist), and Behavior (i.e., pushing, biting, banging head).

To download Social Norms, visit https://www.virtualspeechcenter.com

**FIGURE 5–28.** Virtual Speech Center QR code.

### *Individual Session*

Step 1:  Use social stories when it might be apparent that a client may have a difficult time with an upcoming scenario (i.e., fire drill). They can also be used to create discussion and talk about a better way to behave. *NOTE:* The SLPA should take initial direction from the supervising SLP in regard to clients' ability and targeted objectives.

Step 2:  Choose one of the built-in stories to address the client need.

   a. Tap "START" and select a story from any of the story categories: Behavior, Community, Home, Hygiene/Health, Manners, Safety, or School by tapping the story name.

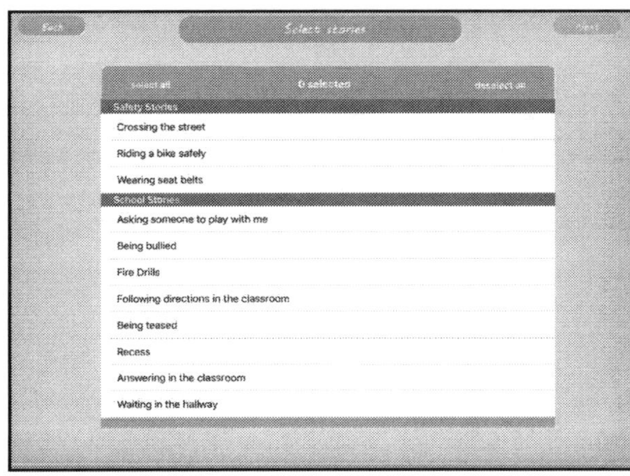

**FIGURE 5–29A.** Virtual Speech Center categories screenshot. Reproduced with permission of Virtual Speech Center.

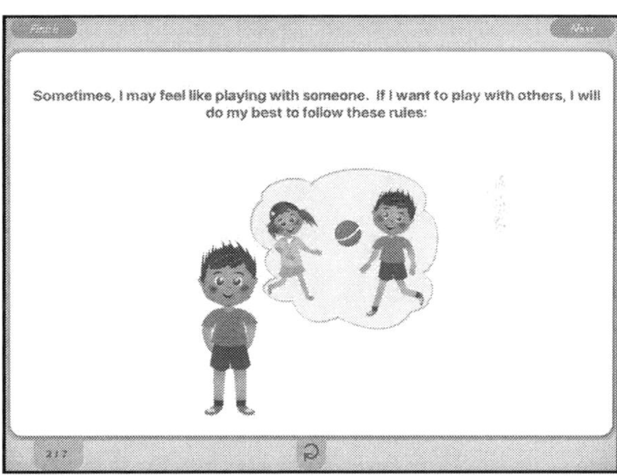


**FIGURE 5–29B.** Virtual Speech Center story page screenshot. Reproduced with permission of Virtual Speech Center.

   b. Tap "Begin" to start the story. *NOTE:* Be sure you have adjusted the settings on the main screen to play the audio of the story or turn it off if you would like to read the story to the client. Another option is for the client to read the story aloud. There is also an option to turn off the display of the story text.

   c. Tap "Next" to advance the pages of the story.

   d. Use this opportunity to discuss the situation with your client.

Step 3: To create a customized story:

    a. Tap "Settings" on the main screen.

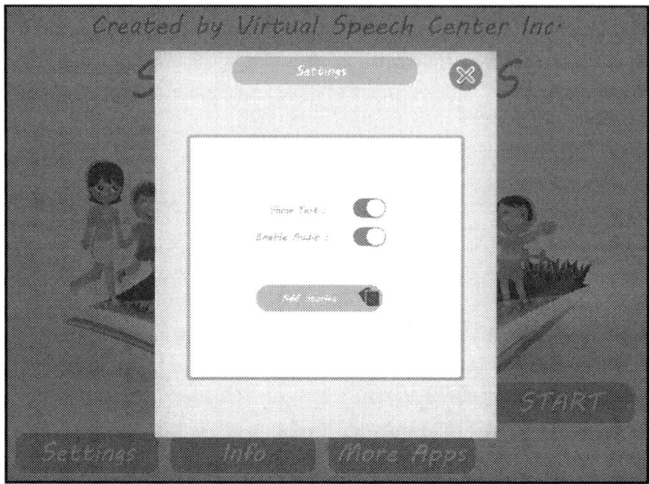

**FIGURE 5–30.** Virtual Speech Center settings screenshot. Reproduced with permission of Virtual Speech Center.

    b. Tap "Add Stories" and "Add New Story."

    c. Tap "dropdown arrow" to display the category you would like your story to be saved to. Tap the category that you would like your story saved to (i.e., Manners).

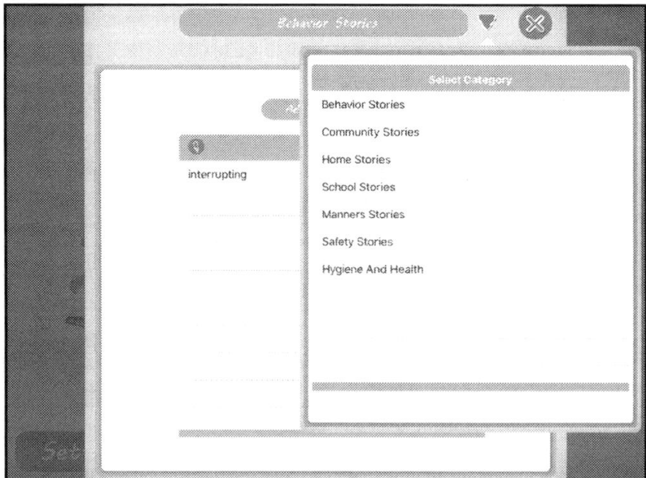


**FIGURE 5–31.** Virtual Speech Center new story dropdown screenshot. Reproduced with permission of Virtual Speech Center.

d. Give the story a title (i.e., interrupting) and tap "Continue." Now you are ready to begin to enter the text and images.

e. Add the text for the first page in the highlighted box. *NOTE:* It's important to keep the text in a positive, matter-of-fact, and first-person format (i.e., Sometimes I . . . I may feel . . . If I want . . . I will . . . ).

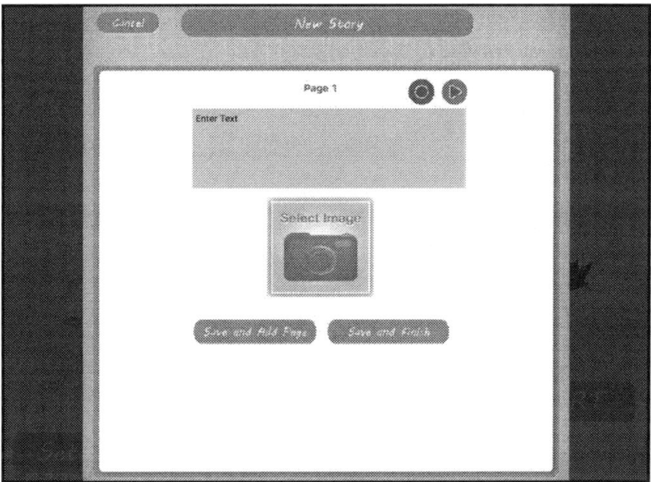


**FIGURE 5–32.** Virtual Speech Center add text, image, recording screenshot. Reproduced with permission of Virtual Speech Center.

f. Select an image from your photo library for the first page. *NOTE:* If you do not have an image you need, take a photograph and add it to your photo library. Be prepared by spending time taking photographs of the client of the undesired and desired behaviors (i.e., shouting out in class, raising hand) and adding them to your photo library.

g. Record the audio for the text you have added. If appropriate, have the client do the recording. Tap the "record button" to begin recording and again to stop the recording. When you are finished and want to listen to the recording, tap the "play arrow."

h. Tap "Save and Add Page" and repeat Steps e to f for additional story pages or tap "Save and Finish" to save your story.

# REFERENCE


American Psychiatric Association. (2013). *Diagnostic and statistical manual of mental disorders* (5th ed.). Arlington, VA: Author.

# 6

# AAC for Complex Communication Needs

Augmentative and alternative communication or AAC may be defined as any tool used to enhance, supplant, or replace verbal speech. Individuals with complex communication needs (CCN) often employ AAC systems to express their thoughts, feelings, needs wants, wishes, and beliefs. These individuals employ AAC to direct others, socialize, express social closeness, ask questions, answer questions, participate in class discussions, make appointments, tease and joke, protest and reject, direct others, advocate, make comments, and provide opinions, among many other essential functions.

AAC systems vary in degree of technology. They can consist of (1) no tech, paper-based, picture icons; (2) low-tech, single-message systems such as paper-overlay devices; and (3) high-tech systems having dedicated dynamic display communication. Many of these high-tech systems consist of iPads housing the latest AAC applications. Regardless of the "system," what is crucial is the availability of core vocabulary (Croos, Baker, Klotz, & Badman, 1997).

The activities included in this chapter will help you address the specific needs of clients with complex communication needs. As you become familiar with these activities (and systems), you will begin to gain confidence working with clients with CCN and, under the guidance of your supervising speech-language pathologist (SLP), can develop your own therapy materials to fit the goals established by the SLP.

## ACTIVITIES FOR AAC FOR COMPLEX COMMUNICATION NEEDS

### Objectives

The following are some sample objectives for clients with complex communication needs:

1. Following a model of target vocabulary, the client will produce a single core vocabulary word (using AAC or natural speech) to control the actions of another (i.e., "more," "stop," "go," "again," or "different") in four of five opportunities across three consecutive data collection points.

2. Using an AAC system or natural speech, the client will make a comment about an activity using a single core vocabulary word (i.e., "like," "good," "bad" "silly") in four of five opportunities across three consecutive data collection points.

3. Given a single verbal prompting, the client will combine two core vocabulary words (using the AAC system or natural speech) to control the actions of another (i.e., "want more," "stop that," "go now," "make go," or "different one") in four of five opportunities across three consecutive data collection points.

> All Aided Language Input (modeled words) throughout these activities will be displayed in CAPS.

## Activity 1

Pop Rocket with Proloquo2Go AAC app for clients 3 to 10 years of age.

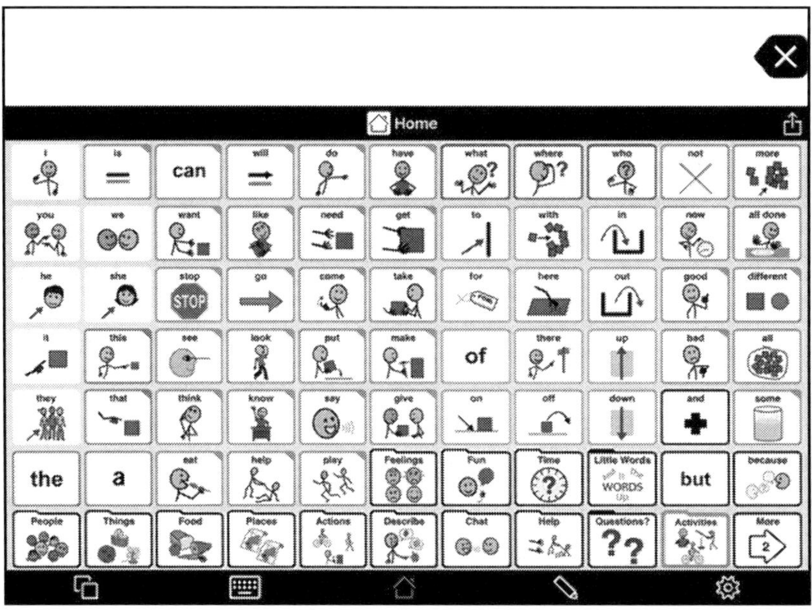

**FIGURE 6–1A.** P2Go Crescendo intermediate 7 × 11 screenshot. Reproduced with permission of ©AssistiveWare, symbols ©SymbolStix, LLC.

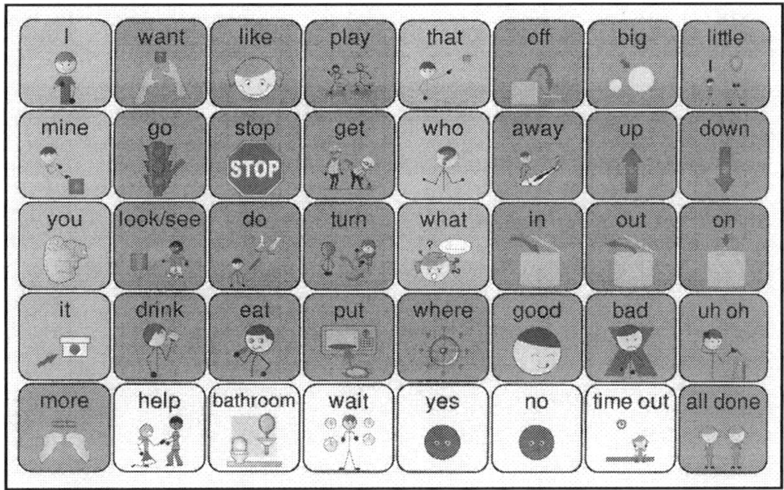

**FIGURE 6–1B.** Core40SS. Reproduced with permission of Smarty Symbols, LLC. All rights reserved.

For purposes of this lesson, P2Go Crescendo Intermediate in the 7 × 11-inch page layout is used. In addition, a paper communication board with core vocabulary created with Smarty Symbols is shown below. These layouts are examples and are presented for illustrative purposes. It's important to note that any type of AAC can be used for this lesson. Proloquo2Go by AssistiveWare is one of several robust symbol-supported communication apps. It is designed to promote growth of communication skills and foster language development using research-based vocabularies.

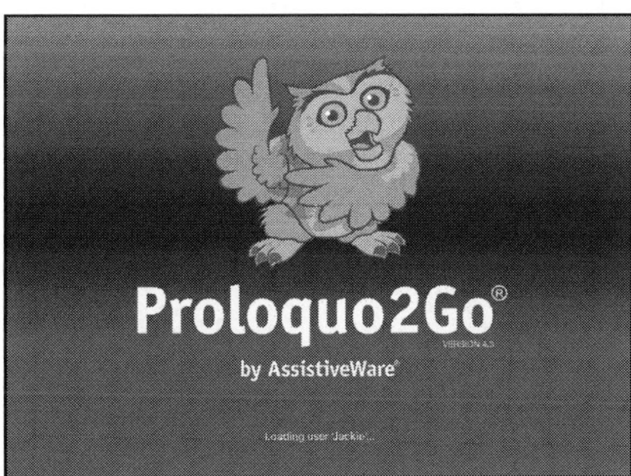

**FIGURE 6–2.** Mainscreen P2G. Reproduced with permission of ©AssistiveWare, symbols ©SymbolStix, LLC.

To download Proloquo2Go by AssistiveWare, visit https://www.assistiveware.com

**FIGURE 6–3.**
AssistiveWare QR code.

Smarty Symbols is an image library containing nearly 17,000 images that are organized according to educational categories such as animals, feelings, transportation, arts, ocean life, occupations, and so on. Visit Smarty Symbols at https://smartysymbols.com to learn more about creating materials with this diverse image library.

**FIGURE 6–4.** Smarty
Symbols QR code.

This AAC lesson does not provide detailed instructions on how to organize the vocabulary within a particular device or app or explain how to use a specific AAC app or device. Rather, the sole purpose is to provide a lesson for you to use in conjunction with any premade AAC board, preprogrammed AAC app, or dedicated device.

### *Materials Needed*

1. An AAC system for each student. Communication systems may be paper-based boards, eye gaze frames, low-tech devices, or high-tech devices (such as dedicated devices or iPads with AAC apps). A wall-sized board or secondary AAC system for modeling is recommended.

2. Foam Toy Rocket Launcher.

3. Option—a secondary iPad or Core Language Board that mirrors the client's communication system for modeling language.

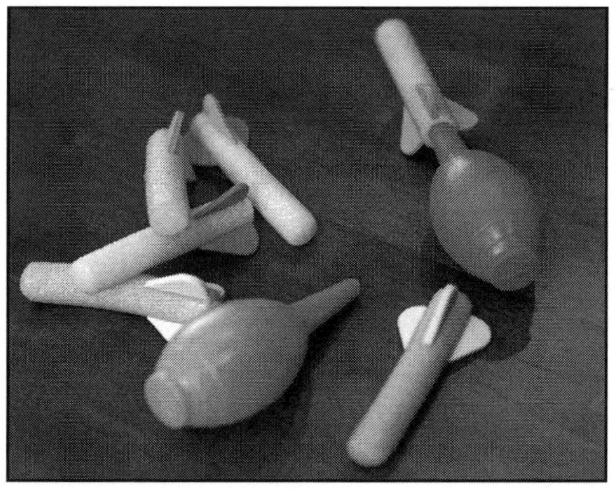

**FIGURE 6–5A.** Image of rocket launcher.

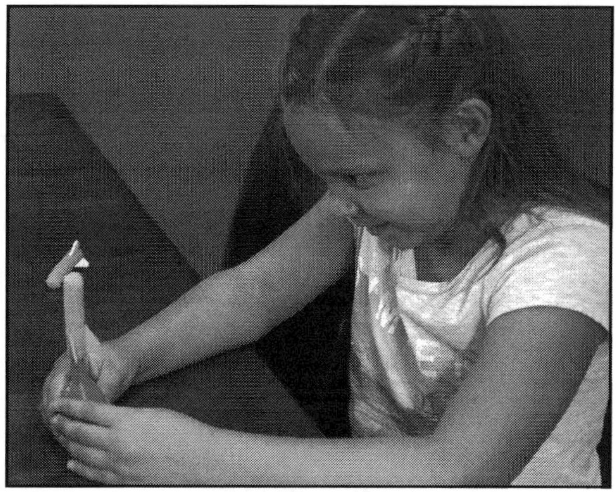

**FIGURE 6–5B.** Ruby Derryberry rocket launcher.

### *Individual or Small Group Session*

Step 1: Instructions

Decide which core words (i.e., WANT, LIKE, UP, DOWN, WHERE, PUT, ON, DO, IT, GIVE, HELP, LOOK, GO, GET, THERE) you are going to model based on the student's current understanding and use, communication goals, and attention span. Practice finding the words on the client's board or device before beginning the activity. Model one word beyond what the client is using (i.e., YES + MORE, PUT + ON, GET + IT, I + WANT).

Step 2: Introduction to Activity

a. With the client sitting next to you and the communication system in front of him or her, show the client the rocket and secure his or her attention. While touching the words on the device, say, "LOOK, let's PLAY!" *NOTE:* The words in CAPS indicate core words to be modeled on the AAC communication system.

b. Squeeze the base of the rocket and make it fly. Pause/wait and watch for a reaction. Say, "Oh, I think YOU LIKE it." Pause/wait. "WHERE did it GO?" Pause/wait. "THERE" "Do you WANT to GET IT?" Pause/wait. "ok GET IT." (If the clients are active, you may want to let them run to get it. Most will bring it back because they want to do it again.)

c. Place the rocket back on the pump or allow client to place the rocket on the pump and use this opportunity to model "HELP" if he or she is struggling to put it on. Say, "Do YOU NEED HELP?" Pause/wait for response/reaction. "HELP PUT ON."

d. Say, "Ready, set." Pause. "GO or UP." "GET IT." *NOTE:* It's important to squeeze the rocket base as soon as the word GO or UP is used so that the client makes the connection between the action and the word. Model for the client, "WANT MORE?" "WANT ALL DONE?" or "WANT DIFFERENT."

e. Depending on the client's response, you may repeat the above steps. Usually three or four cycles are plenty. Each time you go through the steps, pause a little longer after modeling to see if your client will use a new word or expand the length of his or her utterance. Keep it fun and keep it going.

### Essential Resources for Activity

For a flowchart to target vocabulary, visit http://www.speakforyourself.org/tutorials/attachment/building-language-where-do-i-start

**FIGURE 6–6.** SFY flowchart QR code.

## Activity 2

Practicing core vocabulary using wind-up toys targeting all ages (early childhood through adult).

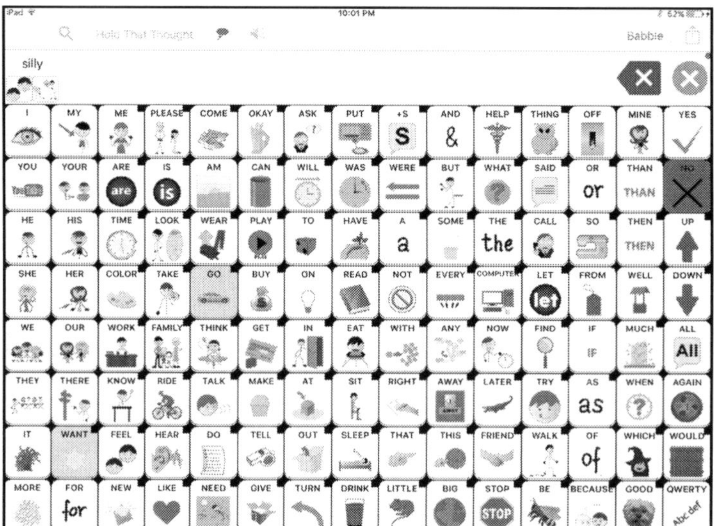

**FIGURE 6–7A.** Speak for Yourself silly screenshot. Reproduced with permission of ©Speak for Yourself, LLC.

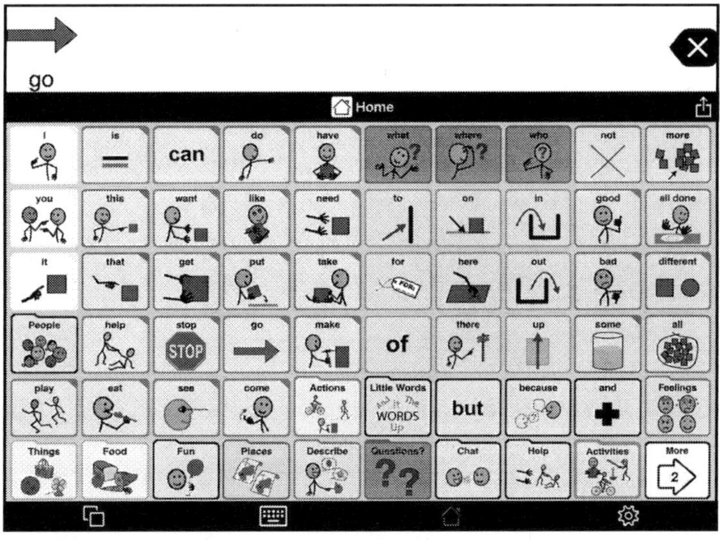

**FIGURE 6-7B.** P2Ggo screenshot. Reproduced with permission of ©AssistiveWare, symbols ©SymbolStix, LLC.

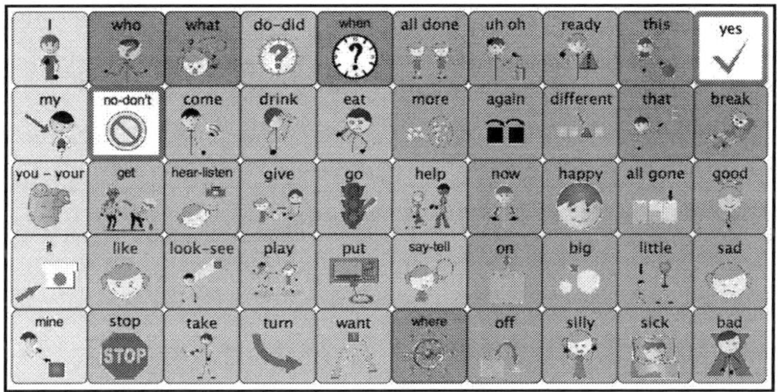

**FIGURE 6-8A.** Smarty Symbols Core Board Full. Reproduced with permission of Smarty Symbols, LLC. All rights reserved.

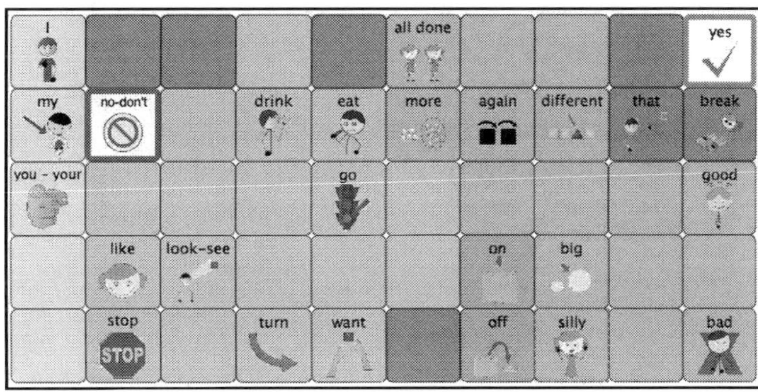

**FIGURE 6-8B.** Smarty Symbols Core Board masked. Reproduced with permission of Smarty Symbols, LLC. All rights reserved.

For purposes of this lesson, we provide screenshots of Speak for Yourself and Proloquo2Go as illustrative examples. In addition, a paper communication board created with Smarty Symbols is also shown below. Any type of AAC can be used for this lesson.

> This AAC lesson does not provide detailed instructions on how to organize the vocabulary within a particular device or app or explain how to use a specific AAC app or device. The sole purpose is to provide a lesson in conjunction with any premade AAC board, preprogrammed AAC app, or dedicated device.

Speak for Yourself is an AAC app that was created by speech-language pathologists. This AAC app turns the iPad into a communication device and gives a voice to those unable to speak or have limited verbal expression.

Speak for Yourself is found at http://www.speakforyourself.org with specific download information and additional resources.

**FIGURE 6–9.** SFY QR code.

Proloquo2Go, by AssistiveWare, is one of several robust symbol-supported communication apps. It is designed to promote growth of communication skills and foster language development using research-based vocabularies.

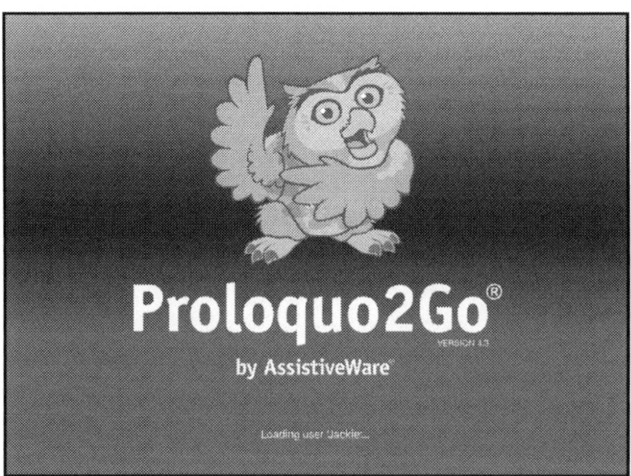


**FIGURE 6–10.** Mainscreen P2G. Reproduced with permission of ©AssistiveWare, symbols ©SymbolStix, LLC.

To download Proloquo2Go, visit https://www.assistiveware.com for specific download information and additional resources.

**FIGURE 6–11.**
ASSISTIVEWARE QR code.

Smarty Symbols is an image library containing nearly 17,000 images that are organized according to educational categories such as animals, feelings, transportation, arts, ocean life, occupations, and so on.

Visit Smarty Symbols at https://smartysymbols.com to learn more about creating materials with this diverse image library.

**FIGURE 6–12.** Smarty
Symbols QR code.

### Materials Needed

1. An AAC system for each student. Communication systems may be paper-based boards, eye gaze frames, low-tech devices, or high-tech devices (such as dedicated devices or iPads with AAC apps). A wall-sized board or secondary AAC system for modeling is recommended.

2. A collection of wind-up toys (works best if the toys are different, with different colors, categories, and actions), and a few duplicates can help teach the concept of SAME (if that is a goal).

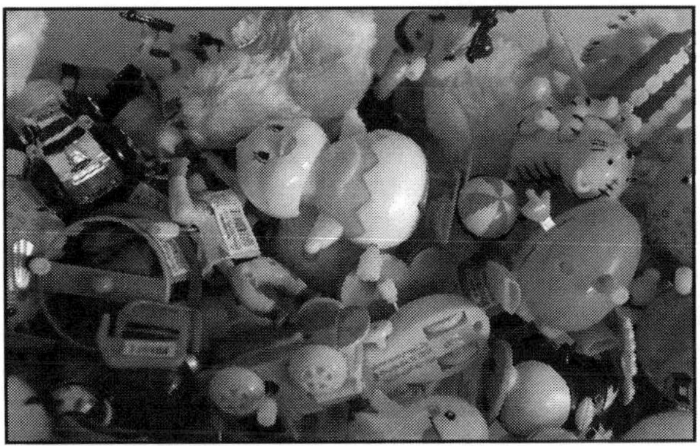

**FIGURE 6–13.** Assorted wind-up toys.

3. A 2 × 2-inch or 3 × 3-inch laminated picture symbol with Velcro on the back to match each of the target core words/symbols for the lesson. (These are optional but can come in very handy for modeling and drawing attention to target words for kids who have trouble attending to communication displays. You will use them often once they are made!)

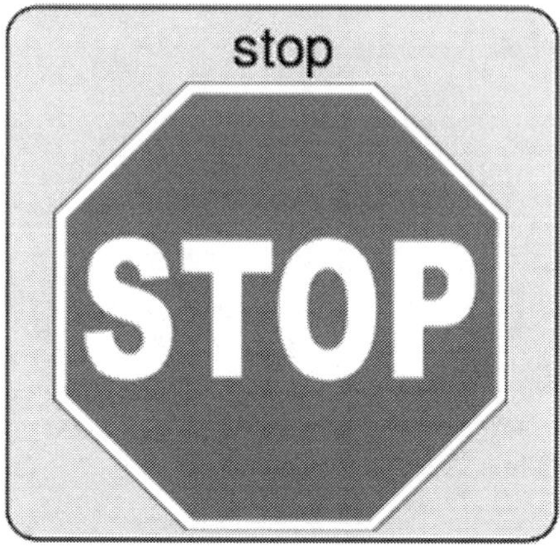


**FIGURE 6–14A.** 2 × 3 stop smarty symbols. Reproduced with permission of Smarty Symbols, LLC. All rights reserved.

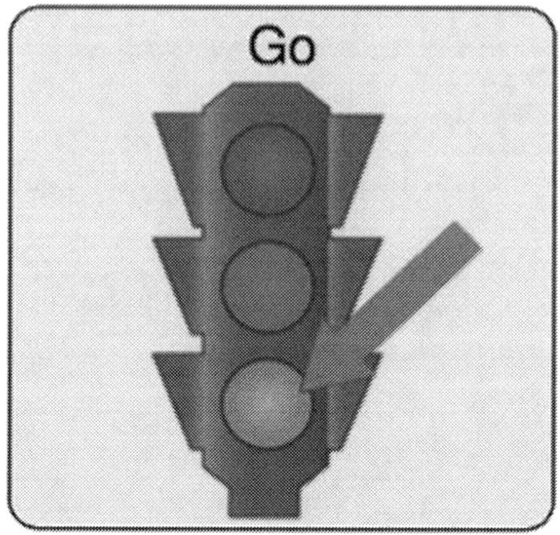


**FIGURE 6–14B.** 2 × 3 go smarty symbols. Reproduced with permission of Smarty Symbols, LLC. All rights reserved.

4. Optional—A small board, piece of cardboard, or strip of Plexiglas with a strip of Velcro that can hold target picture symbols, if needed. If you have a student who will need to eye gaze, a square piece of Plexiglas or a square made from PVC works well. Although optional, this is a key AAC toolkit item for any classroom or therapy room.

5. Optional—A laser pointer or hand pointer. These can be helpful to highlight target words on a board or device while modeling (rather than using your finger). You can often find laser pointers under $3.00 at local department stores. Hand pointers can be found at teacher supply stores, online, or sometimes in the education section at dollar store.

### Individual or Small Group Session

Step 1:  Instructions

Keep an assortment of wind-up toys in a bin that you allow clients to see but not touch. You will be the one winding up the toys at the direction of the clients (via language), so if you allow them to handle a toy, opportunities for language will likely decrease significantly as they may become fixated on playing with the toy.

If clients are able to use vocabulary to select a toy with their AAC system (by naming a color, category, or other attribute of a toy), have them pick a toy. If the clients are emergent communicators who do not yet have vocabulary to make a selection, choose a few toys from the bin and have them select one by pointing or eye gaze. Once the child has selected a toy, begin to model language on his or her system (or a secondary system or wall chart).

Step 2:  Introduction to the Activity—Sample Scripts

"We are going to pick out cool wind-up toys today and make them GO" (pointing to GO on the system). "If you don't like a toy or are tired of a toy, when it's your turn, you will have to tell me to change to a DIFFERENT toy" (while pointing to DIFFERENT on a wall-sized board, their board or system, or a second board or system). "If you really LIKE (pointing to LIKE) a toy and want it to move AGAIN, you can tell me AGAIN and I'll make it GO AGAIN for you" (while pointing to GO and AGAIN on board/system). "You will also get to tell us what you think of these silly toys!" "You can tell me if you LIKE the toy or you DON'T LIKE the toy or even you think it's a GOOD or BAD or SILLY!" (again, pointing to the target core words as you say them).

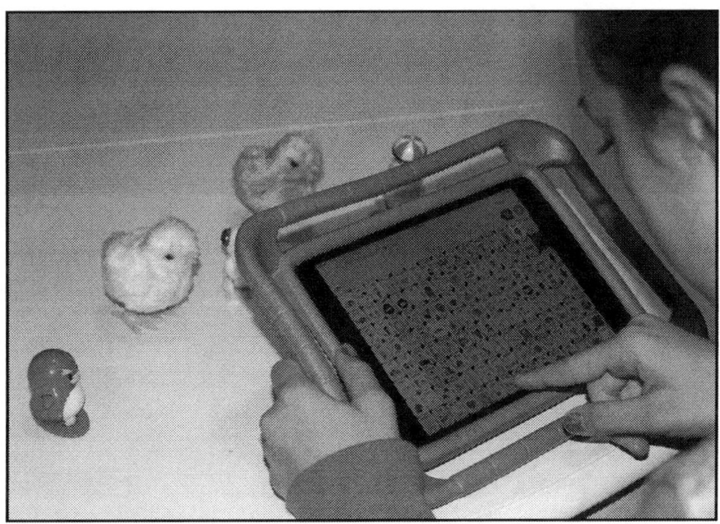

**FIGURE 6–15.** Samantha Enders.

Step 3:  Language During the Activity—Sample Scripts

Discussion during the activity. Every word in quotes should be modeled on the AAC system as you say it. "Should we make him GO?" "Tell me GO and I'll wind him and make him GO! LOOK!" "You said GO and made him GO." "Do you want him to GO MORE or STOP?" "Oh, STOP?" "Ok. You said STOP" (stopping the toy with your hand immediately). "What should we do now?" "Make it GO MORE or pick a DIFFERENT toy?" "Ok, a DIFFERENT toy." "Here's a DIFFERENT toy." "Should we make this toy GO?" (winding it and letting it go as soon as they say GO). "Uh oh! It fell DOWN!" "Should we pick it UP or leave it DOWN on the floor?"

### *Essential Resources for Activity*

For excellent resources on getting started with core words/core vocabulary, check out this helpful post at http://praacticalaac.org/strategy/the-first-12-getting-started-with-core-words from PrAACticalAAC.org.

**FIGURE 6–16.** First12 QR code.

Visit http://praacticalaac.org/praactical/aac-strategies-round-up-aided-language-input to learn more about aided language stimulation or aided language input.

**FIGURE 6–17.** Roundup QR code.

## Activity 3

Introduction to vocabulary (i.e., wh-questions and pronouns) contained within AAC, simultaneously using a variety of highly engaging apps.

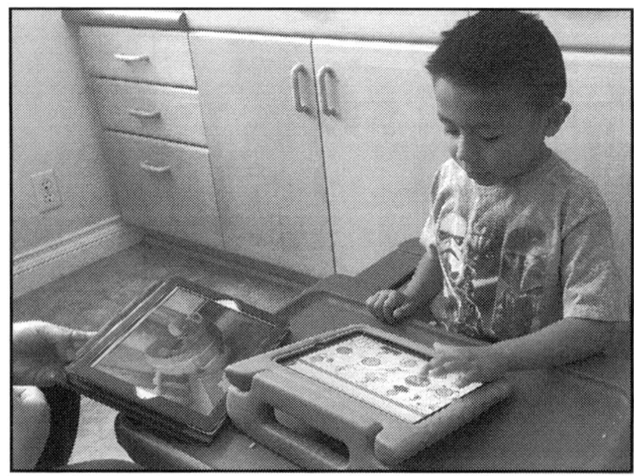

**FIGURE 6–18A.** Jonah Salas TouchChat.

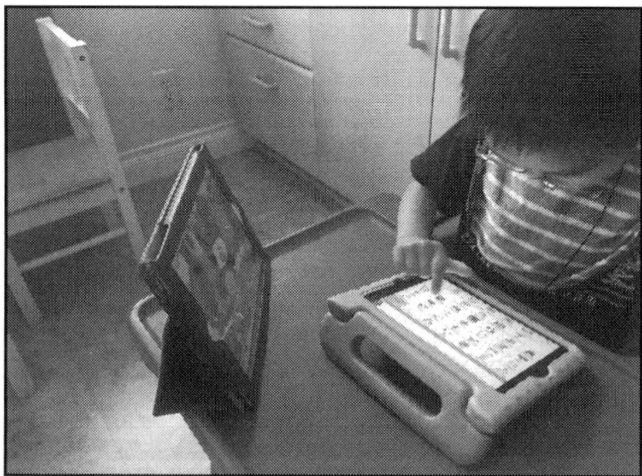

**FIGURE 6–18B.** Timothy Kahn TouchChat.

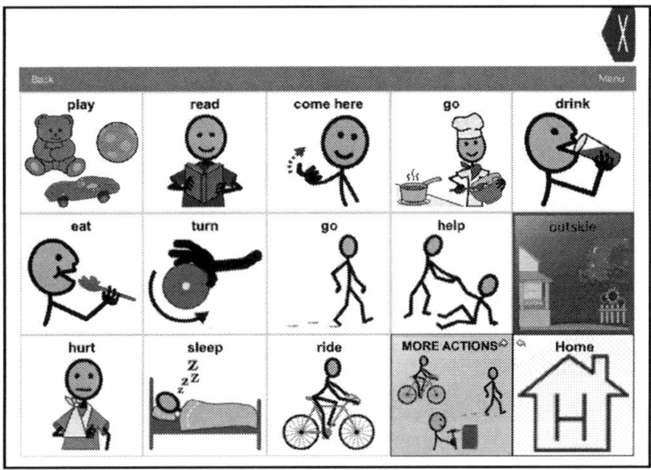

**FIGURE 6–18C.** Multichat15 screenshot. TouchChat app developed by Saltillo Corporation, supported by SilverKite and WordPower-42 Basic and WordPower-108 developed by Inman Innovations.

For purposes of this activity, images of the TouchChat HD–AAC with the WordPower app will be depicted for the AAC. Any AAC app, dedicated device, or paper core board could be used with this activity. Toto's Treehouse by Dr. Panda, What's in the Bag by All4mychild, and Pogg by Ricky Vuckovic will be used to elicit language and engagement from the client. There are many engaging apps that could be used to work on vocabulary, but for illustrative purposes, the above-named apps will be shown as examples.

TouchChat HD–AAC with WordPower by Silver Kite is a full-featured communication solution for individuals who have difficulty using their natural speech. TouchChat is designed for individuals with autism, Down syndrome, ALS, apraxia, stroke, or other conditions that affect a person's ability to use natural speech (retrieved from http://touchchatapp.com/apps/touchchat-hd-aac-with-wordpower).

**FIGURE 6–19.** TouchChat mainscreen. TouchChat app developed by Saltillo Corporation, supported by SilverKite and WordPower-42 Basic and WordPower-108 developed by Inman Innovations.

To download TouchChat apps and for more AAC information, visit http://touchchatapp.com

**FIGURE 6–20.** TouchChat QR code.

Toto's Treehouse by Dr. Panda—The Dr. Panda apps are very popular with younger clients. In this app, the turtle hatches and needs a friend to interact with. This app allows for modeling and use of everyday functional vocabulary. The client can decide what Toto should do: make food, wash, or sleep. Sample vocabulary that can be targeted are bubbles, basketball, eat, drink, sleep, slide, swing, wash swim, cook, foods, places, and feelings.

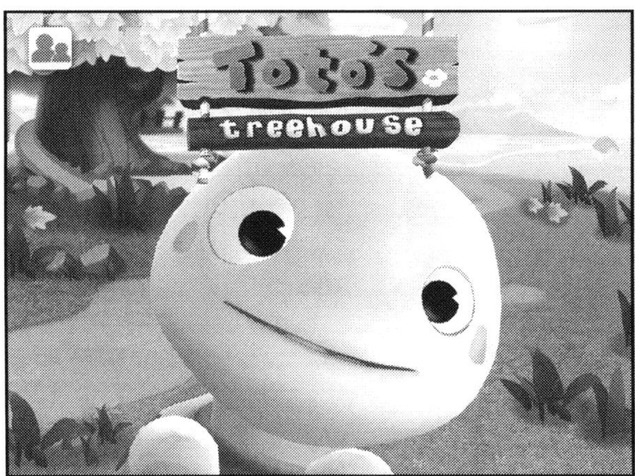


**FIGURE 6–21.** Toto mainscreen. Reproduced with permission of ©Dr. Panda, Ltd. All rights reserved.

To download Toto's Treehouse, visit http://drpanda.com

**FIGURE 6–22.** Dr. Panda QR code.

What's in the Bag by All4mychild—This app works on a variety of skills that can be adapted to the level of the AAC user and also works well in a small group session or push-in with classroom groups. Many skills can be addressed: categorization (with subcategories), verbal description, question asking (sample questions are included in the app), deductive reasoning (similar to 20 questions type of game), same/different, and short-term auditory memory skills.

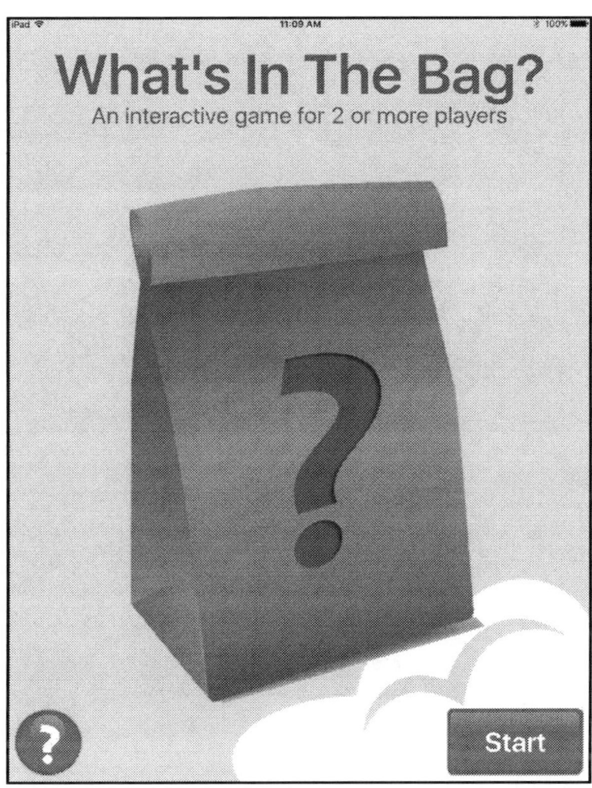


**FIGURE 6–23A.** What's in the Bag mainscreen. Reproduced with permission of all4mychild.

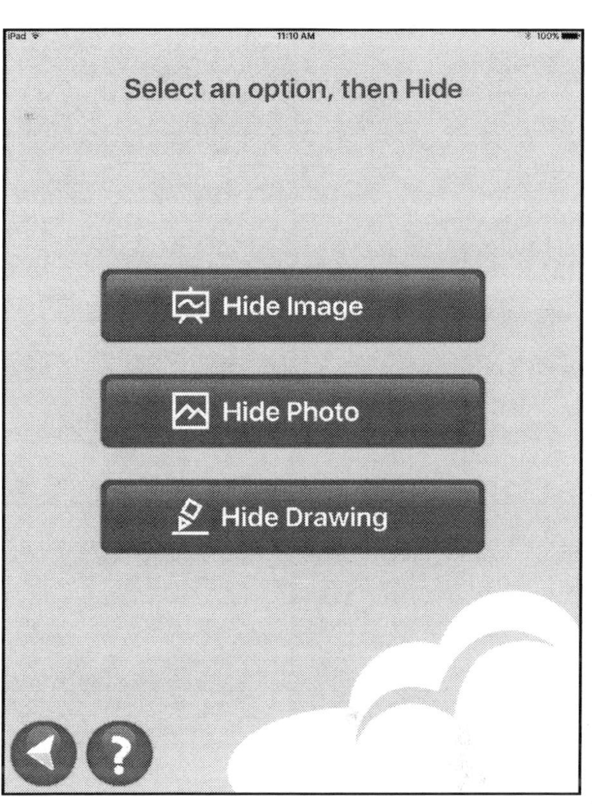


**FIGURE 6–23B.** Hiding screen. Reproduced with permission of all4mychild.

To download What's in the Bag, visit http://all4mychild.com

**FIGURE 6–24.**
All4mychild QR code.

Pogg by Ricky Vuckovic—This app is built on the open question, "What should Pogg do now?" This app is targeted for verb development. Pogg's actions can be viewed through Picture Mode, which presents each action as an easy to touch icon.

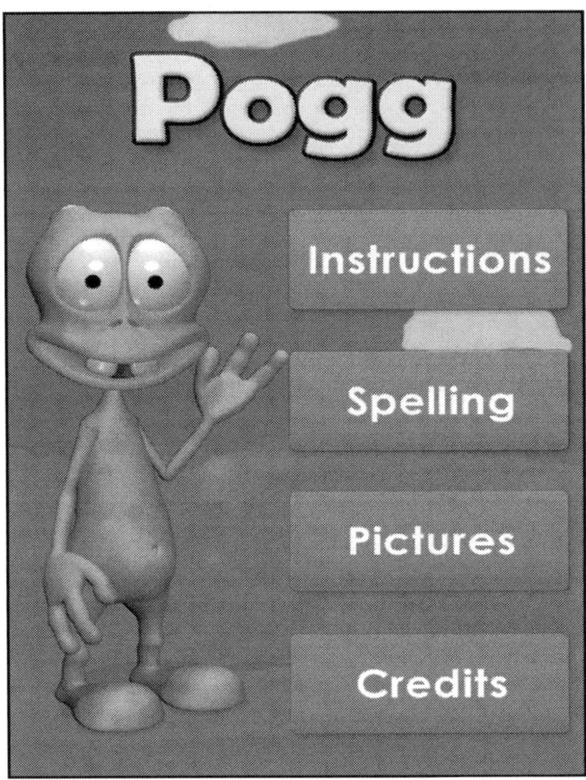


**FIGURE 6–25A.** Pogg main screenshot. Reproduced with permission of Ricky Vuckovic.

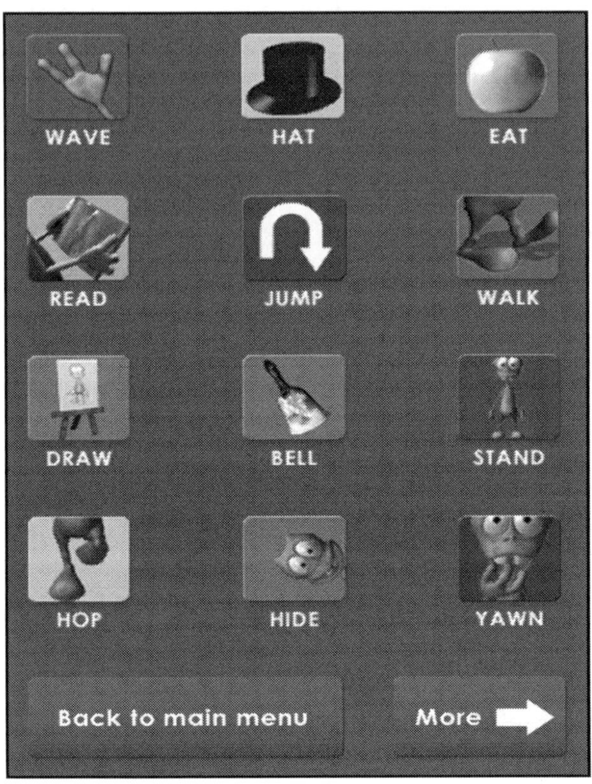


**FIGURE 6–25B.** Pogg verbs actions screen. Reproduced with permission of Ricky Vuckovic.

To download Pogg, visit http://rickyvuckovic.com/apps-for-kids-ipad-iphone-android-osx/pogg-kids-iphone-game

**FIGURE 6–26.** Pogg QR code.

### *Materials Needed*

1. Client with AAC system. A dedicated device, iPad with AAC app, or paper communication board with targeted vocabulary can be used.

2. iPad (in addition to AAC system) with a highly engaging app allowing for a variety of functional core vocabulary. For this lesson, Toto's Treehouse, What's in the Bag, and Pogg will be used. *NOTE:* We recommend that you become familiar with the app prior to the therapy session. See resources at the end of this lesson for a video link for an in-depth tutorial about Toto's Treehouse.

3. Preprogrammed AAC device (iPad with AAC app or dedicated device) with targeted vocabulary or a paper-based communication board.

<table><tr><td>This AAC lesson does not provide detailed instructions on how to organize the vocabulary within a dedicated device or AAC app or explain how to use the specific AAC app or device. The sole purpose is to provide a lesson to use in conjunction with any premade AAC board, preprogrammed AAC app, or dedicated device.</td></tr></table>

### *Individual or Small Group Session*

Step 1:  Open or have the clients open their communication system. If using a paper-based communication board, place in front of the clients.

Step 2:  Using a secondary iPad, choose an app (i.e., Toto's Treehouse, What's in the Bag, or Pogg) to target vocabulary and entice the client. Proceed to the corresponding step for the chosen app.

Step 3:  Toto's Treehouse by Dr. Panda—Sample script by area.

Using the secondary iPad, have Toto's Treehouse open and model how Toto is moved from screen area to screen area.

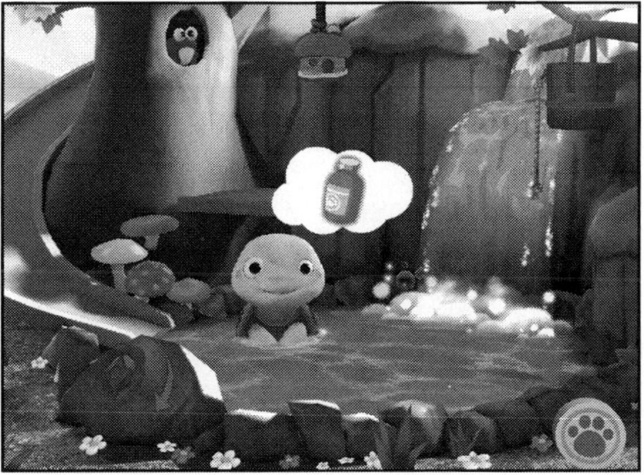

**FIGURE 6–27A.** Toto treehouse bath screenshot. Reproduced with permission of ©Dr. Panda, Ltd. All rights reserved.

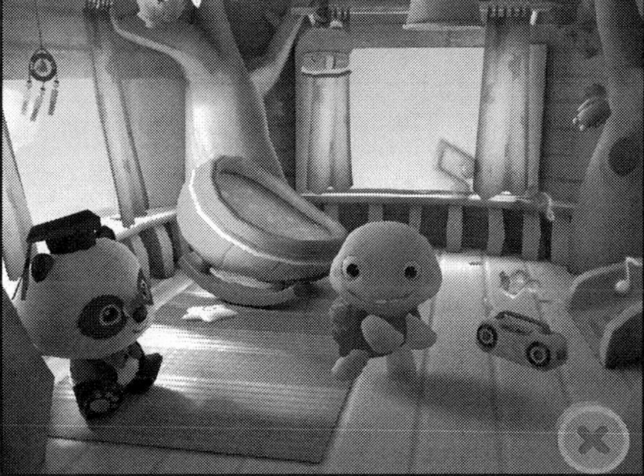

**FIGURE 6–27B.** Toto dancing screenshot. Reproduced with permission of ©Dr. Panda, Ltd. All rights reserved.

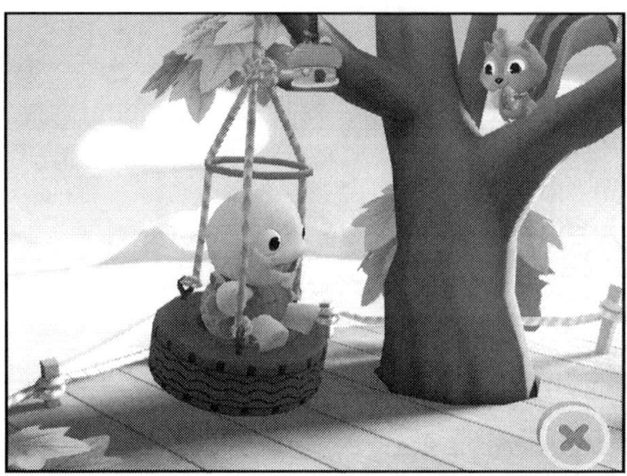

**FIGURE 6–27C.** Toto tire swing screenshot. Reproduced with permission of ©Dr. Panda, Ltd. All rights reserved.

Bedroom screen area:

WHAT is Toto DOING? Sleeping.

WHERE is HE? In bed.

WHAT does HE feel? Tired.

WHAT does HE NEED? The star.

WHAT is HE DOING? Snoring.

Toto is sleeping. WHAT should WE do? Close curtains.

WHAT is wrong? HE is sick.

WHAT does HE need? Medicine.

WHAT does HE WANT? A tickle.

WHAT is Toto doing? Laughing.

Kitchen screen area:

WHAT should HE DO? EAT.

WHY? HE is HUNGRY.

WHAT does HE WANT? BANANA, ice cream, a sandwich.

WHERE does the ice cream GO?

WHAT flavor ice cream do YOU WANT?

DOES Toto WANT sprinkles on his ice cream? YES/NO.

WHO wants to PUT the sprinkles on? I DO.

WHERE does HE need to GO next? To the house.

WHAT is HE doing? Drinking.

I see birds. WHAT are they? HOW MANY? Make them fly. WHAT are THEY doing?

Playground screen area:

WHAT does Toto WANT to PLAY? Ball, bubbles, mouse toy, cups, jump rope, swing.

WHAT should WE do to the swing? Push it.

WHERE is the squirrel? In the tree.

WHERE is Toto? UNDER the cup.

WHO threw the ball? The squirrel.

WHAT should we do? Throw the ball, blow bubbles.

WHAT is Toto doing? Jumping, chasing the mouse.

WHAT happened? HE fell.

WHAT should Toto do? Pop the bubbles.

WHOSE turn is it to blow the bubbles? MY turn.

Pool screen area:

WHY does Toto need a bath? HE is dirty.

WHAT should we use? Soap/shampoo.

WHAT are YOU doing? Washing Toto.

WHAT should WE do? Turn on the BUBBLES.

WHAT is Toto doing? Floating.

WHERE is the frog? In the tree.

WHAT does Toto want to do? HE wants to JUMP.

WHAT toy does Toto want to play with? Boat, duck, panda.

WHERE do the toys go? In the water.

Step 4: What's in the Bag by All4mychild—Instructions and sample scripts. *NOTE:* This same activity can be played with real objects and a bag. Although this app targets many areas, for the purpose of this activity, naming the object is the goal.

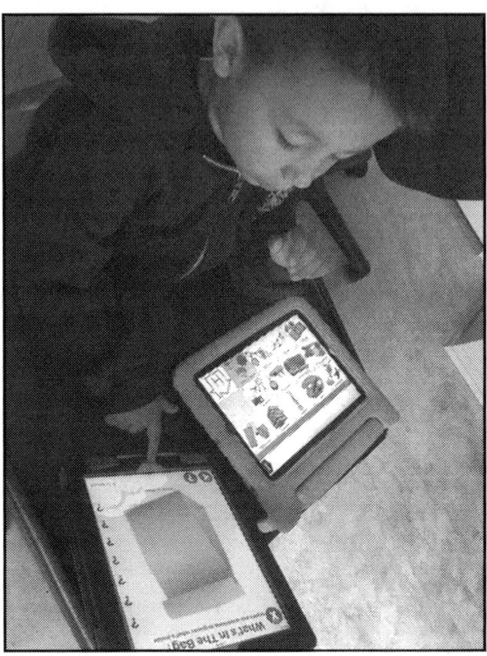

**FIGURE 6–28.** Jonah Salas with What's in the Bag.

Using the secondary iPad with What's in the Bag open, select an image or photo from the photo library and hide it in the bag. A fun customization is to have photos from the therapy room, classroom, or environment already saved into the photo library. Using screenshots of favorite apps is another fun customization and quite motivating. This works well if the AAC clients have picture choices of familiar apps on their communication system.

Once the object (image) is chosen, tap "hide" and it disappears into the bag. Use this opportunity to ask your clients to use their communication system to guess or find the image. This is a great way to teach questions.

WHERE is the _______ ?

WHAT is IN the bag?

Pinch the bag to reveal the image within the bag. Model the sentence: "I SEE the _____. The _____ is IN the bag."

Step 5: Pogg by Ricky Vuckovic—Instructions.

Using the secondary iPad with Pogg open and the client attending, tap "Pictures" and select an action (i.e., walk, wave, jump). A short animation will play.

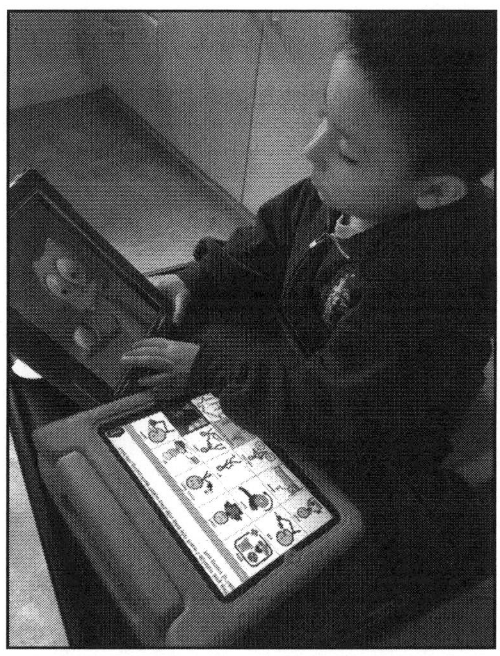

**FIGURE 6–29A.** Jonah Salas with Pogg.

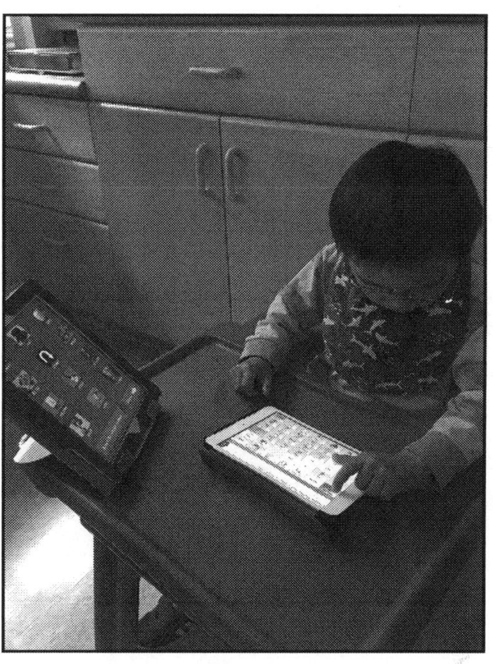

**FIGURE 6–29B.** Timothy Kahn Pogg.

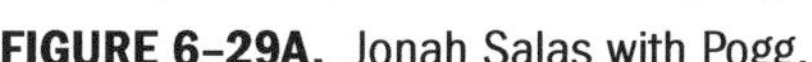

Model the action word you used above on the client's communication system and then select the Pogg action again. Clients choose an action word on their communication system, and allow them to make Pogg do the action.

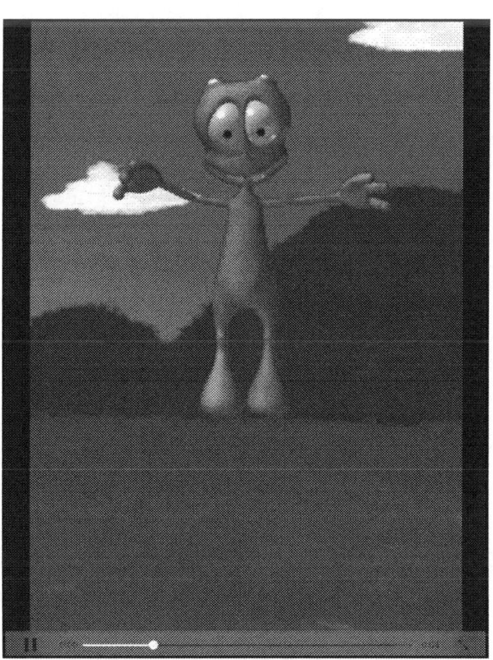

**FIGURE 6–30.** Jumping Pogg screenshot. Reproduced with permission of Ricky Vuckovic.

Options—create individual pictures of each of the action icons from the app. Place in a box, bag, or other enticing container (big, small, medium, round, square, or colors). Clients use their communication systems to specify which container to pull the picture from (i.e., square, red, round, big).

### Essential Resources for Activity

For an in-depth look at Dr. Panda's Toto's Treehouse, visit https://www.youtube.com/watch?v=nQA8fdeNrNA

**FIGURE 6–31.** YouTube video QR code.

## Activity 4

Core vocabulary with toy cars for preschool through second grade. For illustrative purposes, AVAZ Pro Communication App and Clicker Communicator by CrickSoftware will be used in this lesson.

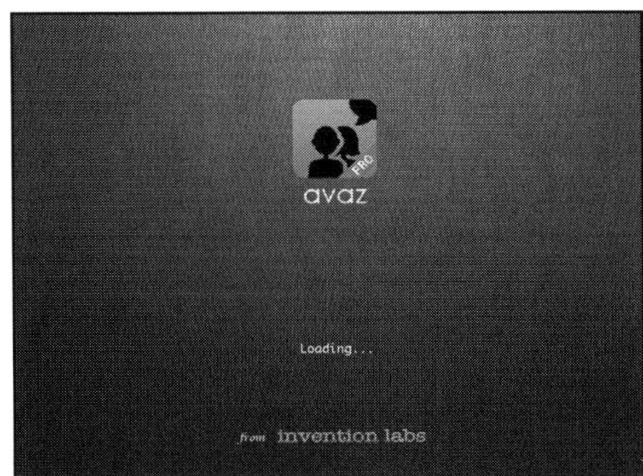

**FIGURE 6–32A.** AVAZ main 1 screenshot. Reproduced with permission of ©Avaz, Inc., http://www.avazapp.com. All rights reserved.

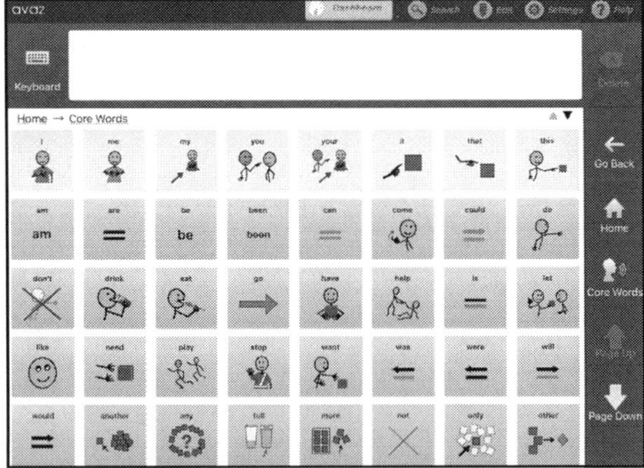

**FIGURE 6–32B.** AVAZ core vocab screenshot. Reproduced with permission of ©Avaz, Inc., http://www.avazapp.com. All rights reserved.

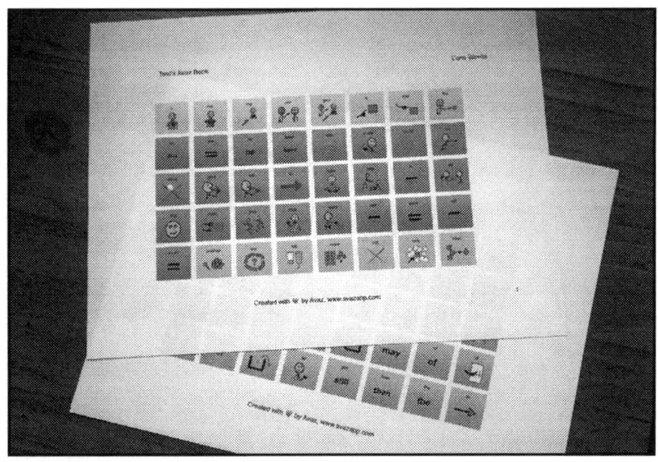

**FIGURE 6–32C.** Printed AVAZ. Reproduced with permission of ©Avaz, Inc., http://www.avazapp.com. All rights reserved.

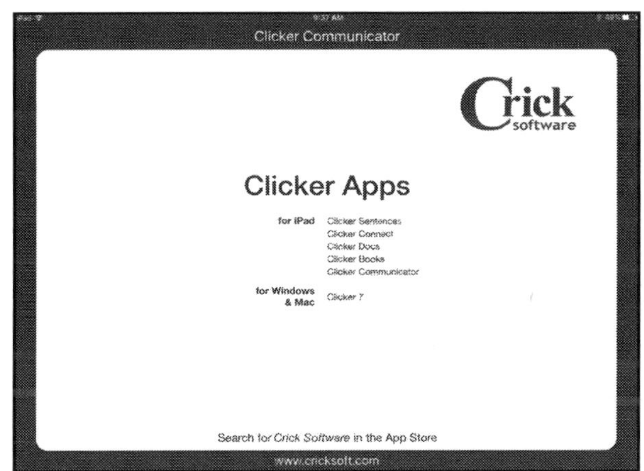

**FIGURE 6–33A.** Clicker Communicator main screenshot. Reproduced with permission of Crick Software, Inc., http://www.cricksoft.com

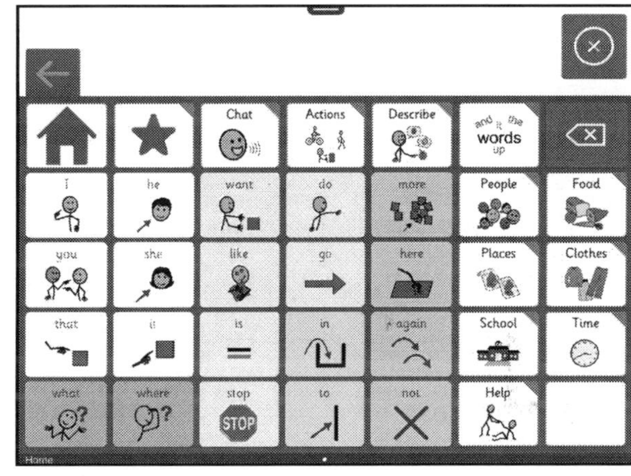

**FIGURE 6–33B.** CC core vocab screenshot. Reproduced with permission of Crick Software, Inc., http://www.cricksoft.com

AVAZ Pro AAC App for Autism (Augmentative Picture Communication Software for Children With Special Needs) is a full-featured AAC app for children who are nonverbal or who have difficulty speaking. AVAZ Pro uses research-based vocabulary and more than 15,000 high-quality SymbolStix images. The ability to import your own images is also available. Vocabulary can be printed so the users may have consistent access to their AAC vocabulary when the iPad is unavailable.

To download AVAZ Pro, visit http://www.avazapp.com

**FIGURE 6–34.** AVAZ QR code.

Clicker Communicator is a user-friendly AAC app that gives a voice to learners with speech and language difficulties. Three, ready-made, core vocabulary sets make it easy to get started. The Clicker Communicator app can be purchased with a main symbol set: SymbolStix, PCS, or Widget. In the app, purchases then can be made for either of the other symbol sets if additional symbols are necessary.

To download Clicker Communicator, visit http://www.cricksoft.com/us/products/communi cator/communicator-home.aspx

**FIGURE 6–35.** Crick Software QR code.

> This AAC lesson does not provide detailed instructions on how to organize the vocabulary within a particular device or app or explain how to use the specific AAC app or device. The sole purpose is to provide a lesson to use in conjunction with any premade AAC board, preprogrammed AAC app, or dedicated device.

### Materials Needed

1. An AAC system for each student. Communication systems may be paper-based boards, eye gaze frames, low-tech devices, or high-tech devices (such as dedicated devices or iPads with AAC apps). A wall-sized board or secondary AAC system for modeling is super helpful too!

2. A variety of toy cars.

3. Option—a secondary iPad or Core Language Board that mirrors the client's communication system for modeling language.

### *Individual or Small Group Session*

Step 1: Instructions

Decide which core words (i.e., WANT, LIKE, DO, IT, GO, STOP, NOT, AGAIN, THAT, MORE) you are going to model based on the student's current understanding and use, communication goals, and attention span. Practice finding the words on the client's board or device before beginning the activity. Model one word beyond what the client is using (i.e., WANT + THAT, GO + AGAIN, LIKE + IT).

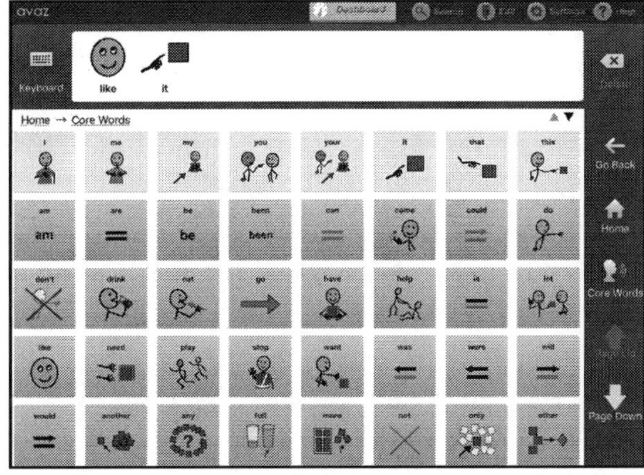

**FIGURE 6–36A.** AVAZ example screenshot. Reproduced with permission of ©Avaz, Inc., http://www.avazapp.com. All rights reserved.

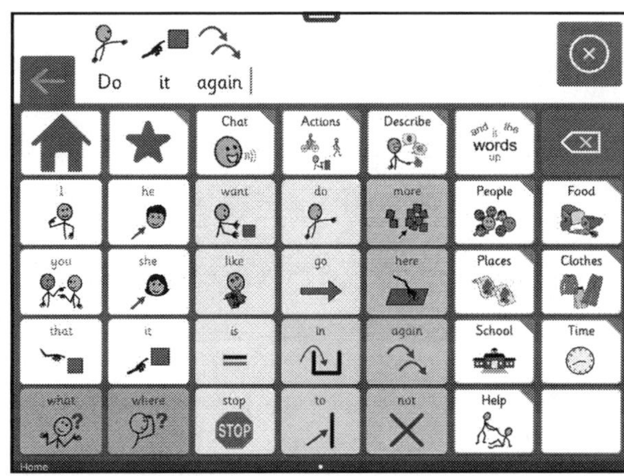

**FIGURE 6–36B.** CC example screenshot. Reproduced with permission of Crick Software, Inc., http://www.cricksoft.com

Step 2: Introduction to the Activity—Sample Scripts

"We are going to play cars and make them GO" (pointing to GO on the system). "If you like a car, you can tell me LIKE IT or if you don't like a car, you can say NOT THAT or you could say WANT THAT." "If I am playing with a car, you can tell me to make the car GO or STOP." "If I do something with the car that you LIKE, you can tell me DO IT AGAIN or MORE" (again, pointing to the target core words as you say them).

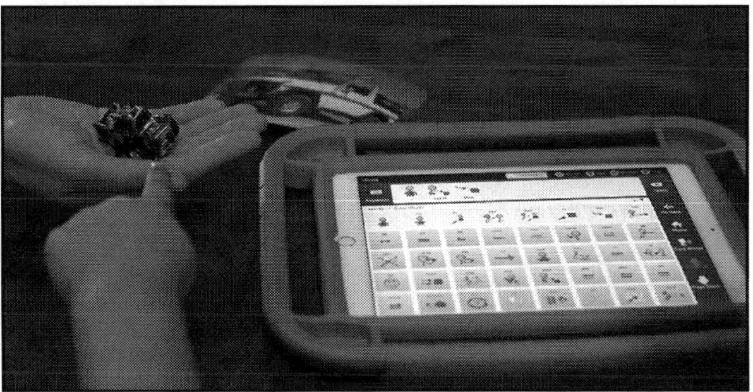

**FIGURE 6–37.** Ruby Derryberry pointAVAZcar.

Step 3:  Language During the Activity—Sample Scripts

Discussion during activity. Each word in CAPS should be modeled on the AAC system as you say it aloud. Displaying a container of cars to the clients as they reach for the car, say, "Oh you LIKE THAT car?" "I LIKE THAT car too." "Should we make the car GO?" Wait for a response. "You want the car to GO?" If no response, model "GO" again and immediately push/move the car. Add "AGAIN" to increase the utterance.

To encourage the client to make a choice, offer a car held out in hand, "Do you WANT IT or NOT?" "Oh, you're looking at the red car, I think you WANT IT." "I'll give IT to you" (handing the car to the client). Immediately offer another car. "Do you WANT IT or NOT?" As you say "not," playfully throw the car into the container to put emphasis on the word "not." Offer another car, modeling WANT or NOT.

Option—to keep client motivated, use some humor and push the car off or under the table or chair. Exaggerate these options modeling, "NOT AGAIN!" as the car goes off the table or under the chair. In small groups (two or more), let the clients use their systems to say "GO" and allow the clients to take turns. Keep it fun and keep it going.

## Activity 5

Targeting positional concepts using core vocabulary and the Sago Mini Boats app. For purposes of this lesson, it is suggested to use a paper-based core board, AAC device or app (i.e. Proloquo2Go) with appropriate core vocabulary.

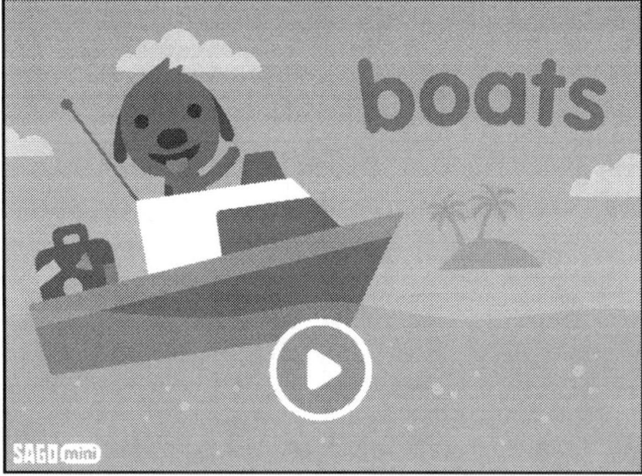


**FIGURE 6–38.** Sago Mini boats mainscreen. Reproduced with permission of Sago Sago.

Proloquo2Go by AssistiveWare is one of several robust symbol-supported communication apps. It is designed to promote growth of communication skills and foster language development through research-based vocabularies. The core board shown below is an example of a paper-based board that can be created using images from Smarty Symbols.

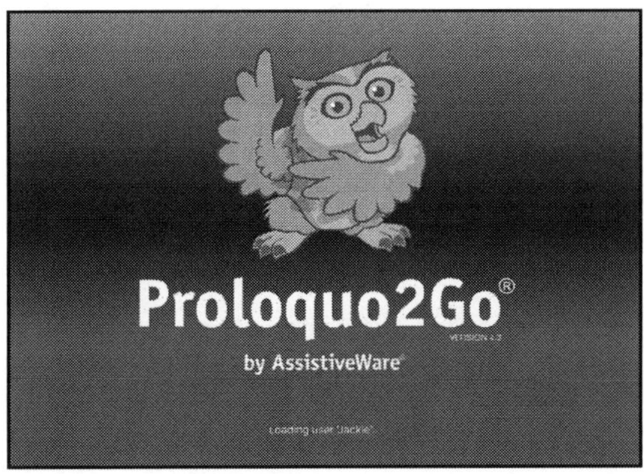

**FIGURE 6–39A.** Mainscreen P2G. Reproduced with permission of ©AssistiveWare, symbols ©SymbolStix, LLC.

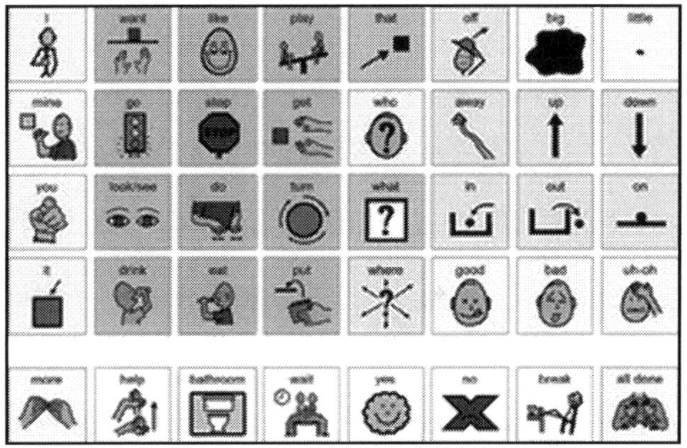

**FIGURE 6–39B.** Paper-based board. Reproduced with permission of Smarty Symbols, LLC. All rights reserved.

To download Proloquo2Go, visit https://www.assistiveware.com /or to find out more about Smarty Symbols visit https://smartysymbols.com

**FIGURE 6–40A.** Assistive Ware QR code.

**FIGURE 6–40B.** Smarty Symbols QR code.

Sago Mini Boats is a highly engaging free-play app with a nautical theme. Clients will pack a suitcase for their voyage, choose a boat, and then head to the high seas. Multiple opportunities to work on vocabulary targeting positional concept is just one example of how this app can be used to introduce and expand vocabulary using AAC.

To download Sago Mini Boats, visit http://www.sagomini.com

**FIGURE 6–41.** Sago Mini QR code.

### *Materials Needed*

1. Client with AAC system. A dedicated device, iPad with AAC app, or paper communication board with targeted vocabulary.

2. iPad (secondary device in addition to AAC system, if an iPad app is being used for AAC) with a highly engaging app that provides a variety of functional core vocabulary words for the client. For this lesson, Sago Mini Boats will be used as an example of how to use an engaging open-ended play app to elicit target words that reflect positional concepts. There are other excellent Sago Sago apps that would work equally well with the same procedures in addition to many other free play apps from other developers. *NOTE:* We recommend you become familiar with the target app prior to beginning your therapy session.

3. Preprogrammed AAC device or iPad with an app having targeted vocabulary. Be sure to locate existing core vocabulary in the system or create a paper communication board.

> This AAC lesson does not provide detailed instructions on how to organize the vocabulary within a dedicated device or AAC app or explain how to use a specific AAC app or device. The sole purpose is to provide a lesson to use in conjunction with any premade AAC board, preprogrammed AAC app, or dedicated device.

### *Individual or Small Group Session*

Step 1:  Open or have the clients open their communication system. If using a paper-based communication board, place in front of the clients.

Step 2:  Using a secondary iPad, open the Sago Mini Boats app to target positional concept words and encourage the client to use the target words as much as possible. Positional concepts are all considered to be core vocabulary words.

Step 3:  As with all vocabulary teaching using AAC (and in natural speech), it's essential that you model the target words extensively within the instructional task. If we hope for the client to learn the word, what it means, and how to use it, you must model, model, model!

Step 4:  Select one of the three available places to go: Packing Screen, Boat Choice, or Voyage.

   a. Packing Screen:  Now you are ready to prepare your character for his trip on the packing screen. Target words on this screen may include IN, OUT, UP, DOWN, LEFT, RIGHT, MIDDLE. Each time you use one of the words, you should model its use by touching, pointing to, or selecting that word on the child's system.

   Sample Script:  "Oh! Look! We need to pick which clothes to pull DOWN from the clothesline for Dog to bring on his trip!" "Which ones should we pull DOWN?" "Should we do the one on the LEFT? RIGHT? MIDDLE?" (each time indicating with your finger which objects are in each of those positions and modeling use of the target words on their system). Encourage the clients to pull DOWN the clothes they want for the trip and put them IN the suitcase.

   Sample Script:  "Ok! This one goes DOWN and IN" (modeling DOWN and IN on the system). "I'm going to pick the one on the LEFT! DOWN and IN it goes! Your turn!" (Encourage them to use their target words and/or model the words that apply to the actions they choose as they do them.) "Wait! I don't want that one! UP and OUT it goes!" "What about the things to the LEFT of the suitcase?" "Which ones should we bring? A fishbowl?" "Yes! UP and IN!" "Is that everything? Ok!" "Let's put DOWN the suitcase lid and get ready to pick our boat."

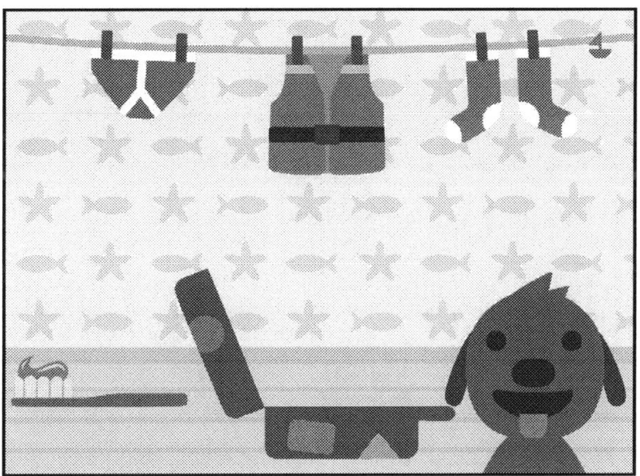

**FIGURE 6–42.** Packing screenshot. Reproduced with permission of Sago Sago.

b. Boat Choice Screen: Target words are RIGHT, LEFT, and DOWN.

Sample Script:  "Time to choose a boat! We need to swipe RIGHT or LEFT to see all of our boat choices!" "RIGHT, RIGHT, RIGHT! I like this one!" "Wait, let's go LEFT!" (Be sure not to actually select the one you want because the app will automatically close the door and advance to the next screen. You want the selection to be the child's selection.) Once the client has practiced LEFT and RIGHT while advancing through the boat options and picks one, you can say, "LOOK! You picked your boat and the door is going DOWN!"

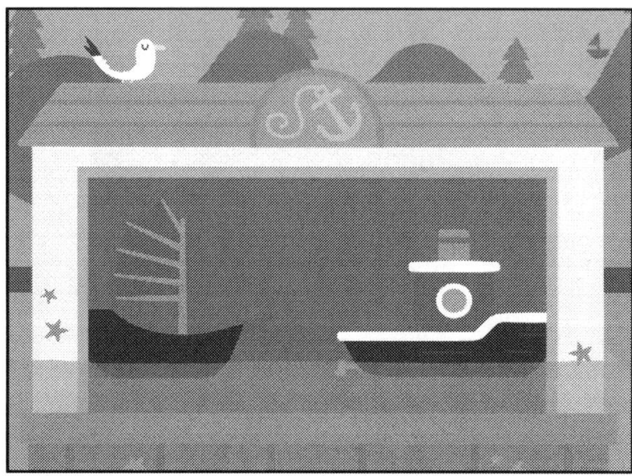

**FIGURE 6–43.** Screenshot of boat choosing screen. Reproduced with permission of Sago Sago.

c. Voyage Screen:  Target words may include UP, DOWN, IN, OUT, UNDER, OVER, FORWARD, BACK, BELOW. (Important: Be sure that the activity requires the CLIENTS to direct YOU to move the character with their use of the positional concepts. If you allow them to access the screen, they will likely get lost in play and not be able to focus on using their system to communicate. If they are incredibly eager to touch the screen themselves, they can earn a minute of free play at the end through hard work.

Sample Script: "Ooh! Look! He can go DOWN and UP, IN the WATER, OUT of the WATER, UP in the air, UNDER the water, FORWARD, BACK, and BELOW the water." (You should be demonstrating each of these by moving the character as you model the target words on their system.) "Where should he go?" "Oh! He should go UP and OUT of the water?" "Funny! Now where should he go?" There are endless opportunities for free play, modeling, and client use of these target words with this screen.

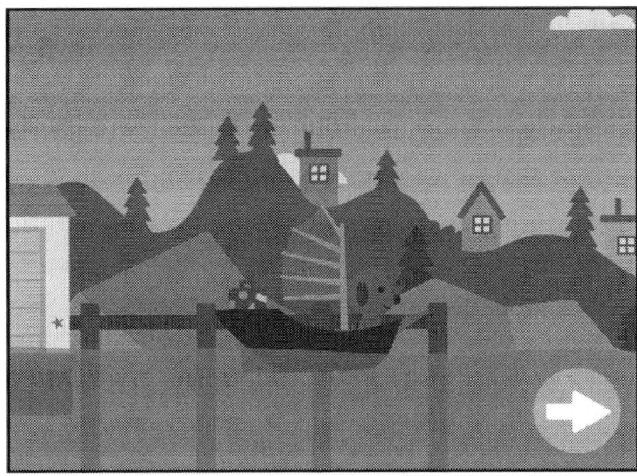

**FIGURE 6–44A.** Screenshot voyage. Reproduced with permission of Sago Sago.

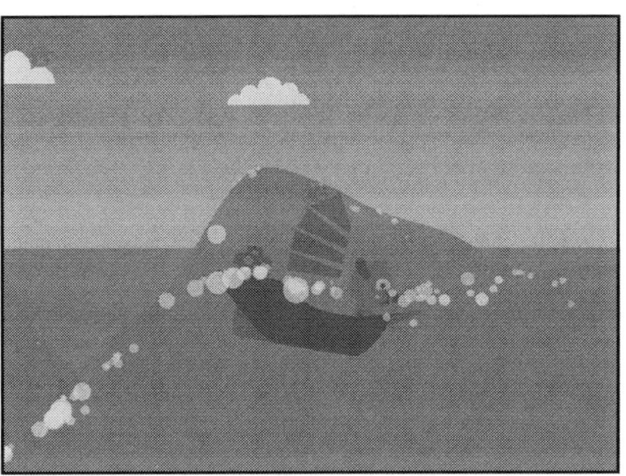

**FIGURE 6–44B.** Screenshot of voyage under. Reproduced with permission of Sago Sago.

Step 5:  End play after this screen by selecting the home button at the top left or return to the home screen and start over with a different place, different packed items, and a different boat.

# REFERENCE

Croos, R. T., Baker, B. R., Klotz, L. S., & Badman, A. L. (1997). Static and dynamic keyboards: Semantic compaction in both worlds. In *Proceedings of the 18th Annual Southeast Augmentative Communication Conference* (pp. 9–17). Birmingham, UK: SEAC Publications.

# 7

# Literacy

Literacy is built by early exposure to the written word through exploration of books via listening during story time, looking at books, or playing with books. The key components to literacy include phonologic awareness (PA), print concepts, alphabet knowledge, and literate language (Paul & Norbury, 2012**)**. PA includes the ability to (1) break words down into smaller parts, (2) recognize similarities between words based on how they sound, and (3) put sounds together to create words. As such, PA is the ability to reflect on and manipulate the structure of an utterance as distinct from its meaning (Paul et al., 2012). Print concepts encompass the structure of the written word. A child must learn that words are made up of letters and words represent ideas. Children must also learn to hold books the right way, and in English, we read from left to right (Paul et al., 2012). Alphabet knowledge (phonics) is the understanding of the phoneme to grapheme correspondence and the configuration of those graphemes to make words (Paul et al., 2012). Literate language is familiarity with narrative genres and understanding decontextualized language. This is the ability to use and comprehend the formal register of the written word. Through the exploration of these components, early literacy is created. Building vocabulary, grammar, verbal reasoning, literacy knowledge, and background knowledge are all examples of positive focal points for language comprehension in creating a strong foundation for literacy. The activities included in this chapter will help you support literacy development for children with language disorders. As you become familiar with these activities, you will begin to gain with confidence working with components of literacy and, under the guidance of your supervising speech-language pathologist (SLP), can develop your own therapy materials to fit the therapy goals established by the SLP.

7<br>Pre & Early<br>Literacy

## ACTIVITIES FOR PRE- AND EARLY LITERACY

### Objectives

The following are some sample objectives for pre- and early literacy within a therapy session:

1. Client will correctly identify the number of phonemes in verbally presented words in 9 of 10 opportunities across three consecutive data collection points.

2. Client will correctly produce at least three rhyming words for a given word in 8 of 10 opportunities across three consecutive data collection points.

3. Client will correctly manipulate specified sounds within verbally presented words in 8 of 10 opportunities across three consecutive data collection points.

## Activity 1

Tiggly Words for ages 4 to 8 years to introduce long and short vowels, phonics, nouns and verbs, and word building using optional letter manipulatives (interactive vowel toys can be purchased separately). Choose one or all of the app activities (1A, 1B, 1C, 1D) to target client objectives.

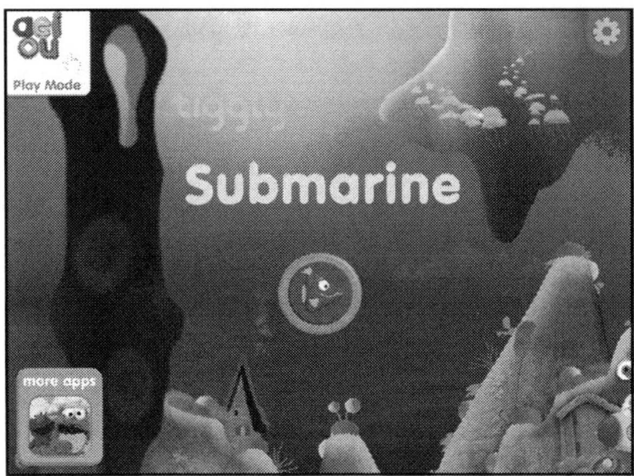

**FIGURE 7–1A.** Tiggly Submarine screenshot. Reproduced with permission of Tiggly.

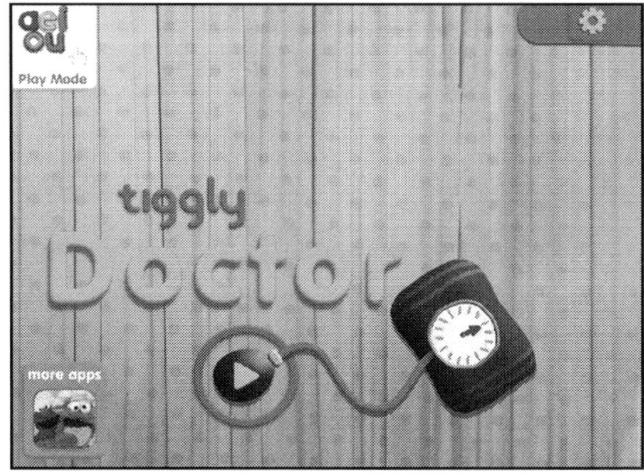

**FIGURE 7–1B.** Tiggly Doctor screenshot. Reproduced with permission of Tiggly.

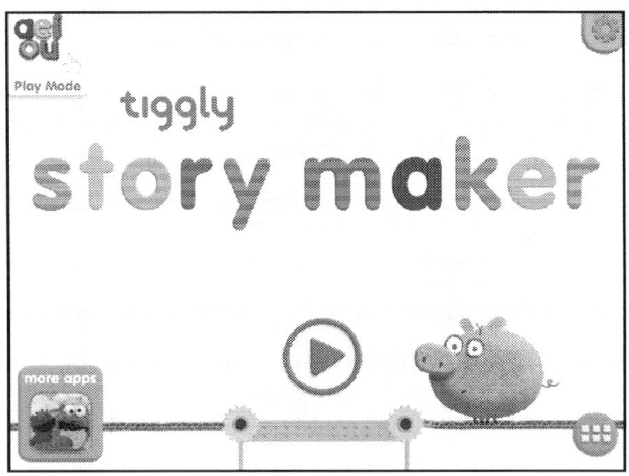

**FIGURE 7–1C.** Tiggly Story Maker screenshot. Reproduced with permission of Tiggly.

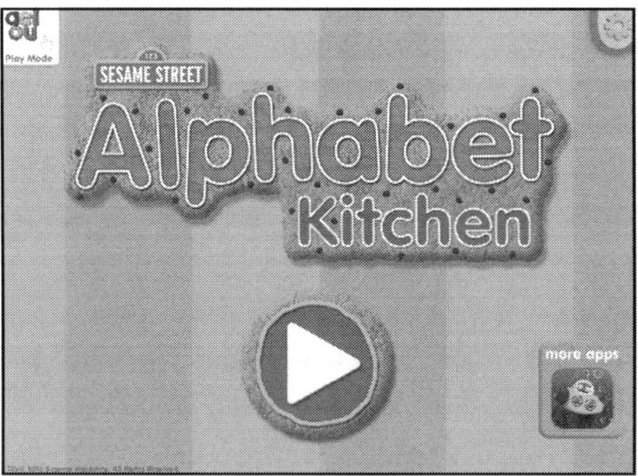

**FIGURE 7–1D.** Sesame Street and Tiggly Alphabet Kitchen screenshot. Reproduced with permission of Tiggly and Sesame Workshop®. Sesame Workshop®, Sesame Street®, and associated characters, trademarks, and design elements are owned and licensed by Sesame Workshop®. ©2016 Sesame Workshop®. All rights reserved.

To download the individual apps (Tiggly Submarine, Tiggly Doctor, Tiggly Story Maker, Sesame Street Alphabet Kitchen®) or purchase the interactive vowel toys, which include all of the apps below, visit http://www.tiggly.com

**FIGURE 7–2.** Tiggly QR code.

## Activity 1A

Tiggly Submarine aids in providing fun interactive activities in an underwater theme that will engage clients in identifying short vowel sounds (letter/sound identification) at the beginning or middle of words. This app can be used with or without the interactive vowel toys.

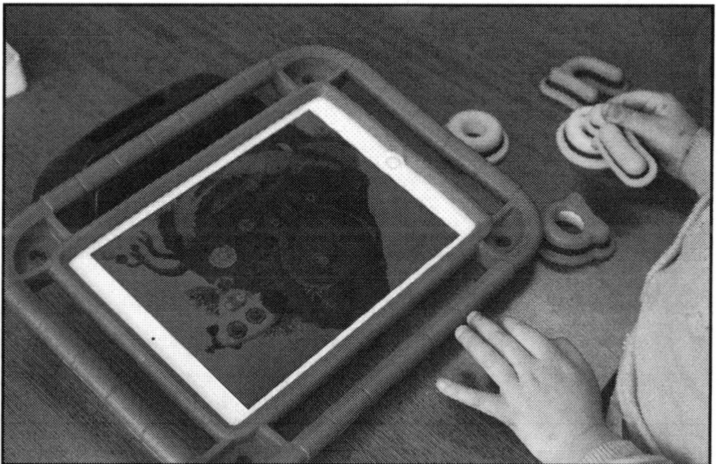

**FIGURE 7–3.** Hannah Clark Submarine.

### *Individual or Small Group Session*

Step 1:  With the client sitting aside or across from you, explain that the client will be using an app during this session to help with recognizing vowel sounds and words.
*NOTE:* The speech-language pathology assistant (SLPA) should take initial direction from supervising SLP in regard to the client's ability to use this lesson and modify as needed.

Step 2:  Open the app Tiggly Submarine and proceed.

    a.  Tap the white icon in the upper left corner to choose the "Play Mode." The colored vowel letters will be displayed when tapped for using the interactive vowel toys, or a hand image will be displayed when tapped for using the app without the interactive vowel toys.

    b.  Tap the "gear" image located in the top right corner to access options for turning off music, sounds, and voiceover.

Step 3:  Tap the arrow to begin. A yellow submarine will appear. This submarine will be dragged using your finger through the ocean to get to various island activities. *NOTE:* When using the app for the first time, allow the client to become familiar with the different island areas. Model how to move the submarine to get to each activity island (i.e., "Let's practice and find all the islands in the ocean where we can play and learn").

Step 4:  Keeping within the target area of client need and ability, guide the client to one or more activity areas by dragging the submarine toward the hungry octopus, the underwater coral island, or the undersea elevator.

    a.  To engage with the hungry octopus, tap any of the vowels with a finger or use the interactive vowel toys by placing the vowel on the tablet screen to hear a pronunciation of the vowel sound, create a word and object, and watch animation of the octopus eating the object. If repeating this activity, a new word will appear and is based on the vowel chosen. *NOTE:* For clients with reading ability or if SLPA would prefer to say the vowel sound, read the word, or ask client questions (which one is "eh" or which vowel is in the word "cat"?), turn off the sound in the settings on the main screen when the app is opened.

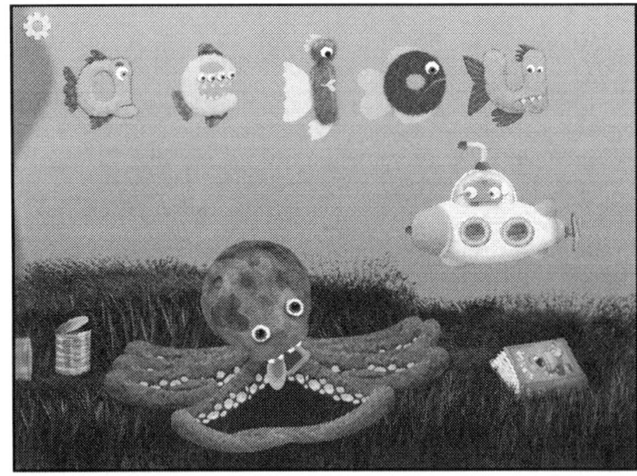

**FIGURE 7–4A.**  Tiggly octopus fingerplay screenshot. Reproduced with permission of Tiggly.

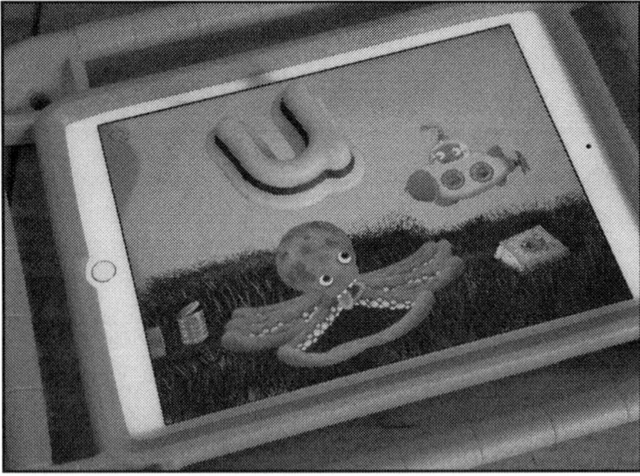

**FIGURE 7–4B.**  Octopus vowel toy.

b. To activate the hose suction in the ocean cave, place your finger on the corresponding vowel or place the appropriate vowel toy on the screen tablet that matches the vowel in the word or object shown until the word and object are sucked into the submarine. If the child isn't familiar with the name of the object shown or the name of the vowel (i.e., "gem" or "a"), the SLPA should say the word or the appropriate vowel to prompt the client; "That is a gem," or "What vowel sound do you hear in the word 'gem'?" or "Choose 'a'" or say the short vowel sound that you would like them to choose.

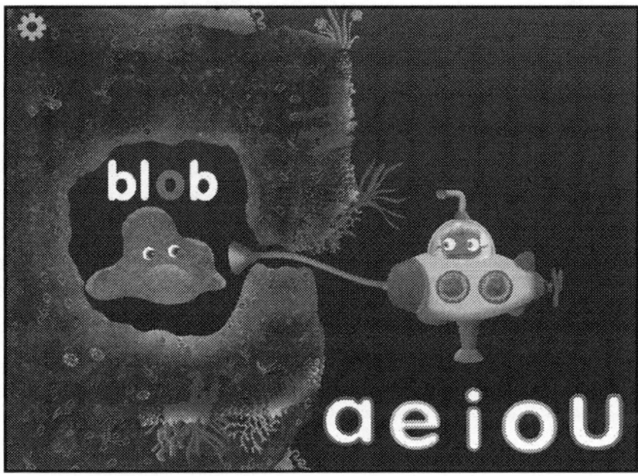


**FIGURE 7–5A.** Tiggly cave fingerplay screenshot. Reproduced with permission of Tiggly.

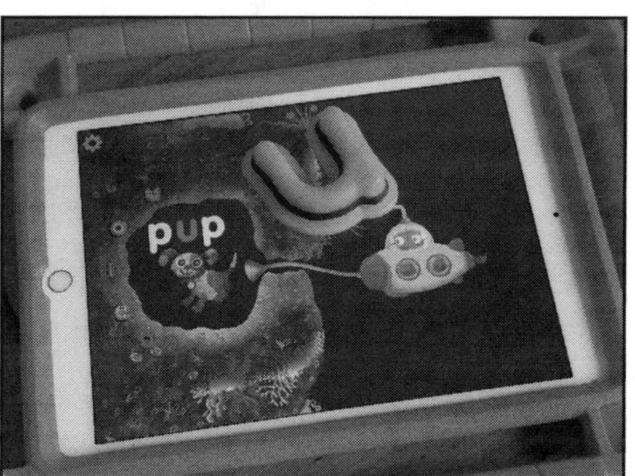


**FIGURE 7–5B.** Cave vowel toy.

c. To open the wooden door on the underwater coral island, tap one of the vowels above the door or place an interactive vowel toy on the tablet screen. Use this opportunity to ask the client to recall or repeat the word or use the word in a sentence to increase his or her MLU (mean length of utterance ).

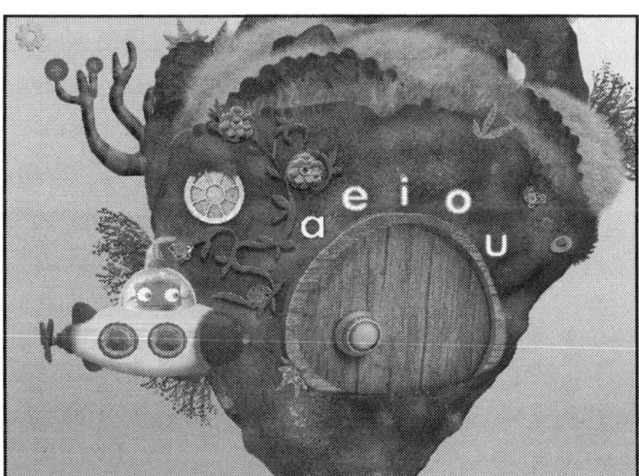


**FIGURE 7–6A.** Tiggly door fingerplay screenshot. Reproduced with permission of Tiggly.

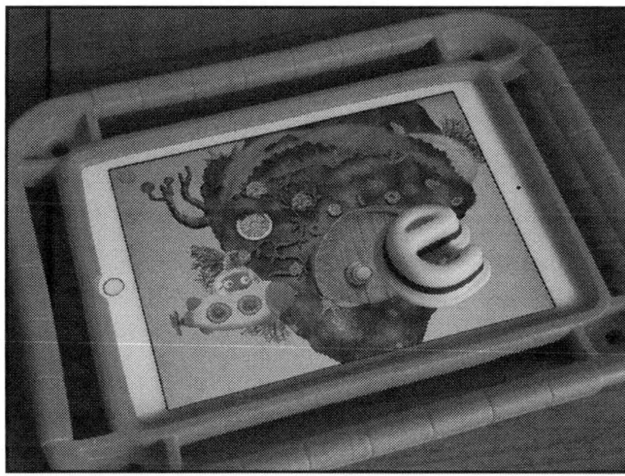

**FIGURE 7–6B.** Door vowel toy.

d. To open the elevator doors on the underwater cave, tap one of the vowels above the doors or place an interactive vowel toy on the tablet screen. Use this opportunity to ask the client to recall word or repeat the word or use the word in a sentence to increase his or her MLU. Give oral instructions to client (i.e., "Choose the vowel letter 'a'" or "Choose the vowel that is in the word 'cat'").

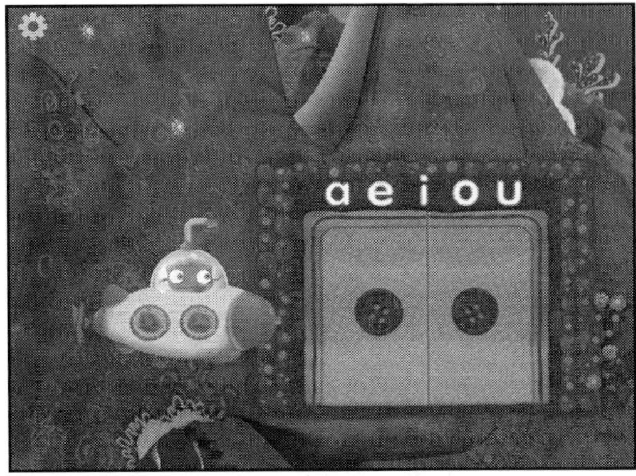

**FIGURE 7–7A.** Tiggly elevator fingerplay screenshot. Reproduced with permission of Tiggly.

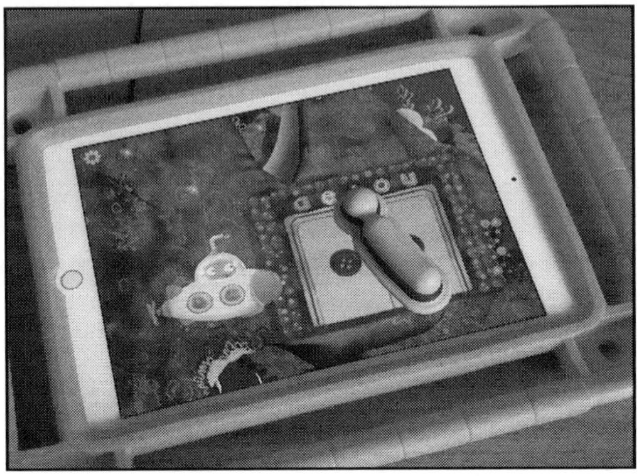

**FIGURE 7–7B.** Elevator vowel toy.

e. If using the interactive vowel toys, there is the ability to free play and place the vowels anywhere in the ocean to make vowel fish appear and hear the vowel sound.

> If the client does not or cannot tap or pick up one of the vowels, prompt with a gesture (i.e., pointing) or, if needed, a full physical prompt (i.e., hand over hand).

## Activity 1B

Tiggly Doctor aids in learning verbs, multisyllabic words, vocabulary building, and spelling patterns for long and short vowel words while taking care of three patients and their ailments. This app can be used with or without the interactive vowel toys.

### *Individual or Small Group Session*

Step 1: With the client sitting aside or across from you, explain that the client will be using an app during this session to help with his or her individual goals (i.e., "Johnny, you will work on multisyllabic words, and Sally, you will work on learning new action words"). *NOTE:* The SLPA should take initial direction from the supervising SLP in regard to the client's ability to use this lesson and modify as needed.

Step 2: Open the app "Tiggy Doctor" and proceed.

    a. Tap the white icon in the upper left corner to choose the "Play Mode." The colored vowel letters will be displayed when tapped for using the interactive vowel toys or a hand image will be displayed when tapped for using the app without the interactive vowel toys.

    b. Tap the "gear" image located in the top right corner to access options for turning off music, sounds, and voiceover.

    c. Tap the "arrow" to begin and proceed to the three characters in the "waiting room."

Step 3: Keeping within the target area of the client's need and ability, guide the client to one or more activity areas by tapping one of the three characters.

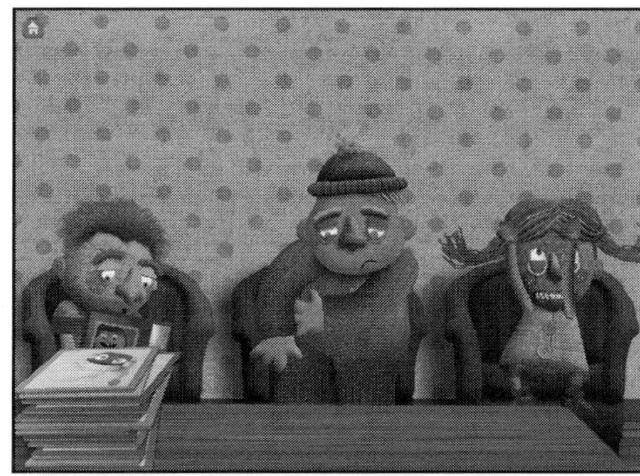

**FIGURE 7–8A.** Tiggly doctor waiting room screenshot. Reproduced with permission of Tiggly.

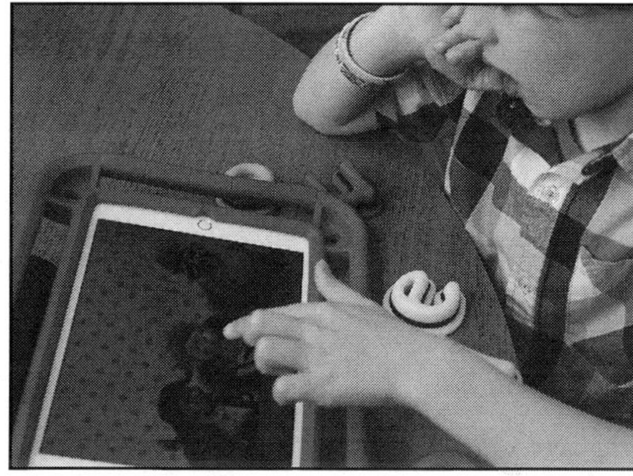

**FIGURE 7–8B.** Riley Clark doctor.



    a. To work on verbs and become familiar with spelling patterns to build vocabulary, tap "the character with blue skin" or "the character with purple skin." Tap with a finger or use an interactive vowel toy to fill in the missing letters to create an action word and engage in the activity. The client may use a finger to move the "Dr. Tool" to help take care of the patient. Use this opportunity to ask clients to use the word in a sentence, retell what they are doing, think of another word (synonym) that means the same thing, and recall or tell of a similar experience they have had.

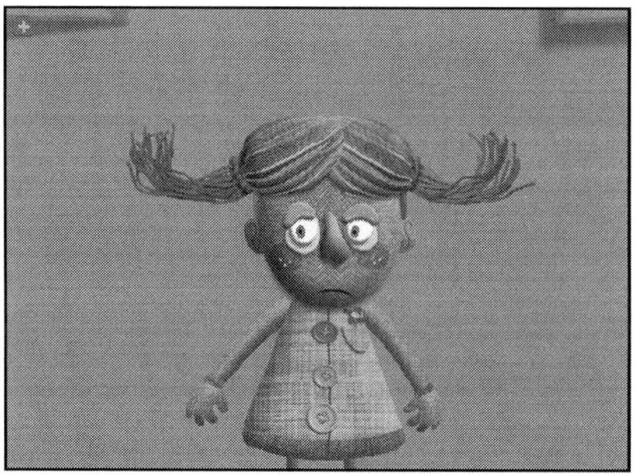

**FIGURE 7–9A.** Tiggly doctor girl screenshot. Reproduced with permission of Tiggly.

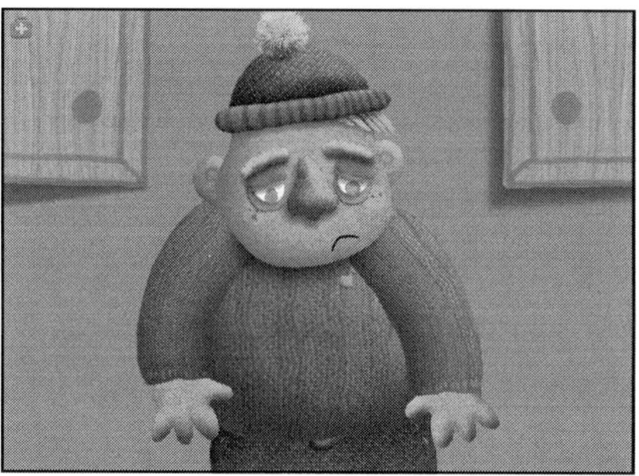

**FIGURE 7–9B.** Tiggly doctor boy hat screenshot. Reproduced with permission of Tiggly.

b.  To work on multisyllabic words with definitions, tap "the character with the screen skin and orange hair." Tap a vowel with your finger or use an interactive vowel toy in any order to fill in the missing letters to spell a multisyllabic word and hear the definition. Use this opportunity to allow the client to use the word in sentence, recall the definition or write the word on a separate piece of paper, or practice counting the number of syllables in the word.

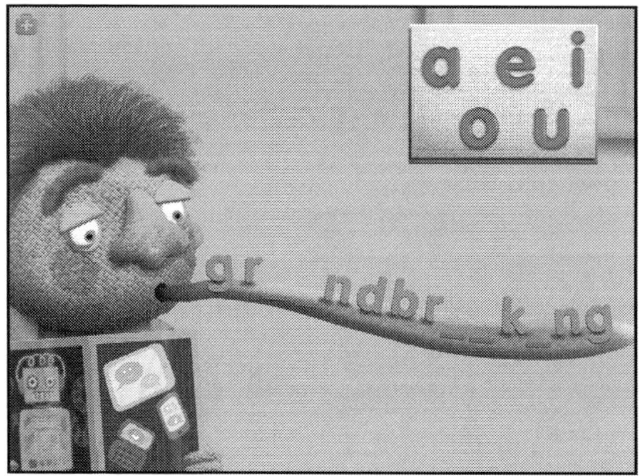


**FIGURE 7–10A.** Tiggly multisyllabic word screenshot. Reproduced with permission of Tiggly.

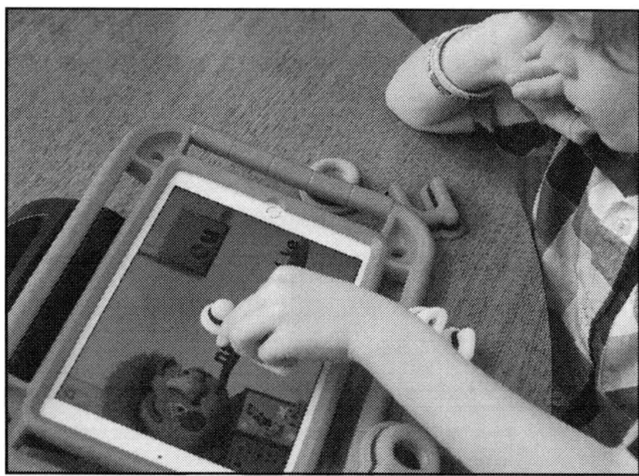

**FIGURE 7–10B.** Riley Clark doctor.

## Activity 1C

Tiggly Story Maker aids in creating words by replacing the vowel. Practice CVC (consonant, vowel, consonant) patterns, short vowel sounds, word building, and storytelling with built-in recording. This app can be used with or without the interactive vowel toys.

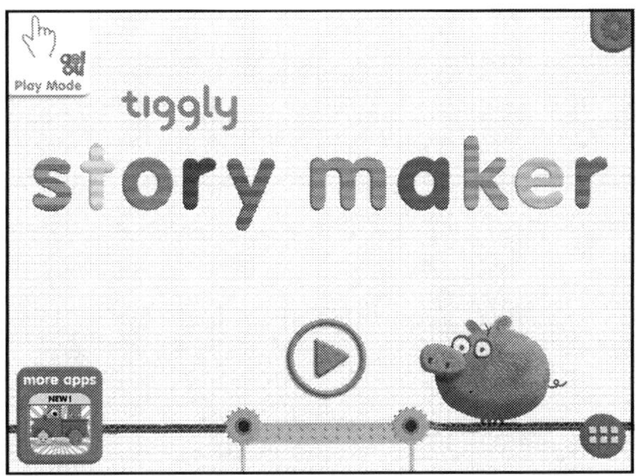

**FIGURE 7–11.** Tiggly storymaker main screenshot. Reproduced with permission of Tiggly.

### *Individual or Small Group Session*

Step 1:  With the client sitting aside or across from you, explain that the client will be using an app during this session to help with his or her individual goals (i.e., "Today we will work on making up and telling stories"). *NOTE:* The SLPA should take initial direction from the supervising SLP in regard to the client's ability to use this lesson and modify as needed.

Step 2:  Open the Tiggly Story Maker app and proceed:

a.  Tap the white icon in the upper left corner to choose the "Play Mode." The colored vowel letters will be displayed when tapped for using the interactive vowel toys, or a hand image will be displayed when tapped for using the app without the interactive vowel toys.

b.  Tap the "gear" image located in the top right corner to access options for turning off music, sounds, and voiceover.

c.  Tap the lower right corner to access any stories that have been previously saved.

d.  Tap the "arrow" to begin.

Step 3: To create CVC words, tap the vowel image with your finger or use an interactive vowel toy to fill in the vowel to create a word and see an animation. Use the "pull tool" above the first and last consonants to change beginning and ending sounds. Tap the letters to hear sounds. Repeat to create new CVC words. *NOTE:* For clients with reading ability or if the SLPA would prefer to say the vowel sound, read the word, or ask client questions (i.e., "Which one is 'eh'?" or "Which vowel is in the word?"), turn off the sound in the settings on the main screen when the app is opened.

Step 4: To create, animate, and narrate stories, tap the "star" in the upper left corner of the screen. A drop-down icon menu appears; tap the "video" icon. *NOTE:* Be certain the app has access to the microphone for recording purposes. Use this opportunity to help guide clients to use specific words in their story and might provide visual cues by using the words on index cards or sticky notes (i.e., first, then, next, last).

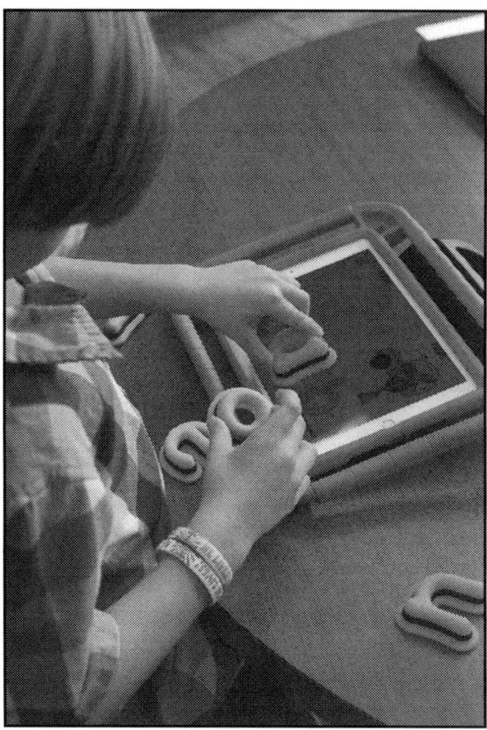

**FIGURE 7–12.** Riley Clark storymaker.

a. To add animation and narration to your story screen, drag additional images into the background from the bottom of the screen (optional), move the images around to animate (i.e., up, down, left, and right), and begin talking.

b. Tap the "video" icon to stop the recording. There are 3 minutes available for each recording.

c. Tap the "arrow" to watch and hear a playback of the story. The story will be saved and dated and can be accessed later from the home screen.

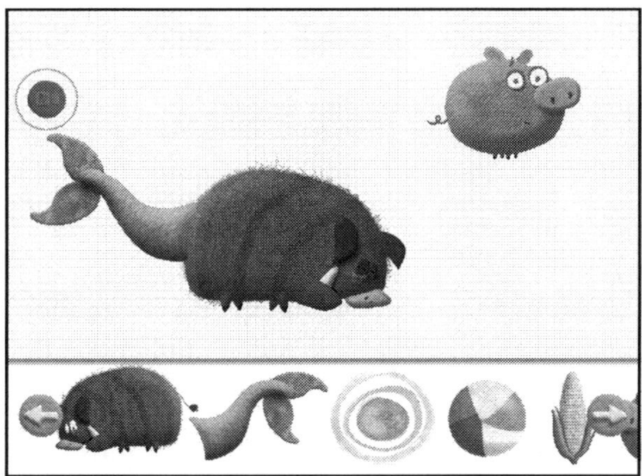

**FIGURE 7–13.** Tiggly storymaker recording screenshot. Reproduced with permission of Tiggly.

## Activity 1D

Sesame Street Alphabet Kitchen® aids in vocabulary building for early literacy skill practice by blending sounds to create three- and four-letter words or learning vowel names with corresponding letters. This app can be used with or without the interactive vowel toys.

**FIGURE 7–14.** Sesame Street® and Tiggly Elmo/Cookie Monster screenshot. Reproduced with permission of Tiggly and Sesame Workshop®. Sesame Workshop®, Sesame Street®, and associated characters, trademarks, and design elements are owned and licensed by Sesame Workshop®. ©2016 Sesame Workshop®. All rights reserved.

### *Individual or Small Group Session*

Step 1:  With the client sitting aside or across from you, explain that the client will be using an app during this session to help with his or her individual goals (i.e., "Today we are going to learn to blend sounds to create three- and four-letter words"). *NOTE:* The SLPA should take initial direction from the supervising SLP in regard to the client's ability to use this lesson and modify as needed.

Step 2:  Open the Sesame Street Alphabet Kitchen® app and proceed:

    a. Tap the white icon in the upper left corner to choose the "Play Mode." The colored vowel letters will be displayed when tapped for using the interactive vowel toys, or a hand image will be displayed when tapped for using the app without the interactive vowel toys.

    b. Tap the "gear" image located in the top right corner to access options for turning off music and sounds. Built-in character voices cannot be turned off; however, volume can be turned off on the tablet in order for the client or SLPA to read and sound out words.

    c. Tap the "arrow" to begin.

Step 3:  Tap the Cookie Monster to blend letters to create three- and four-letter words.

    a. Tap the vowel or use interactive vowel toys to fill in the missing letter.

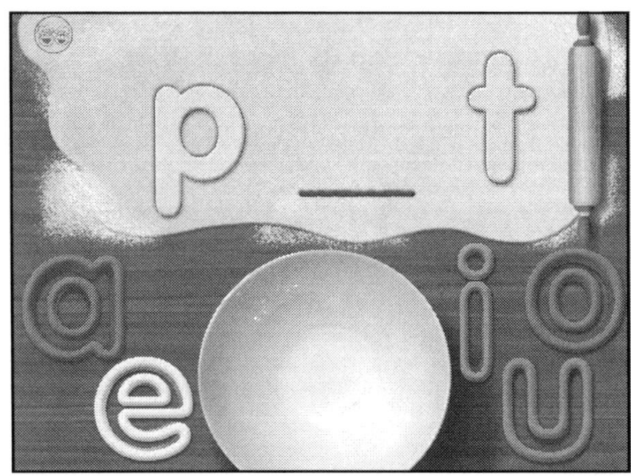

**FIGURE 7–15A.** Sesame Street® and Tiggly alphabet kitchen word screenshot. Reproduced with permission of Tiggly and Sesame Workshop®. Sesame Workshop®, Sesame Street®, and associated characters, trademarks, and design elements are owned and licensed by Sesame Workshop®. ©2016 Sesame Workshop®. All rights reserved.

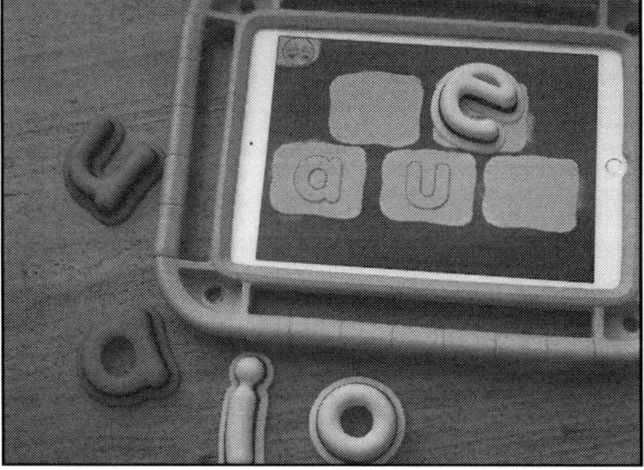

**FIGURE 7–15B.** Sesame Street® and Tiggly alphabet kitchen toy screengrab. Reproduced with permission of Tiggly and Sesame Workshop®. Sesame Workshop®, Sesame Street®, and associated characters, trademarks, and design elements are owned and licensed by Sesame Workshop®. ©2016 Sesame Workshop®. All rights reserved.

b. Tap colored frostings and mix by circling a finger on the bowl. Any combination of colors may be added. This allows for an opportunity to experience color mixing (i.e., red plus yellow makes orange). Giving the client directions at this point adds another element of learning and listening (i.e., first, add green; next/second, add pink; or last/then/third, add red).

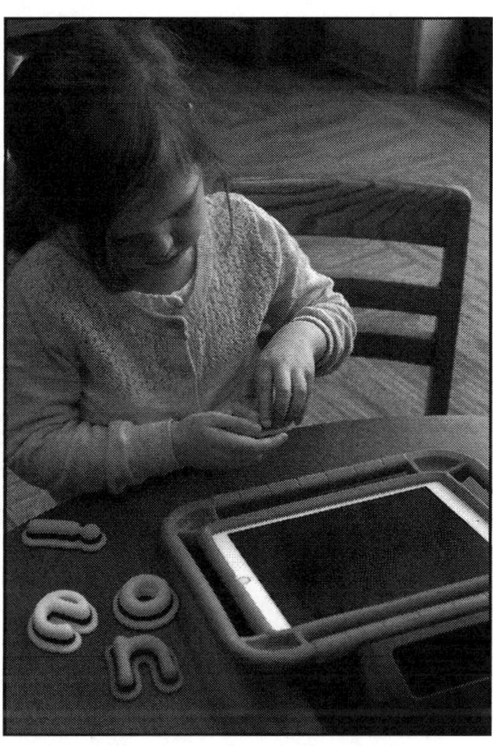

**FIGURE 7–16.** Sesame Street® and Tiggly and Hannah Clark alphabet kitchen. Reproduced with permission of Tiggly and Sesame Workshop®. Sesame Workshop®, Sesame Street®, and associated characters, trademarks, and design elements are owned and licensed by Sesame Workshop®. ©2016 Sesame Workshop®. All rights reserved.

c. Listen to the character sound out the word or turn off the tablet volume to have the client or SLPA read aloud.

d. Drag the rolling pin across dough to change the letter arrangement if needed.

e. Repeat four times to watch the animation and interact with the character. *NOTE:* A graph with completed cookies will appear in the bottom left of the screen. When working in small groups, this makes for an appropriate place to have clients take turns.

f. Drag cookies to "share" with a character or tap the cookie to pretend to eat. When working in small groups, give all clients an opportunity to "eat" or "share" the cookie word.

g. Tap the circle icon with "character faces" in the upper left to return to the main screen to choose the other character.

Step 4:  Tap Elmo to experience vowel names and with the corresponding letter images.

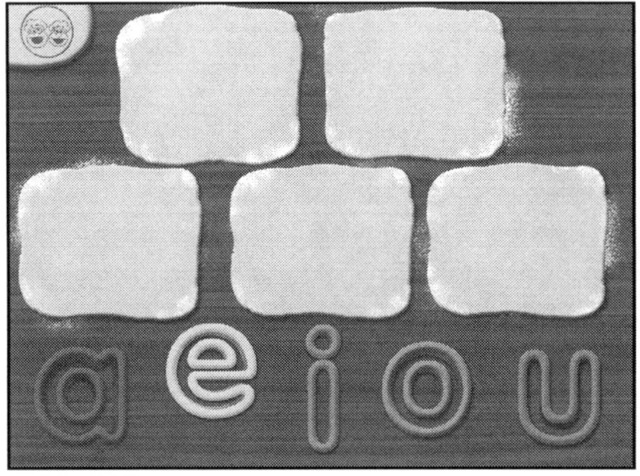

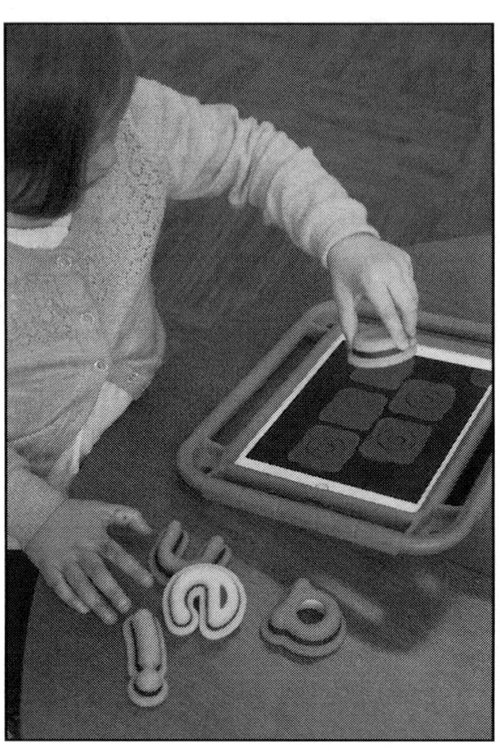

**FIGURE 7–17A.**  Sesame Street® and Tiggly alphabet kitchen screenshot. Reproduced with permission of Tiggly and Sesame Workshop®. Sesame Workshop®, Sesame Street®, and associated characters, trademarks, and design elements are owned and licensed by Sesame Workshop®. ©2016 Sesame Workshop®. All rights reserved.

**FIGURE 7–17B.**  Hannah Clark alphabet kitchen vowel and Sesame Street® and Tiggly screengrab. Reproduced with permission of Tiggly and Sesame Workshop®. Sesame Workshop®, Sesame Street®, and associated characters, trademarks, and design elements are owned and licensed by Sesame Workshop®. ©2016 Sesame Workshop®. All rights reserved.

a.  To work on identification of vowel names and corresponding letters, tap a vowel for it to appear on a dough square or use interactive vowel toys placed directly on a dough square. Use this opportunity to request the client to use a specific vowel toy or tap a specific vowel to check comprehension (i.e., choose the vowel "a" or choose the one that makes the short sound "eh," or choose the one that makes the sound in "hot").

b.  Repeat until all dough squares are filled. *NOTE:* Turn the tablet volume to mute or off to silence the character voices. This is helpful for when you want the client to imitate the vowel sound without cues.

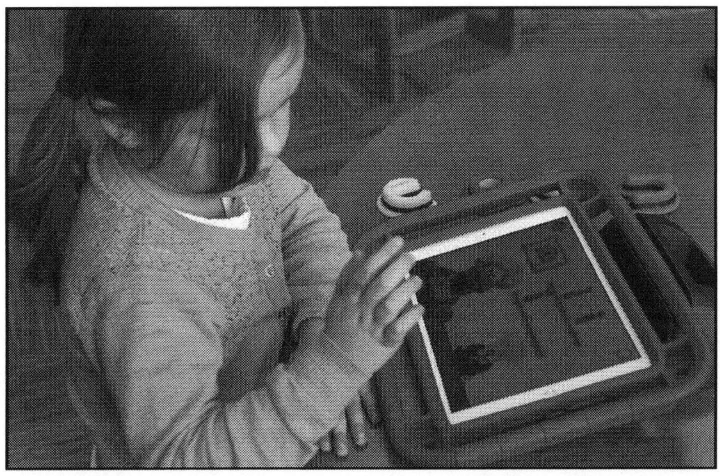

**FIGURE 7–18.** Hannah Clark alphabet kitchen and Sesame Street® and Tiggly screengrab. Reproduced with permission of Tiggly and Sesame Workshop®. Sesame Workshop®, Sesame Street®, and associated characters, trademarks, and design elements are owned and licensed by Sesame Workshop®. ©2016 Sesame Workshop®. All rights reserved.

c.  Decorate the cookie letters using the icing and toppings. Scroll through the choices at the bottom of the screen by using a swipe motion and drag the item to the specific cookie letter. Use this opportunity for clients to take turns, following directions or requesting the client give instructions to a peer or SLPA (i.e., first use green icing, next choose a topping that is a fruit, a pink sugary topping, a lemon, etc.). Any combination of icing or toppings can be used.

d.  Tap the "bell" icon to finish decorating and proceed to the next screen. Tap the cookies to pretend to eat or drag the cookies to share with the characters. Use this opportunity to continue taking turns for small group therapy sessions. Request the clients to say a word or model a word for the clients with the cookie letter sound before they pretend to "eat" or "share" the cookie.

e.  Tap the circle icon with "character faces" in the upper left to return to the main screen to choose the other character.

## Activity 2

Targeting alphabet knowledge, phonologic awareness, or rhyming using the Word Wizard app by L'Escapadou for ages 4 to 10 years.

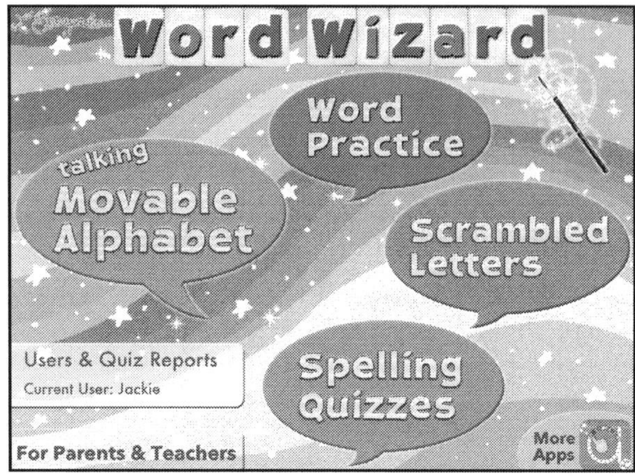


**FIGURE 7–19A.** L'Escapadou Word Wizard main screenshot. Reproduced with permission of L'Escapadou.

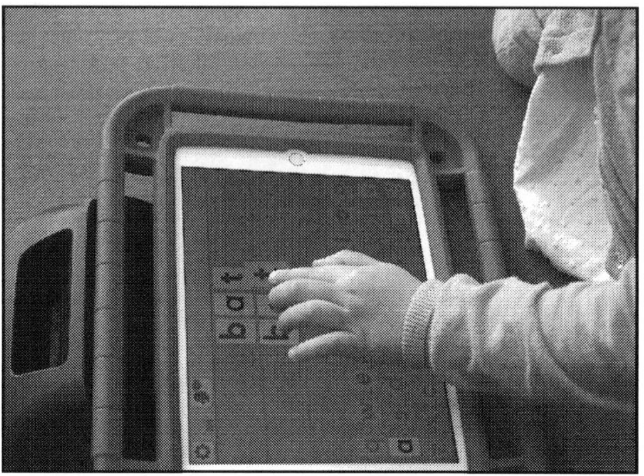

**FIGURE 7–19B.** Hannah Clark Word Wizard.

> To make for a more effective therapy session, create a user (client) list, determine settings, choose a built-in word list, or customize a word list prior to the therapy session.

Word Wizard by L'Escapadou offers several unique reading and spelling activities.

- A talking movable alphabet that allows kids to experiment with phonics and word building.

- Three spelling activities that increase in difficulty with a list of more than 1,400 questions and answers: word practice, scrambled letters, spelling quizzes.

- 184 built-in word lists: beginners, Dolch words, most frequently used words, body parts and more. Ability to customize and create your own word lists.

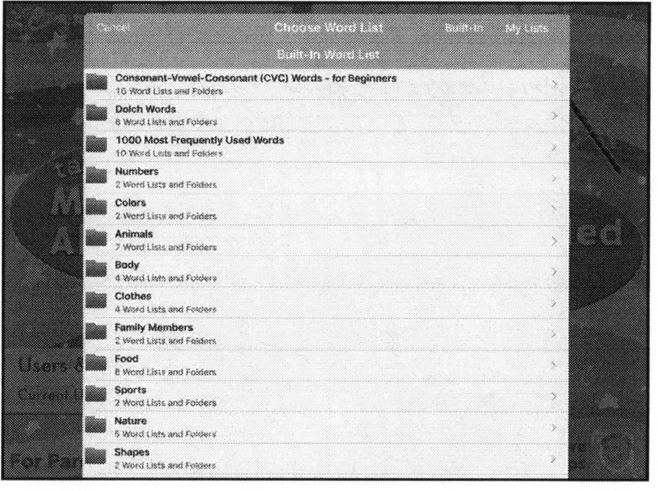

**FIGURE 7–20.**  L'Escapadou word list screenshot. Reproduced with permission of L'Escapadou.

- Track client progress with detailed reports. Can have unlimited number of users.

- Retrieved from http://lescapadou.com

To download Word Wizard, visit http://lescapadou.com

**FIGURE 7–21.**
L'Escapadou QR code.



### *Individual or Small Group Session*

Step 1:  Create a user list. This is where you will enter client names prior to therapy session time. Settings can also be customized as needed.

Step 2:  With the client sitting aside or across from you, explain that you will be using Word Wizard to practice his or her target goals (i.e., creating rhyming words). Based on the client's targeted objectives, tap one of the four areas to work in:

a.  Talking Movable Alphabet—Use this area for targeting alphabet recognition and manipulating letters to make real and/or nonsense words.

b.  Word Practice—Use this area for customizing word lists or using the built-in lists. Practice word families, rhyming, and spelling patterns. Consider this app for clients also working on articulation and creating specific phoneme lists (i.e., /s, r, l/).

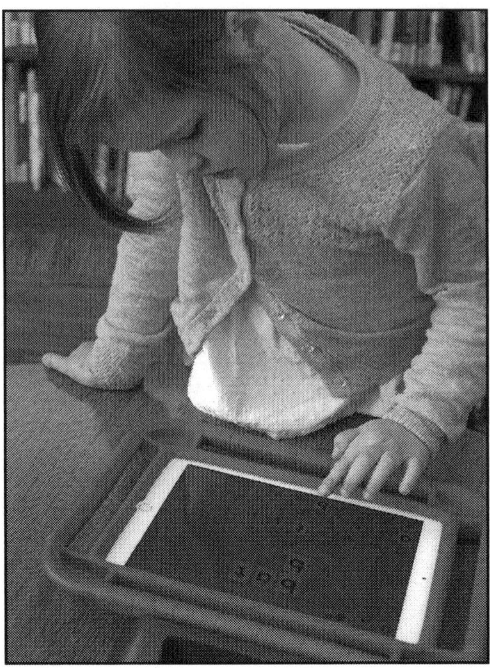

**FIGURE 7–22.** Hannah Clark movable alphabet.

   c. Scrambled Letters—Use this area to target comprehension of word families and spelling patterns already learned. Customized lists can also be created.

   d. Spelling Quizzes—Use this area to hear a word and then spell it. Includes visual cues if needed. Customize lists or use the built-in lists.


## Activity 3

Targeting print concept ideas, using "Brown Bear, Brown Bear," by Eric Carl and accompanying app Writing Wizard by L'Escapadou. *NOTE:* This activity may be used with any print text.

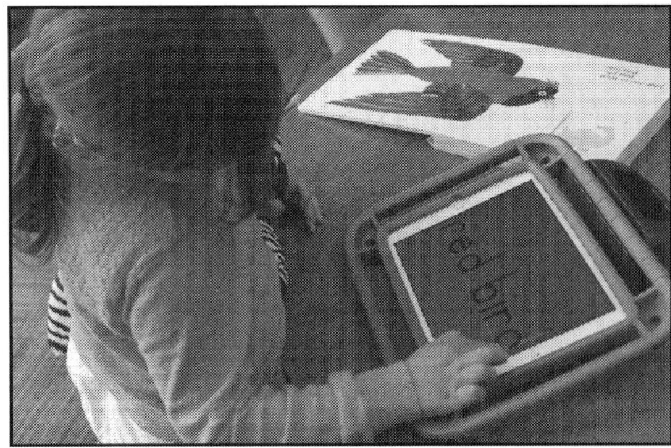

**FIGURE 7–23A.** Hannah Clark Writing Wizard.

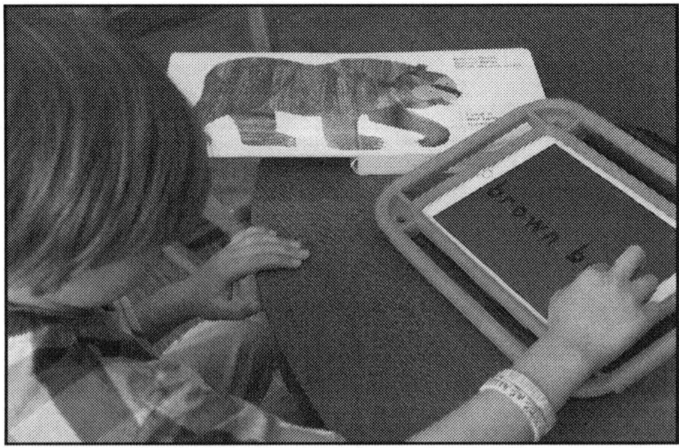

**FIGURE 7–23B.** Riley Clark Writing Wizard.

Writing Wizard is a unique app that allows users to practice writing on a screen using their finger or a stylus. In addition, an option for printing paper worksheets within the app is offered. Pairing Writing Wizard with a favorite book can help in developing literacy skills while engaging clients with the interactivity of writing.

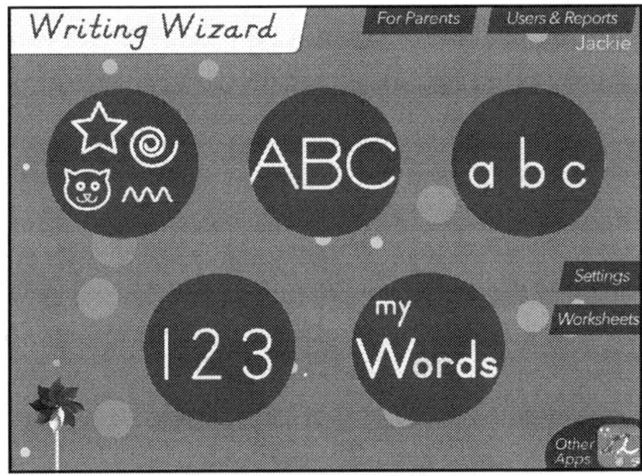

**FIGURE 7–24A.** L'Escapadou Writing Wizard main screenshot. Reproduced with permission of L'Escapadou.

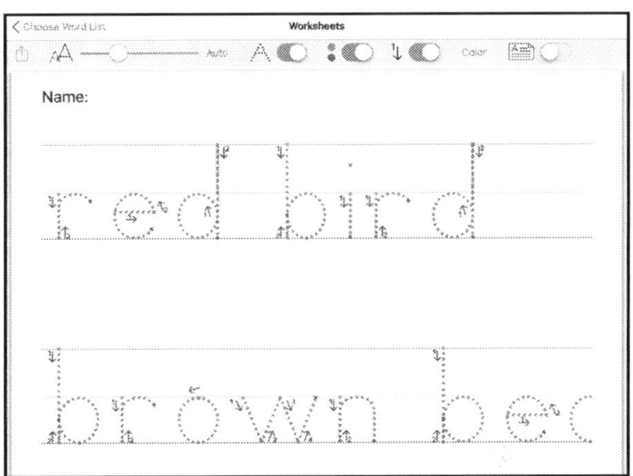

**FIGURE 7–24B.** L'Escapadou worksheet screenshot. Reproduced with permission of L'Escapadou.

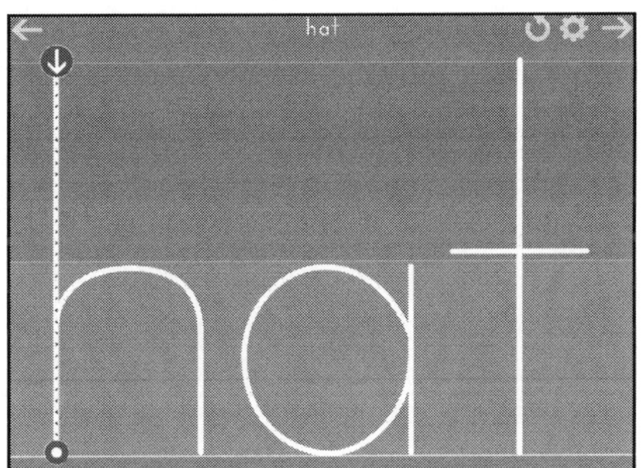

**FIGURE 7–24C.** L'Escapadou writing screenshot. Reproduced with permission of L'Escapadou.

To download Writing Wizard, visit http://lescapadou.com

**FIGURE 7–25.**
L'Escapadou QR code.

### *Individual or Small Group Session*

Step 1:  Prior to the session, create a custom word list that corresponds with text from a book.

    a.  To create a word list, open the Writing Wizard app and tap on "my Words." In the upper right-hand corner, tap on "Word Lists."

    b.  Tap on "New List" in upper left-hand corner.

    c.  Type the desired name of list. For purposes of this lesson, name the list "Brown Bear" and tap "Save."

    d.  Tap "Add Word," type word(s) in the text area, and tap "Save." *NOTE:* It is optional to add a voice recording for each word if desired.

    e.  Repeat "Add Word" for as many words needed for this lesson (i.e., brown bear, red bird, blue horse, etc.).

Step 2:  With the client sitting aside or across from you, explain that you will be reading and using the app Writing Wizard to practice words and phrases from the book.

Step 3:  Choose two or three pages of the book for focus to target client goals and objectives and open Writing Wizard.

    a.  Read aloud a chosen page or have the client take turns reading the page.

    b.  Tap "my Words" to choose a previously created word list in Writing Wizard and allow the client to find the word or phrase that corresponds with what was read (i.e., red bird). Tap on the chosen word to have it appear on the screen. If a recording was made during word list creation, the narrated voice will be audible. *NOTE:* Tap on the settings gear in the upper right-hand corner to change the writing color. To change color, tap on the "circle" icon in the "Style" row. Choose a color to write with by tapping the colored circle. For purposes of this lesson, try to coordinate the color with the word (i.e., choose red for "red bird" or choose yellow for "yellow duck").

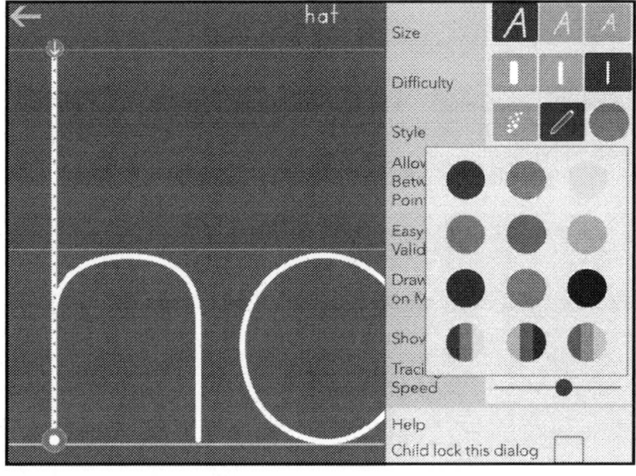


**FIGURE 7–26.** L'Escapadou style color screenshot. Reproduced with permission of L'Escapadou.

c. Allow client to write the word with his or her finger or an appropriate tablet screen stylus. To repeat writing the same word or phrase, tap the "circular arrow" on the top of the screen. This is beneficial if you are working in small groups and want each client to have a turn with the same word or phrase.

d. To return to the word list, tap the "back arrow" in the upper left-hand corner of the screen.

e. Continue reading pages and practice identifying and writing words or phrases from the created word list.

---

Consider using the Writing Wizard app for an articulation word list (i.e., initial /s/ word list) or for a category or vocabulary lesson (i.e., a list of fruits, vegetables, clothing, occupations, etc.).

---

## ACTIVITIES FOR SCHOOL-AGE LITERACY

## Objectives

The following are some sample objectives for literacy for the school-age client within a therapy session:

1. Client will correctly identify and sort words based on prefix and/or suffix patterns in 8 of 10 opportunities across three consecutive data collection points.

2. Client will correctly identify the order of events in literature and informal text 80% of the time across three consecutive data collection points.

3. Client will correctly identify and sort words based on reading patterns such as word families, vowel teams, or syllabic patterns in 9 of 10 opportunities across three consecutive data collection points.

## Activity 1

WordQuations app by Communication APPtitude for building verb vocabulary and meaning for older school-age clients by exposing them to the motivation and emotion behind the word.

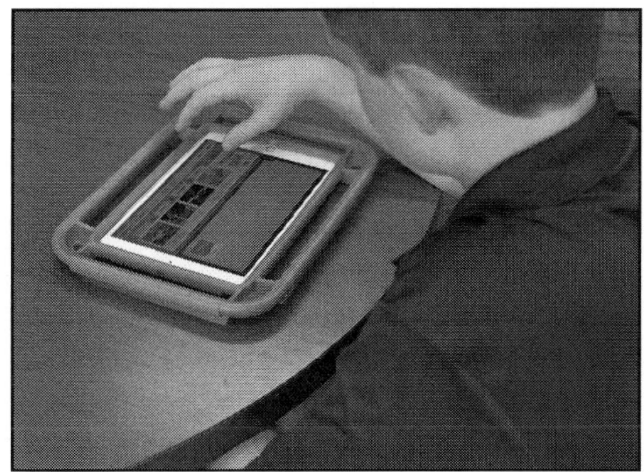

**FIGURE 7–27A.** Ethan Dworak WordQuations 1.

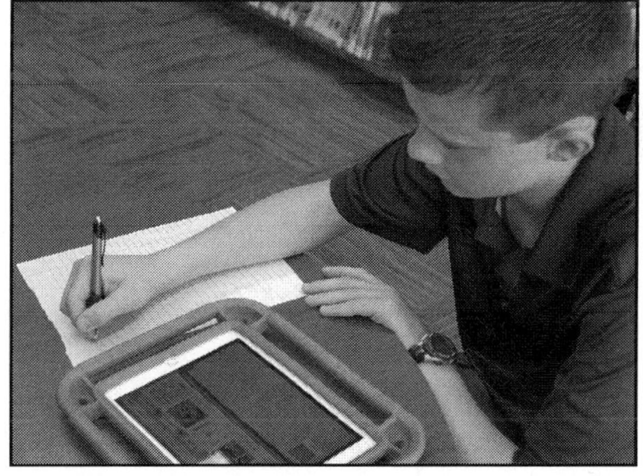

**FIGURE 7–27B.** Ethan Dworak WordQuations 2.

WordQuations is an iPad app designed to help students master the subtle meanings of verb synonyms. It helps older students understand the distinctions between synonyms such as plod, trudge, meander, and slink. The theme presented throughout the app provides clues about character motivation and feelings for improved reading comprehension. Students can also use the app to improve verb choices in their writing, eliminating random thesaurus choices. Retrieved from http://www.communicationapptitude.com

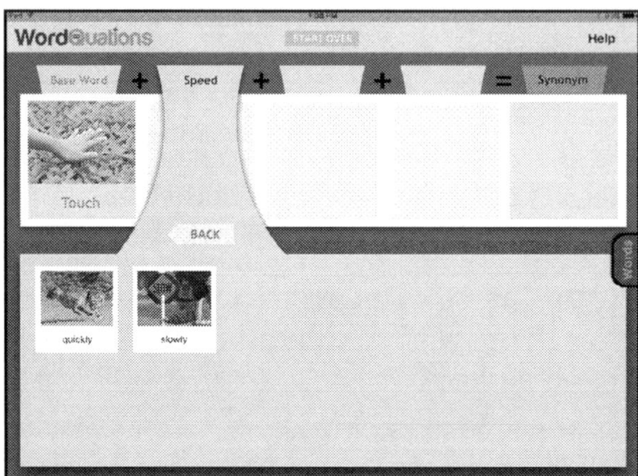

**FIGURE 7–28.** Communication APPtitude WordQuation touch screenshot. Reproduced with permission of Communication APPtitude, LLC. Copyright ©2017–2018. All rights reserved.

To download WordQuations by Communication APPtitude, visit http://www.comunication apptitude.com

**FIGURE 7–29.**
Communication APPtitude
QR code.

### *Individual or Small Group Session*

Step 1:  Open the WordQuations app and proceed:

    a. Tap one of the base words that appears at the bottom of the screen to begin setting up the word equation: Drink, Eat, Look, Put, Sit, Talk, Think, Touch, Understand, Walk, or Write.

    b. Tap a corresponding speed to go with the base word chosen: Quickly or Slowly.

    c. Tap a corresponding volume, intensity, or heaviness to go with the base word chosen: Slowly or Powerfully.

d. Tap a corresponding motive or emotion to go with the base word (i.e., tired, sad, old, deep in thought, etc.).

e. Tap on one of the synonyms at the bottom of the screen. There may be more than one. Choose the synonym with the definition that is appropriate for your "idea." Once selected, the synonym will appear at the far right of the word equation.

f. Read the definition and tap the "arrow" within the synonym tile to play a video that depicts the word in a fun and meaningful way.

Step 2:  To see a list of synonyms and their definitions, tap the word to see the equation and a video.

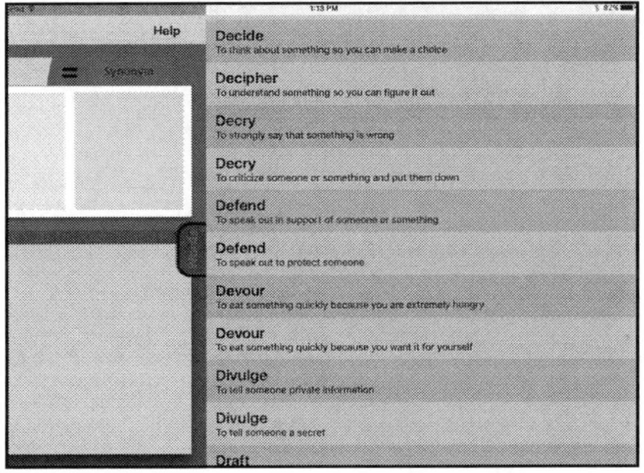

**FIGURE 7–30A.** Communication APPtitude decide list screenshot. Reproduced with permission of Communication APPtitude, LLC. Copyright ©2017–2018. All rights reserved.

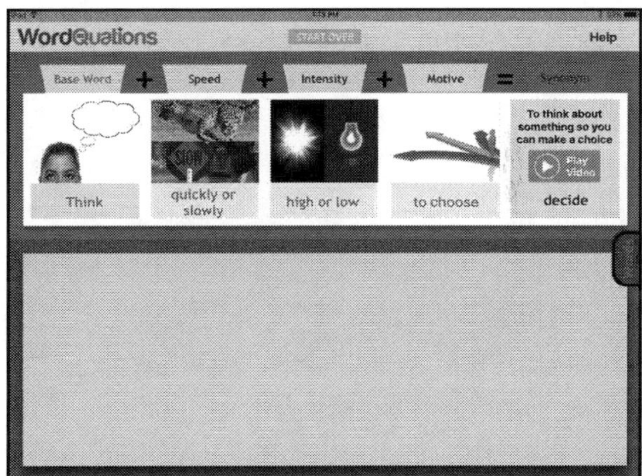

**FIGURE 7–30B.** Communication APPtitude equation screenshot. Reproduced with permission of Communication APPtitude, LLC. Copyright ©2017–2018. All rights reserved.

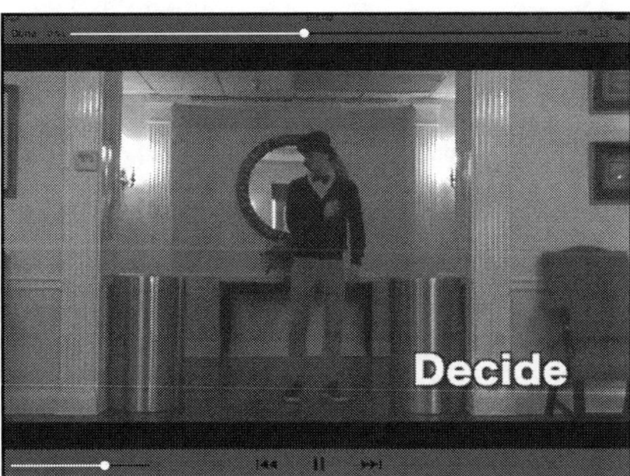

**FIGURE 7–30C.** Communication APPtitude decide video screenshot. Reproduced with permission of Communication APPtitude, LLC. Copyright ©2017–2018. All rights reserved.

Step 3:  Use this opportunity to create meaningful sentences for new verbs learned. For words that create more than one synonym, have the client explain the differences and how that word could be used in writing or speaking.

## Activity 2

InferCabulary 1, InferCabulary 2, or InferCabulary 3 by Communication APPtitude for working on core curriculum vocabulary words for elementary through high school-age clients.

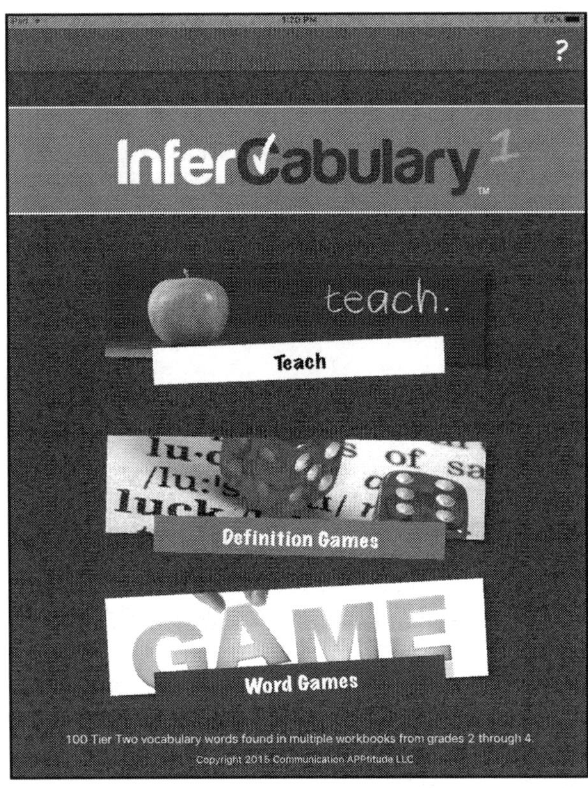


**FIGURE 7–31A.**  Communication APPtitude InferCabulary 1 screenshot. Reproduced with permission of Communication APPtitude, LLC. Copyright ©2017–2018. All rights reserved.

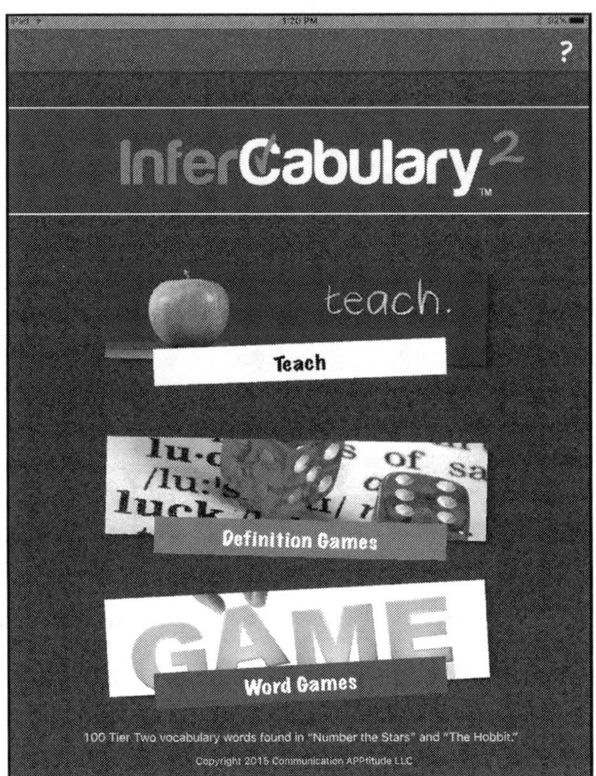


**FIGURE 7–31B.**  Communication APPtitude InferCabulary 2 screenshot. Reproduced with permission of Communication APPtitude, LLC. Copyright ©2017–2018. All rights reserved.

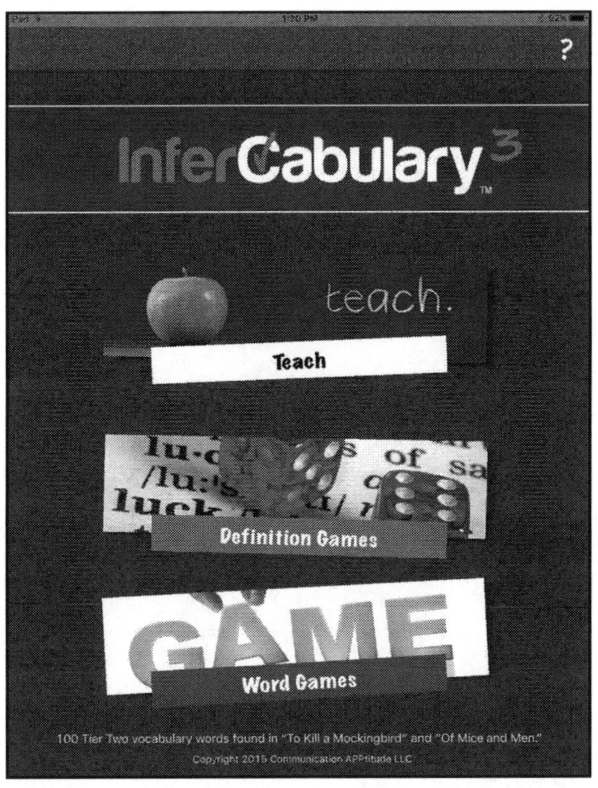

**FIGURE 7–31C.** Communication APPtitude InferCabulary 3 screenshot. Reproduced with permission of Communication APPtitude, LLC. Copyright ©2017–2018. All rights reserved.

InferCabulary is a vocabulary app requiring students to visually infer the meaning of core curriculum vocabulary words. Definitions are presented in simple language with beautiful photos further solidifying the meaning for students. Students can use a teach mode and/or game mode to reinforce and support vocabulary understanding. Versions include vocabulary from specific literary works used in school systems across the country. Retrieved from http://www.communicationapptitude.com

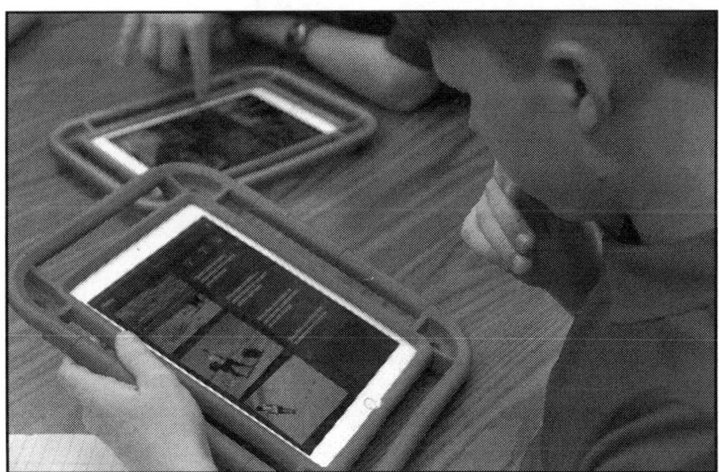

**FIGURE 7–32.** Jordan Potter.

To download any of the InferCabulary apps or for additional resources, visit http://www
.communicationapptitude.com

**FIGURE 7–33.**
Communication APPtitude
QR code.

### *Individual or Small Group Session*

Step 1:  Open the appropriate InferCabulary app based on client needs and objectives. InferCabulary 1 includes 100 Tier Two vocabulary words for clients in elementary school. InferCabulary 2 includes 100 words from popular literature (*Number the Stars* and *The Hobbit*) used in middle school. InferCabulary 3 includes 100 words from popular literature (*Of Mice and Men* and *To Kill a Mockingbird*) used in high school.

Step 2:  Tap one of the play areas: TEACH, DEFINITION GAMES, or WORD GAMES.

a.  TEACH to display five corresponding photographs for a word. The client can visually take in the meaning of the word, tap each photograph to get a simple explanation, tap the speaker to hear the word read aloud, tap the word to

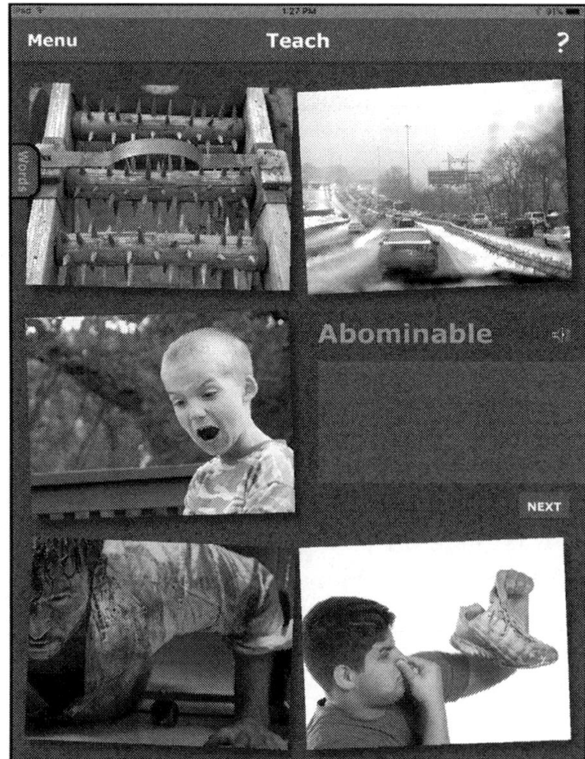


FIGURE 7–34.  Communication APPtitude image of teach screenshot. Reproduced with permission of Communication APPtitude, LLC. Copyright ©2017–2018. All rights reserved.

display a definition, or tap "next "to move to the next word. Choose the "words tab" to reveal a list and tap a specific targeted word to display the photographs and word. Use the TEACH section to give clients opportunities to visually absorb the different aspects of a word. Ask questions of the client before tapping the image to get the explanation (i.e., "What do you think Active might mean?"). Give the clients an opportunity to use the word in a sentence or share a time when they were "Active."

b. DEFINITON GAMES—four game areas to target definitions for vocabulary words. Two pictures are presented with five definitions. Read and/or listen to the definitions and choose the one that matches the two pictures. If the correct definition is chosen, earn points. If the incorrect definition is chosen, a third picture will appear with the chance to earn more points. Use this area to have the client practice new definitions and words learned in a fun, interactive way.

- Novice—Tap the pictures to get an audio and text clue.
- Speed—Try to answer before time (90 seconds) runs out.
- Sudden Death—One wrong answer and the game is over.
- 3 Lives—Three wrong answers and the game is over.

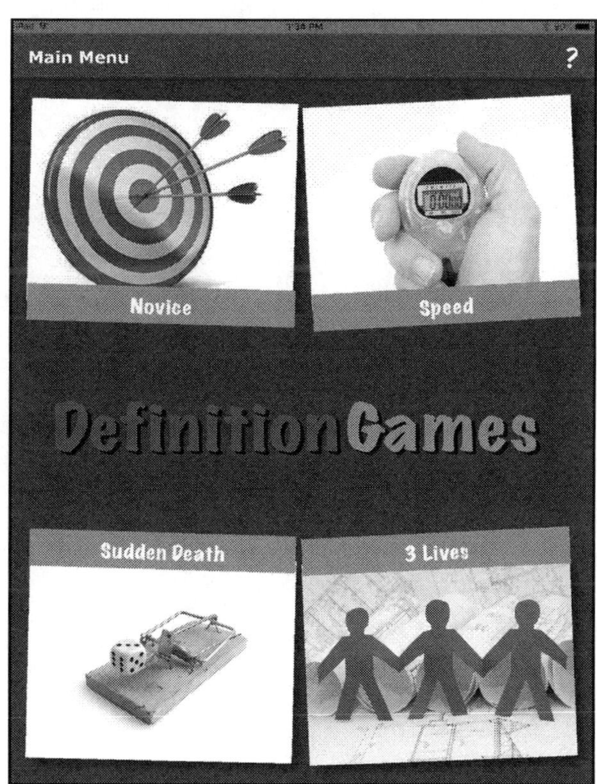


**FIGURE 7–35A.** Communication APPtitude definitions screenshot. Reproduced with permission of Communication APPtitude, LLC. Copyright ©2017–2018. All rights reserved.

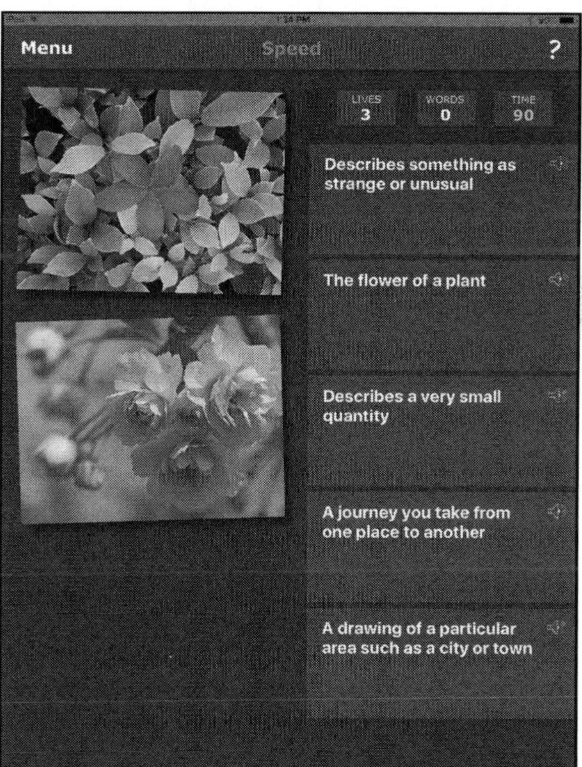


**FIGURE 7–35B.** Communication APPtitude speed screenshot. Reproduced with permission of Communication APPtitude, LLC. Copyright ©2017–2018. All rights reserved.

c. WORD GAMES—Analyze the five photographs, then choose the correct word out of four that best represent all the pictures. Read and/or listen to the word read aloud. Tap the photographs for a simple explanation with audio and text. Use this area to have the client practice new definitions and words learned in a fun, interactive way.

- Novice—Tap the pictures to get an audio and text clue.
- Speed—Try to answer before time (90 seconds) runs out.
- Sudden Death—One wrong answer and the game is over.
- 3 Lives—Three wrong answers and the game is over.

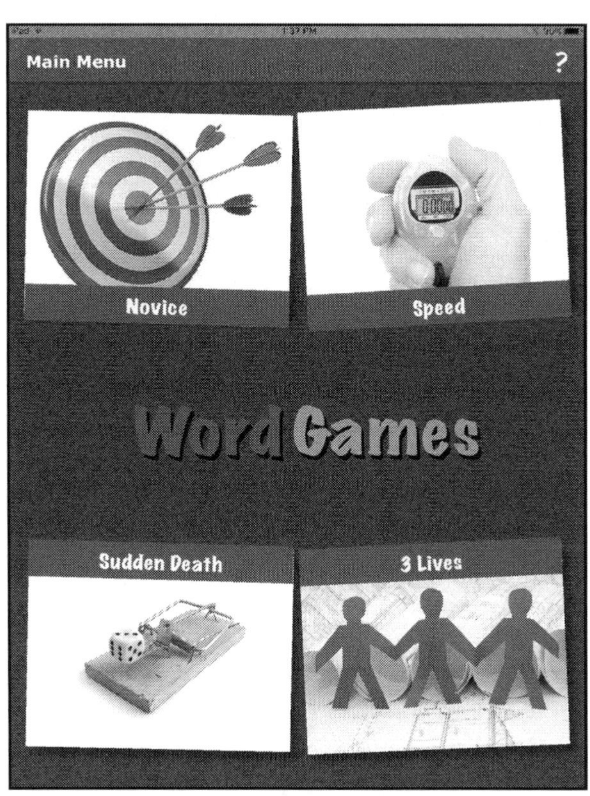


**FIGURE 7–36A.** Communication APPtitude word game screenshot. Reproduced with permission of Communication APPtitude, LLC. Copyright ©2017–2018. All rights reserved.

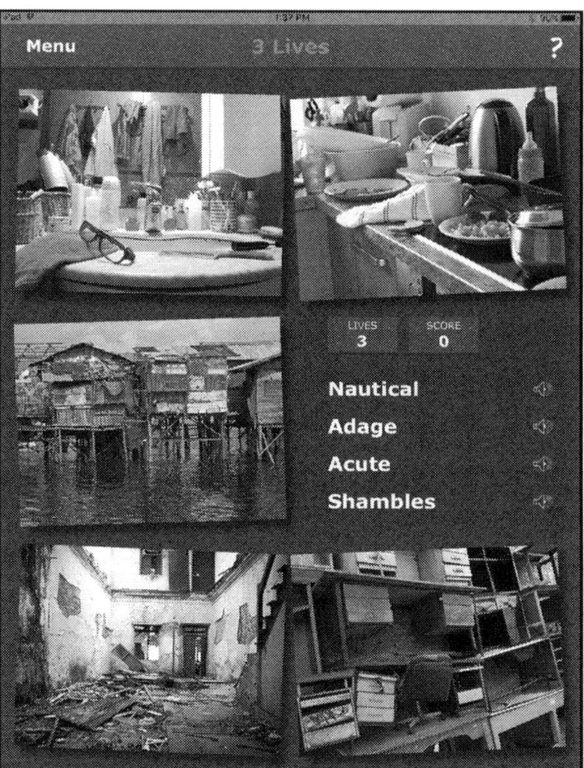


**FIGURE 7–36B.** Communication APPtitude 3 lives screenshot. Reproduced with permission of Communication APPtitude, LLC. Copyright ©2017–2018. All rights reserved.

## Activity 3

This lesson targets phonologic awareness skills, print concepts, and word recognition using the app Mystery Word Town by Artgig Apps for school-aged children 6 through 12 years of age.

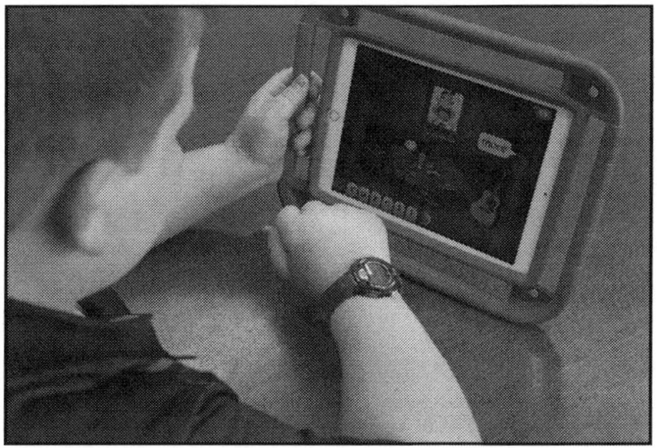

**FIGURE 7–37A.** Emmit Dworak Mystery Word Town.

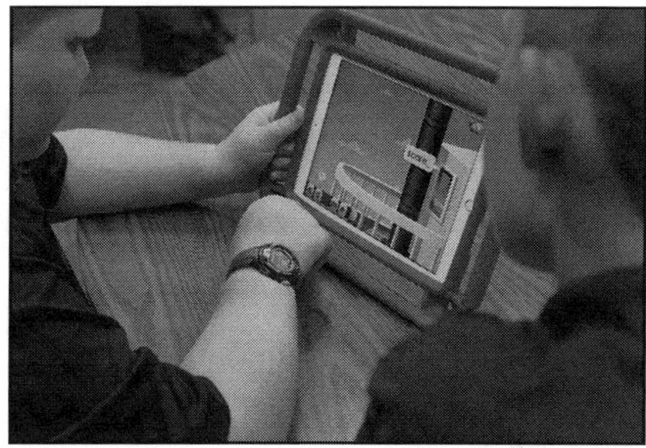

**FIGURE 7–37B.** Emmit Dworak and Ethan Dworak Mystery Word Town.

Mystery Word Town integrates spelling practice and word recognition with a rich, immersive game experience. It's highly customizable, has flexible learning within three skill levels, and offers scaffolding with visual hints for more challenging words and two modes of play: listen and spell or create a word from your collected letters. Retrieved from http://artgigapps.com/apps/mystery-word-town

Create unlimited user accounts for working with multiple clients and their targeted goals and objectives (i.e., words with specific spelling patterns, commonly misspelled words, verbs, or adjectives). Two modes of play offer the ability to create your own words, spell your own words from a selected arrangement of collected letters, and listen and then spell.

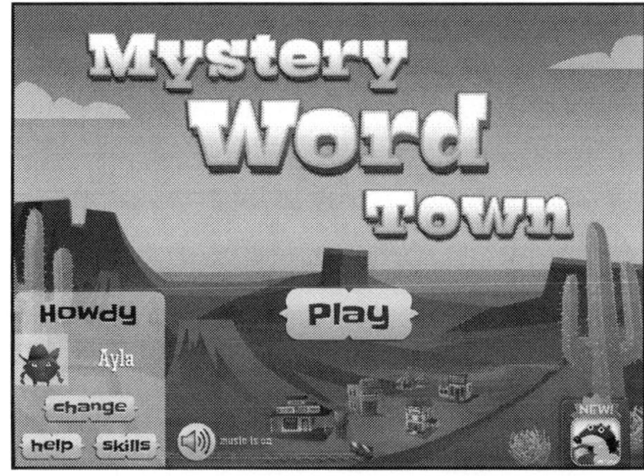


**FIGURE 7–38A.** Artgig Apps Mystery Word Town main screenshot. Reproduced with permission of Artgig Studio.

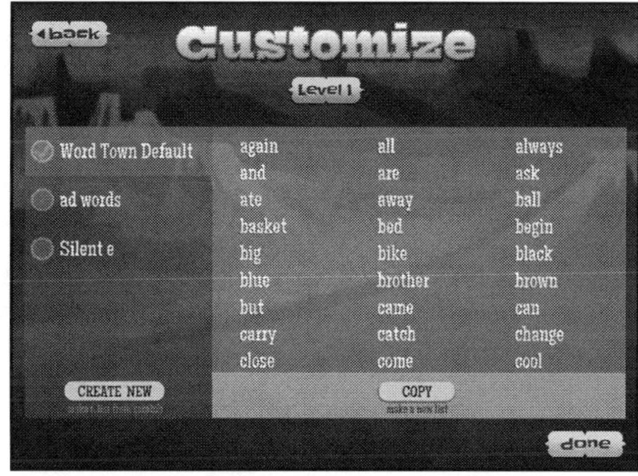


**FIGURE 7–38B.** Artgig Apps mystery word lists screenshot. Reproduced with permission of Artgig Studio.

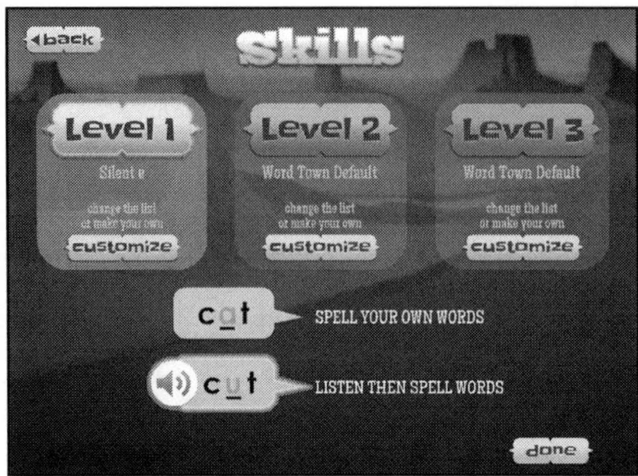


**FIGURE 7–38C.** Artgig Apps skills screenshot. Reproduced with permission of Artgig Studio.

To make for more effective and efficient therapy sessions, enter specific client data (i.e., client names, initials, or group names) and customize settings as needed prior to the therapy session.

To download Mystery Word Town, visit http://artgigapps.com

**FIGURE 7–39.** Artgig Apps QR code.

### *Individual or Small Group Session*

Step 1:  Prior to the therapy lesson, create client user name or group names and avatars, customize word lists if needed, and choose an appropriate level. Use this opportunity to create individualized lists for your clients. To keep track of word lists, name each appropriately (i.e., misspelled words, word families, new vocabulary, verbs, and adjectives). When working in small groups, consider creating a group name (i.e., vocab group) that will allow for more than one client to work on the same word list while turn taking. *NOTE:* Clients will enjoy the opportunity to customize their avatar; however, all customized word lists should be previously input.

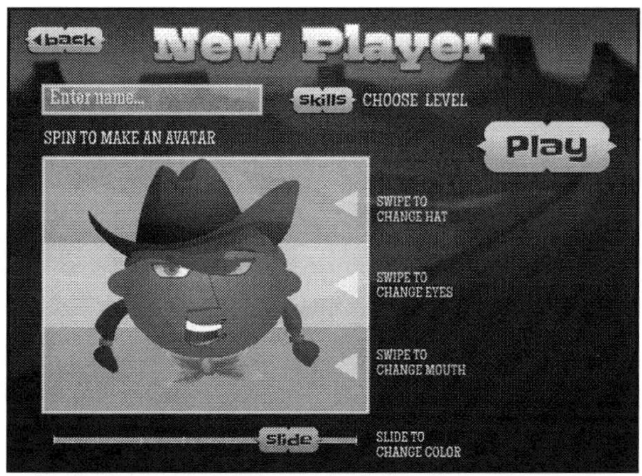


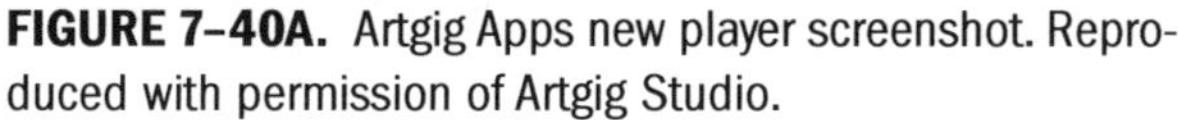

**FIGURE 7–40A.** Artgig Apps new player screenshot. Reproduced with permission of Artgig Studio.

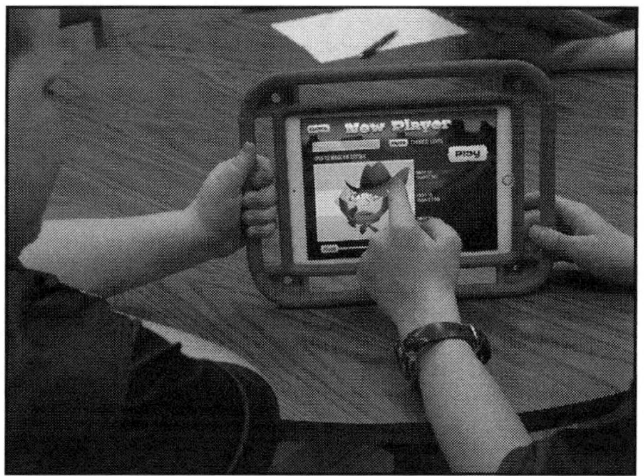

**FIGURE 7–40B.** Emmit Dworak Mystery Word Town.

Step 2: With the client sitting aside or across from you, explain that the client will be using an app during this session to help with his or her targeted goals. *NOTE:* The SLPA should take initial direction from the supervising SLP in regard to the client's ability to use this lesson and modify as needed.

Step 3: Using the "Guest" user name, model and explain how to collect letters and move about the game. There is a built-in Help option for reference, if needed.

Step 4: Choose the individual user or group user name that was previously set up to begin and tap "play."

Step 5: Tap on an unlocked building. *NOTE:* Buildings become unlocked as the client proceeds through each building. Buildings may be revisited at any time once unlocked.

Step 6: Tap on each letter to begin collecting letters and they will be added to the tool belt at the bottom of the screen. These letters will move along from room to room. Replace or trade letters by tapping the unwanted letter onto the screen and tapping the wanted letter into the tool belt at the bottom of the screen.

Step 7: Tap on any one of the exit areas (door, window, ladder, stairs) to display or hear a word to spell and identify. The ghost character will need to be dragged in and out of doors, up and down ladders, and in and out of windows. The bag shown in the upper right-hand corner in each room will show how many gold nuggets need to be collected to complete the building.

Step 8: Tap the letters in the appropriate order to finish the incomplete word and then drag the ghost character into the next room. Use this opportunity to ask the client what letters are needed or prompt as necessary. Have the client use the word in a sentence, write the word down, define the word, or spell the word aloud before moving on to the next area. *NOTE:* Critical thinking skills are used along the way; at times, a user may have to go back into a previous room to collect or trade out a needed letter need to complete the word.

Step 9: When working in small groups, let clients each have a turn to identify or define a word when moving from room to room.

Step 10: When all the gold is collected, the next building will be unlocked. Tap on the "gold nuggets." The upper right corner of the screen will display how many nuggets are still needed (i.e., 6/10) to unlock the next building.

Step 11: Track data as needed for clients (words used in a grammatically correct sentence, spelling patterns identified, etc.).

## Activity 4

Developing phonologic awareness (i.e., word families, rhyming), practicing directional tracking, reading fluency, or oral narrative with recording while using the engagement of the Explain Everything Interactive Whiteboard app.

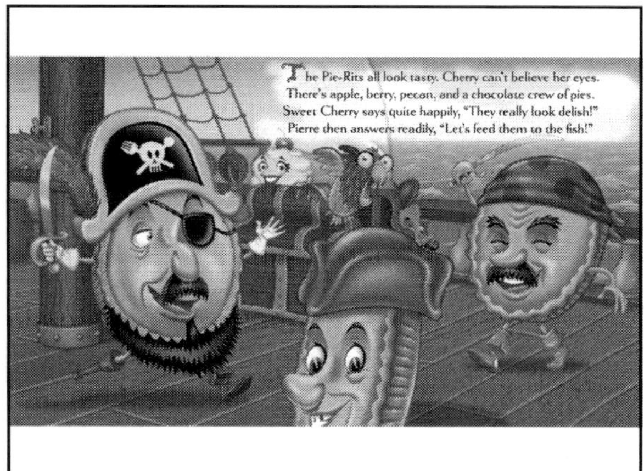


**FIGURE 7–41A.** Kite Readers Pie-Rits screenshot. Reproduced with permission of Kite Readers.

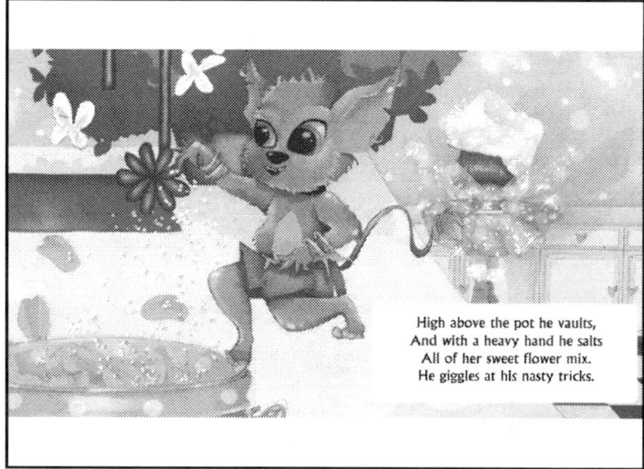


**FIGURE 7–41B.** Kite Readers Caarina the Cooking Fairy. Reproduced with permission of Kite Readers.

For purposes of this lesson, screenshots from KiteReader e-books (Pie-Rits and Caarina the Cooking Fairy, authored by Julia Dweck) will be used; however, any book app, e-book, or image from a paper book can be used by adding it to the tablet photo library.

> e-books are separate material typically contained within apps such as Kindle or iBook.

Create an interactive page of text from an e-book, book app, or paper book using Explain Everything Interactive Whiteboard by uploading images (screenshots or photos of text). This app has the ability to import multiple images and save individual recordings for each image, and it provides fun interactive engagement with built-in tools for directional tracking and annotations (i.e., laser/arrow pointers, highlighting). Explain Everything Interactive Whiteboard is a powerful tool that offers many more features; this lesson will focus on using the recording and annotation features.

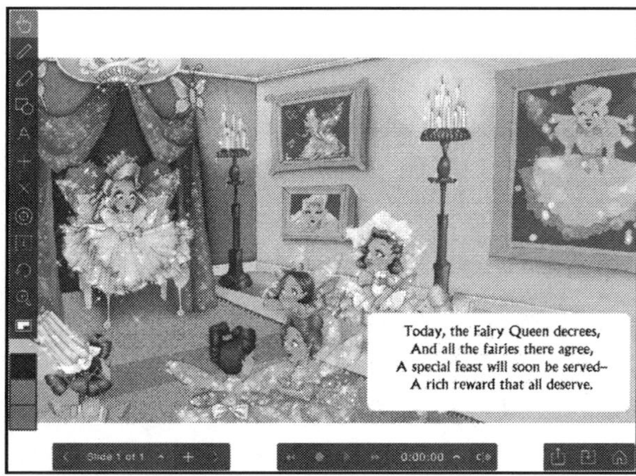



**FIGURE 7–42.** Explain Everything and Kite Reader (Caarina) screenshot. Reproduced with permission of Explain Everything and Kite Readers.

Visit http://explaineverything.com/ to download Explain Everything Interactive Whiteboard or view a comprehensive tutorial.

**FIGURE 7–43.** Explain Everything QR code.

### Individual or Small Group Session

Step 1:  Prior to the therapy session, prepare by having all images available (screenshots or e-book, book app, or clear photographs of text from a print book) in your photo library on the tablet. If using text documents saved elsewhere (i.e., Dropbox, Google drive), they also may be uploaded into the app. The focus is to have clear, readable text that is at the client's appropriate reading level or a suitable image for an oral narrative. The SLPA should take direction from the supervising SLP in choosing appropriate material that targets a specific client's goals and objectives.

a.  Open the Explain Everything Interactive Whiteboard app and tap the small document icon in the top left of the screen. *NOTE:* Backups and projects will also display on the home screen.

b. On the "New Project from File or Images" screen, tap the icon where the images or text files will be retrieved from. If using photos (already saved screenshots or photographs), tap the "Photos" icon to retrieve them. If using text that has been saved elsewhere, tap on the appropriate icon (i.e., Dropbox) to retrieve the file.

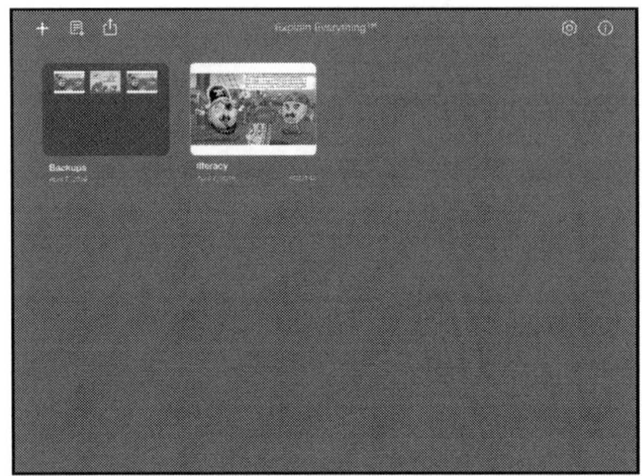

**FIGURE 7–44A.** Explain Everything home screenshot. Reproduced with permission of Explain Everything.

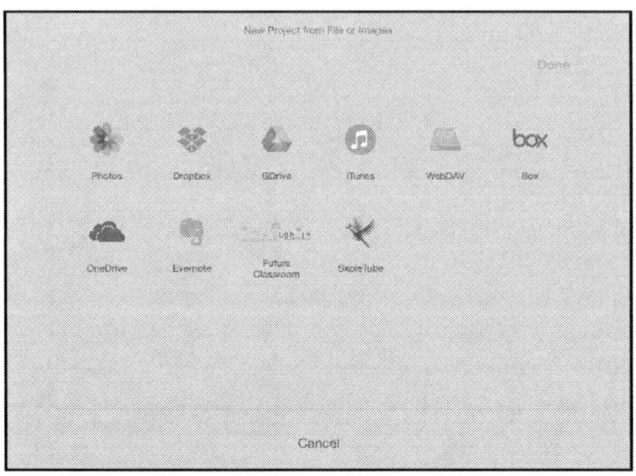

**FIGURE 7–44B.** Explain Everything new project screenshot. Reproduced with permission of Explain Everything.

c. Choose the image(s) or text files to import for the project. They will be converted into slides, and the number of slides will appear at the bottom of the screen (i.e., Slide 1 of 4). *NOTE:* It is important to consider the session type (individual or small group). For small group sessions, images should be in the order that clients will be taking turns (i.e., book app screenshot for Client 1, photograph of a page of a book for Client 2, etc.).

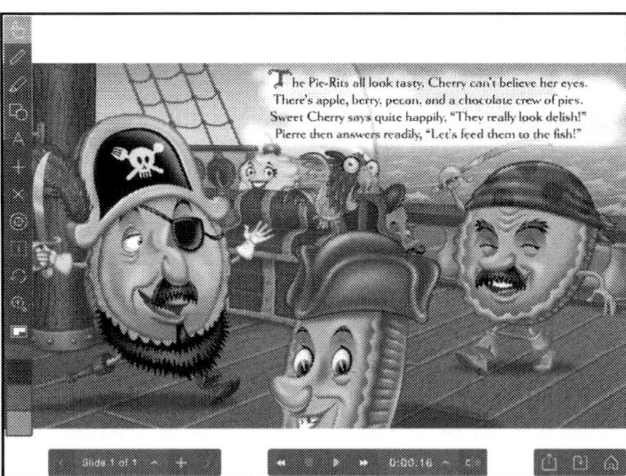


**FIGURE 7–45.** Explain Everything screenshot of imported Kite Readers (Pie-Rits) book page. Reproduced with permission of Explain Everything and Kite Readers.

d. Tap the small up arrow "^" next to the slide numbers to open the "Template change" window. Drag the images to appear in the order that the images should be presented. Tap "2X" to duplicate an image (i.e., if you would like the same image/text for more than one client or for recording text multiple times [trials] for one client and having the option to compare). Tap the small up arrow "^" to close the "Template change" window.

e. Tap the "Home" icon in the bottom right of the screen to title and save the project. The project is now saved to use during a therapy session time.

Step 2:  With the client sitting aside or across from you, explain that the client will be using an app during this session to help with his or her targeted goals. *NOTE:* The SLPA should take initial direction from the supervising SLP in regard to the client's ability to use this lesson and modify as needed.

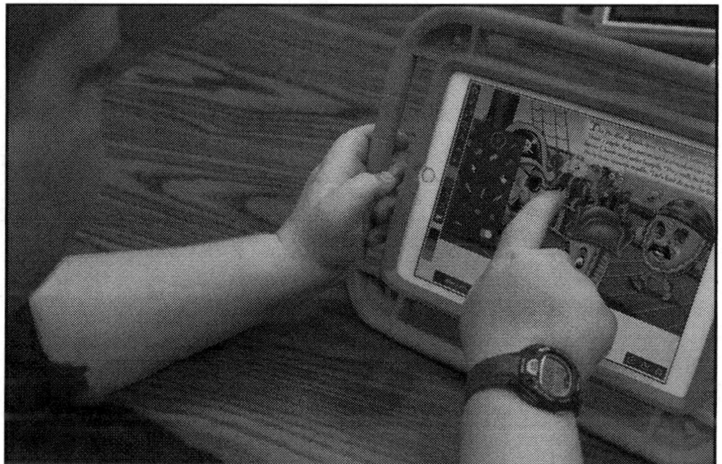

**FIGURE 7–46.** Emmit Dworak Explain Everything.

Step 3:  Open the Explain Everything Interactive Whiteboard app and select the appropriate project for the therapy session.

Step 4:  Target client goals and objectives: phonologic awareness, directional tracking, reading fluency, or oral narrative (using an image without text).

a. To record a client reading the text or providing an oral narrative for an image, tap the "red record dot" to begin. Tap the "red record dot" a second time to end the recording. The recording will be saved to review immediately or at a later time. To record over a recording, hold the "back arrow" to bring the time to 0:00 and tap the "Overwrite" arrow. Use this opportunity for client self-monitoring if appropriate. When working in small groups, a client may independently be using the project to record while you are working with other clients on different activities.

b. To add an interactive reading experience for directional tracking to the recording, tap the the "target" icon to open the "tracking tools," choose a "tracking tool," and turn the "Offset" to on. Take this opportunity to experiment with what works best to engage the client (i.e., laser point, saber, arrow). The recording will also "screencast" and the client's "tracking tool" use will be recorded along with the narration. This is very helpful for using popular interactive book apps where "directional finger tracking" causes the built-in interactivity to be activated (i.e., tapping or touching activates a hot spot within the book app). Observe and take note how the client is simultaneously tracking and reading.

c. To provide an interactive experience for building literacy skills, tap the "pencil" or "highlighter" icon. Choose one of the colors by tapping the color blocks at the left side of the screen. This can be helpful and allows for text from a print book to be highlighted/underlined/circled.

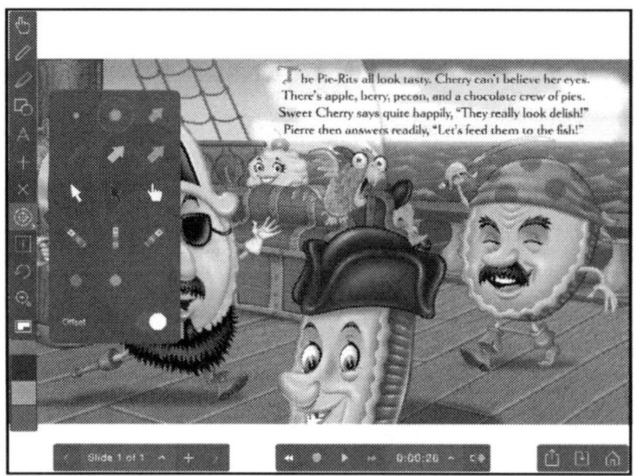


**FIGURE 7–47A.** Explain Everything tool window screenshot of imported Kite Readers (Pie-Rits). Reproduced with permission of Explain Everything and Kite Readers.

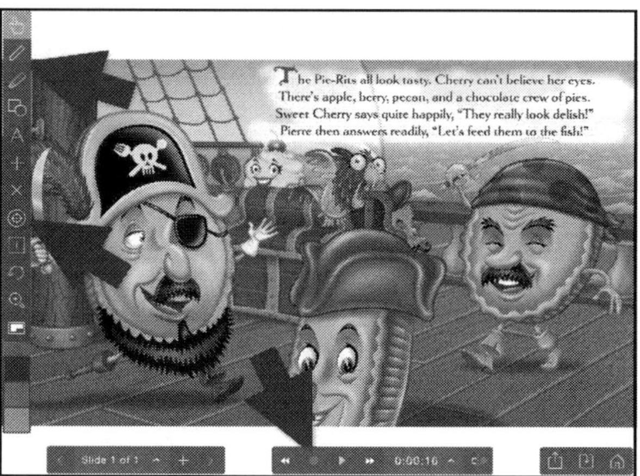


**FIGURE 7–47B.** Explain Everything pencil highlight screenshot with imported Kite Readers (Pie-Rits). Reproduced with permission of Explain Everything and Kite Readers.

Step 5: Record data as needed in the client file.

> Consider modifying this activity to use with clients targeting articulation or voice/fluency. In addition, recordings and screencasts can be shared with supervising SLPs (i.e., via e-mail).

## Activity 5

Targeting phonologic awareness for pre-K through third grade using the TPT product Summer Fun with Phonological Awareness by The Reading Speechie.

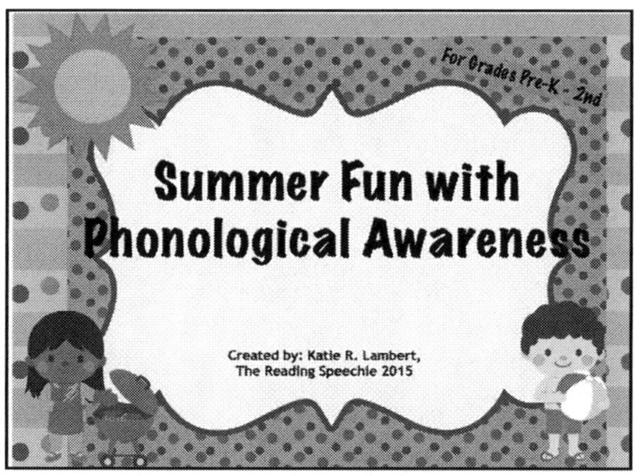


**FIGURE 7–48A.** Katie Lambert Reading Speechie Summer Fun title screenshot. Reproduced with permission of The Reading Speechie.

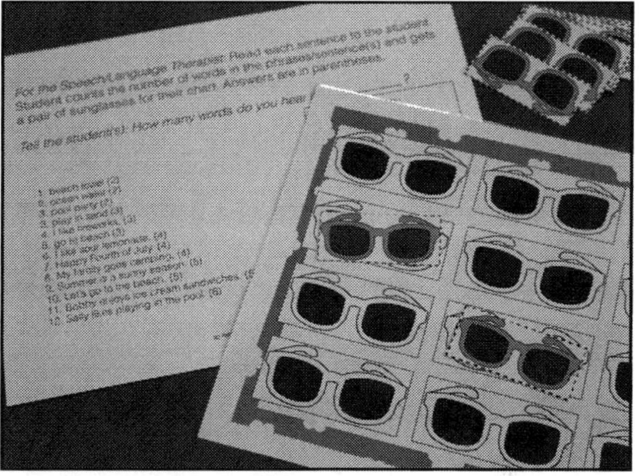

**FIGURE 7–48B.** Katie Lambert Reading Speechie Summer Fun example screenshot. Reproduced with permission of The Reading Speechie.

This TPT product focuses on listening skills, including following directions and phonologic awareness (sentence segmenting, syllable segmenting, sound segmenting, and rhyming).

To download Summer Fun with Phonological Awareness, visit https://www.teacherspayteachers.com/Product/Summer-Fun-with-Phonological-Awareness-1988273

**FIGURE 7–49.** Reading Speechie QR code.

It is suggested that this activity be printed on cardstock and laminated for durability prior to session time.

### Individual or Small Group Session

Step 1:  Select the appropriate level to begin for each client. *NOTE:* The SLPA should take initial direction from the supervising SLP in regard to the client's ability and targeted objectives.

Step 2:  With the client sitting aside or across from you, explain the directions as written on each activity page.

Step 3:  It may be necessary to use manipulatives such as blocks, counters, and so on to represent the words, syllables, or sounds as a support for the client with the segmenting task.

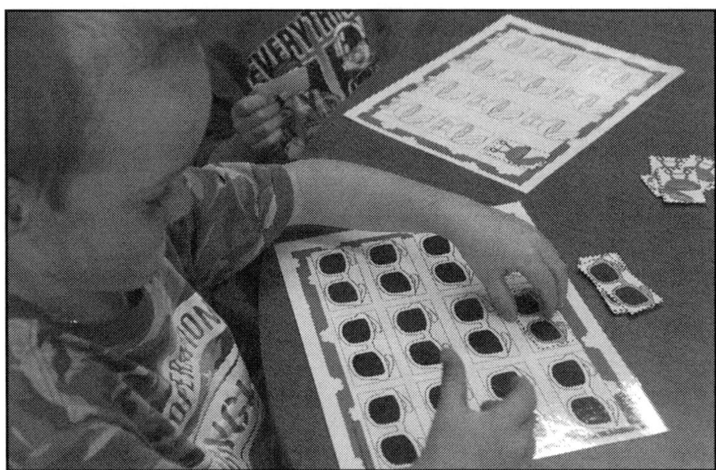

**FIGURE 7–50.** Jason and Dillon Allen segmenting match.

## Activity 6

Targeting word families for kindergarten through third grade using the TPT product Mugz 'N Mallows by the Reading Speechie.

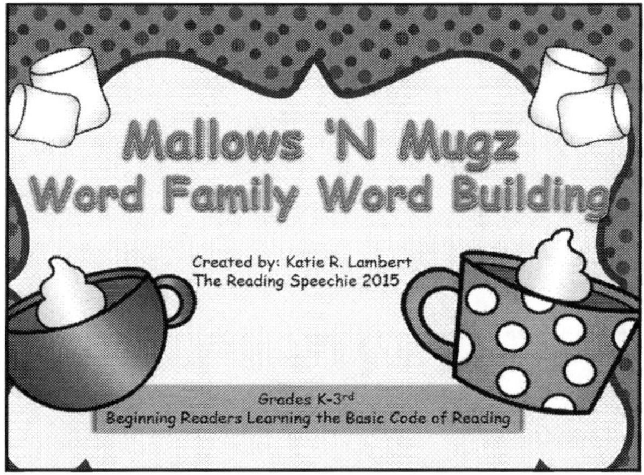


**FIGURE 7–51.** Katie Lambert Reading Speeching Mugz 'N Mallows title screenshot. Reproduced with permission of The Reading Speechie.

This product focuses on generating words containing word families by adding the onset (marshmallow) to the word family (mug), reading the word and locating the picture matching the word. In addition, vocabulary skills are increased.

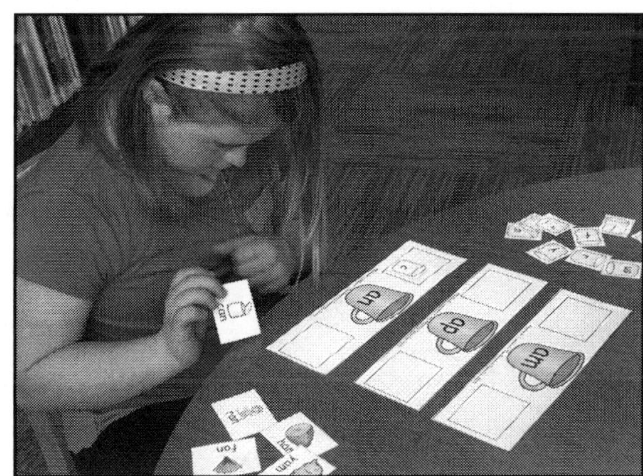

**FIGURE 7–52A.** Elizabeth Giese Mugz 'N Mallows.

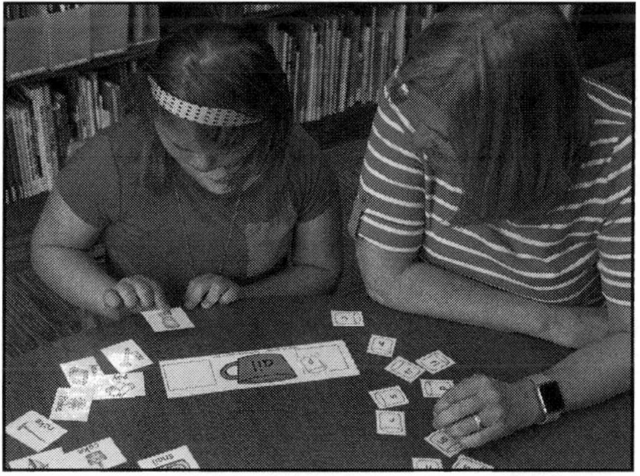

**FIGURE 7–52B.** Elizabeth Giese Mugz 'N Mallows.

To download Mugz 'N Mallows, visit https://www.teacherspayteachers.com/Product/Mugz-N-Mallows-2273809

**FIGURE 7–53.** Reading Speechie QR code.

It is suggested that this activity be printed on cardstock and laminated for durability prior to session time.

### *Individual or Small Group Session*

Step 1: With the client sitting aside or across from you, explain that he or she will be building words and then finding the picture that goes with the word that was built.

Step 2: Scatter the marshmallows out on the table along with the pictures; be sure to keep the letters and pictures on separate side of the workspace.

Step 3: Pass out a mug to each client and have the client start building words and finding matching pictures. Use this opportunity to specify a word or have the clients explore and create their own. *NOTE:* Be aware of the client's skill level and provide prompts, if needed.

## Activity 7

Identifying events with literature and information text using Story Telling is a Hoot by the Reading Speechie for kindergarten through third grade.

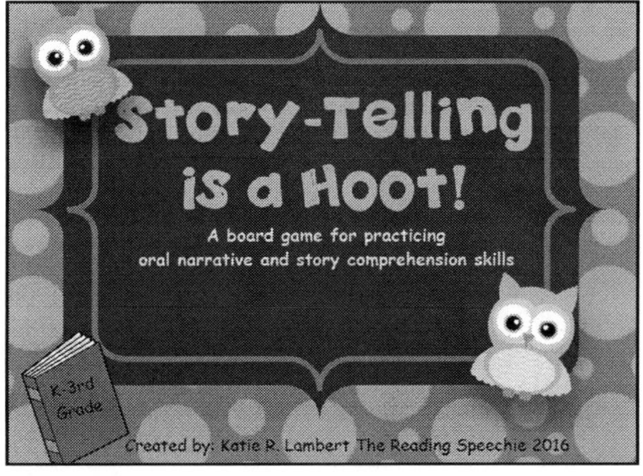


**FIGURE 7–54A.** Katie Lambert Reading Speechie Hoot title screenshot. Reproduced with permission of The Reading Speechie.

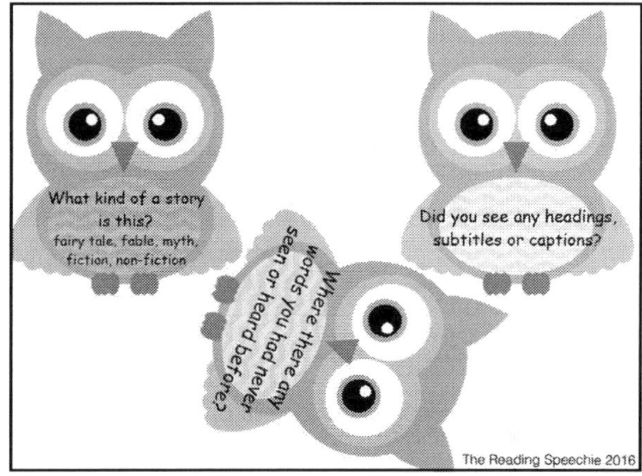


**FIGURE 7–54B.** Katie Lambert Reading Speechie sample owls screenshot. Reproduced with permission of The Reading Speechie.

This activity is a board game that aids in practice for oral narrative and story comprehension skills aligned with Common Core Standards for reading literature. Any storybook can be used with this game.

To download Story Telling is a Hoot, visit https://www.teacherspayteachers.com/Product/Story-Telling-is-a-Hoot-2350434

**FIGURE 7–55.** Reading Speechie QR code.

It is suggested that this activity be printed on cardstock and laminated for durability prior to session time.

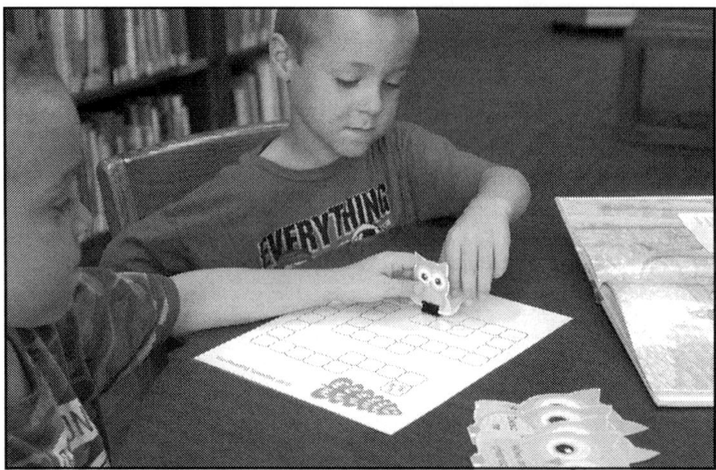

**FIGURE 7–56.** Jason and Dillon Allen hoot.

### *Individual or Small Group Session*

Step 1: Read the story first and explore the story and language presented within the story. *NOTE:* Any story or classroom curriculum can be used for this activity.

Step 2: With the client sitting aside or across from you, explain that he or she will play a game while answering questions about the story you just read together.

Step 3: Lay out the board game in the middle of the table and let the client choose his or her owl marker. Use a paper clip to provide a stand for the owl markers.

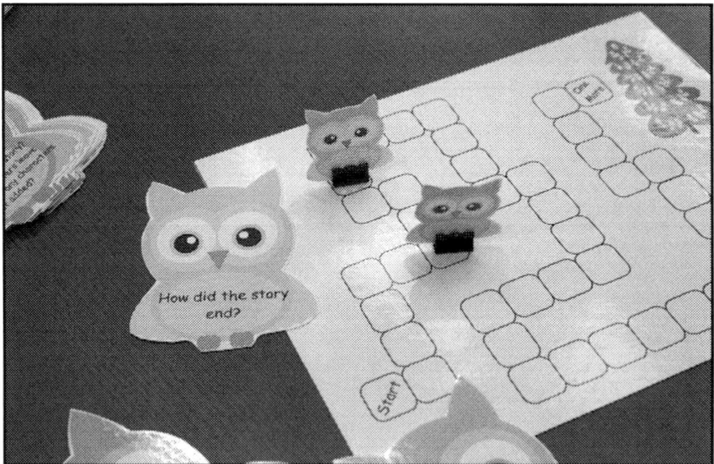


**FIGURE 7–57.** Owl clip game.

Step 4: Each client rolls a die, moves the marker that number of spaces, and then answers a question from the deck of cards. *NOTE:* Keep in mind that clients are not penalized for incorrect answers. Instead, validate the answer given and then guide toward the correct answer. The game is over when the owls reach the end of the game board.

Step 5: Take client data as needed.

## REFERENCE

Paul, R., & Norbury, C. (2012). *Language disorders from infancy through adolescence.* St. Louis, MO: Elsevier Mosby.

# 8

# Voice and Fluency Disorders

A voice disorder is described by the abnormal production of vocal pitch, loudness, quality, resonance, and/or duration that is likely improper for an individual's sex or age. In the general population, the prevalence is estimated to be from 3 to 10% (Stemple, 2014). An abnormally functioning larynx is due to functional, structural, and/or neurologic origins causing the distortions we hear in speech (Stemple, 2014). The voice may sound hoarse, breathy, bumpy (glottal fry), whispered (aphonia), abnormally high (falsetto voice), or like there are two pitches (diplophonia). A few types of voice disorders are primary muscle dysphonia, vocal cord nodules, and vocal cord paralysis (Stemple, 2014). It is recommended that a voice client be seen by an otolaryngologist (ENT) prior to speech therapy to rule out a life-threatening pathology and to ensure speech therapy is the correct course of action.

A fluency disorder (or, stuttering) is often characterized by primary (speech) and secondary (concomitant) behaviors. Primary behaviors typically include repetitions of sounds, syllables, whole words, prolongation of single sounds, blocks of airflow, and voicing during speech. Secondary behaviors consist of negative reactions, physical tension in the body, avoidance tactics, and body movements. Some examples of secondary behaviors include frequent eye blinks, facial grimaces, circumlocution, tensing of muscles, and avoiding situations related to stuttering. Fluency disorders can have a negative impact on communication beyond transmitting a message. It can be the reason a person restricts his or her participation in certain situations (American Speech-Language-Hearing Association [ASHA], 2016).

The activities included in this chapter will help you address voice and fluency disorders your may come across in your caseload. Among the nine activities presented in this chapter, only one (Activity 5) addresses voice. This is due to the fact that speech-language pathologists (SLPs) commonly work with voice clients who are under an ENT's care. School-aged children with voice problems (hoarseness) due to abuse (yelling!) often participate in a vocal hygiene program developed by the SLP. The app in Activity 5 will enable you to work with these children and help them use appropriate voicing.

As you become familiar with these activities, you will begin to gain confidence working with clients with voice and fluency disorders and, under the guidance of your supervising SLP, can develop your own therapy materials to fit the therapy goals established by the SLP.

## ACTIVITIES FOR VOICE AND FLUENCY

### Objectives

The following are some sample objectives for voice therapy:

1. Client will identify abnormal vocal quality in three-syllable words during 9 of 10 opportunities when describing pictures across three consecutive data collection points.

2. Client will identify abnormal vocal quality in phrases during 9 of 10 opportunities when describing pictures opportunities across three consecutive data collection points.

3. Client will identify abnormal vocal quality in sentences during 9 of 10 opportunities when describing social picture scenes across three consecutive data collection points.

The following are some sample objectives for fluency therapy:

1. Client will use easy onset and vowel prolongation in unison with the SLPA to facilitate fluent speech during 9 of 10 opportunities across three consecutive data collection points.

2. Client will use easy onset and vowel prolongation after a model of the word, phrase, or sentence to facilitate fluent speech during 9 of 10 opportunities across three consecutive data collection points.

3. Client will use easy onset and vowel prolongation in response to questions from the SLPA to facilitate fluent speech during 9 of 10 opportunities across three consecutive data collection points.

## Activity 1

Speech Pacesetter app by Aptus Speech and Language Therapy for all ages working on pacing based on client reading ability.

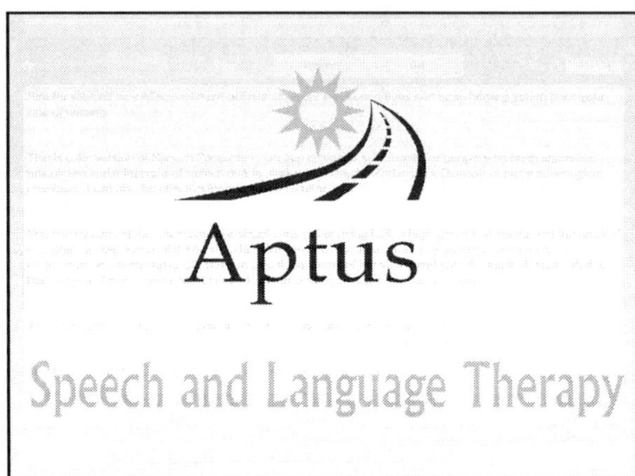


**FIGURE 8–1.** Aptus Speech Language screenshot. Reproduced with permission of Aptus Speech & Language Therapy.

For the purposes of this lesson, we will only be using the "Pasteboard" tab within the app. It is designed specifically for those who have imprecise articulation and a fast rate of speech. The client uses a visual cue of a bouncing ball, a highlighted text cursor, or the gradual appearance of the text to pace his or her reading rate. The Pasteboard feature allows readers of all ages the ability to customize reading levels and choose high-interest topics. The users simply copy the text of their choice and paste it on the Speech Pacesetter screen, with the option to save their stories to the app. Additionally, Speech Pacesetter has a number of stories to choose from, including phonemically balanced texts and Aesop's fables. The app also has the option of adding a metronome sound cue.

To download Speech Pacesetter or the free Speech Pacesetter Lite by Aptus Speech & Language Therapy, visit http://www.aptus-slt.com

**FIGURE 8–2.** Aptus SLT QR code.

To make for more effective and efficient therapy sessions, paste the reading content on the Pasteboard prior to the therapy session.

### *Task Setup*

Step 1:  Retrieve a reading selection from an appropriate Internet site, select one of your own saved stories, or create your own text in a separate document. If you are working with a younger client, you will need to choose the text. Older clients may prefer to choose text that interests them. Keep in mind the topic should be appropriate in nature.

> Skill level may be chosen by using functional words, phrases, questions ("How are you?" "My brother's name is Carl." "I need my book."), or leveled reading passages. If you are using reading passages, we recommend those of high interest and of the client's choosing. The use of text below clients' reading level is recommend to ensure you are not penalizing clients due to poor reading skills. The purpose of this lesson is to focus on speech fluency, not reading fluency.

Step 2:  Open the Speech Pacesetter app and proceed. To view built-in instructions, tap on the "Info" at the bottom of the screen. *NOTE:* The SLPA should take initial direction from the supervising SLP in regard to the client's receptive and expressive language skills, reading level, reading speed, frequency of pausing, length of the pause, and other options on the app. The SLP will have determined therapy goals and settings based on the results of a complete fluency evaluation.

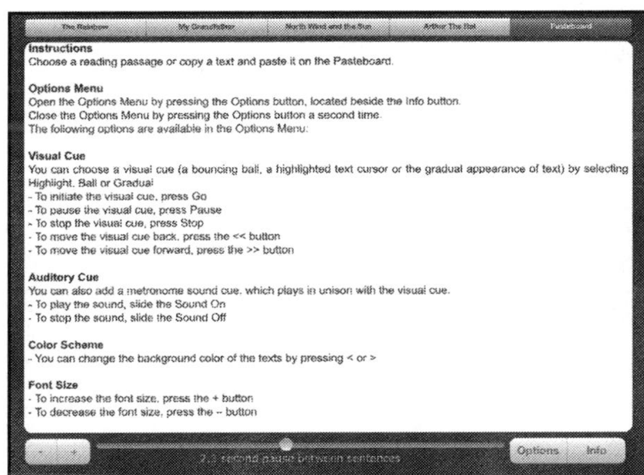

**FIGURE 8–3A.** Pacesetter Instruction screenshot. Reproduced with permission of Aptus Speech & Language Therapy.

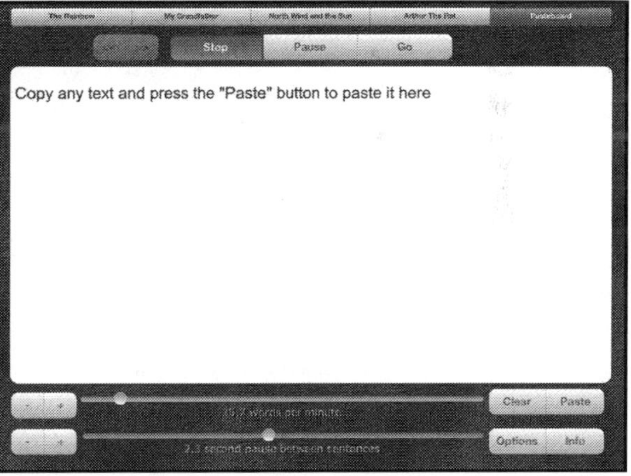

**FIGURE 8–3B.** Pacesetter add text screenshot. Reproduced with permission of Aptus Speech & Language Therapy.



a.  Paste a reading selection into Pasteboard, select one of your own saved stories, or choose from a list of provided stories.

b.  Slide the top slider bar by moving your finger left to right. This sets the words per minute. Choose the setting based on client objectives. If your goal is a slower speech rate, set it at 30 words per minute.

c.  Set the bottom slider bar by moving your finger left to right. The app provides the option of setting pauses from 1 to 5 seconds after each period. For client comfort, it is recommended to set the delay to the maximum of 5 seconds.

d.  Select "Option" to adjust font size and background colors to accommodate your clients' comfort level. Font sizes range from 14 to 40 with a variety of combinations of text and background colors.

e.  The "Option" setting in Speech Pacesetter offers a visual cue of "Highlight," "Ball," or "Gradual." For the purposes of this activity, select "Ball."

f.  Set the option to "Sound Off."

> Consider using a language hierarchy, along with functional vocabulary and frequently used sentences, to develop treatment materials. If your client is preparing a class presentation or reading an interesting book, use these items to create meaningful therapy materials combined with the Pacesetter app.

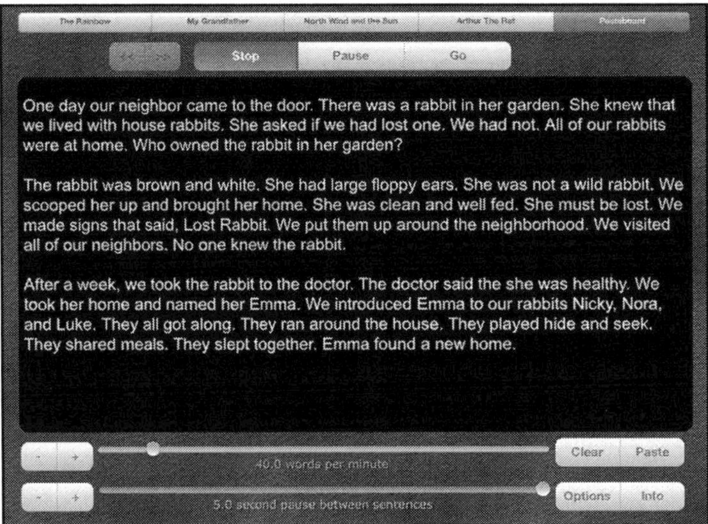



**FIGURE 8–4.** Pacesetter reading selection screenshot. Reproduced with permission of Aptus Speech & Language Therapy.

### *Individual or Group Session*

Step 1:  With the client sitting across from you and the app displaying the reading selection in front of him or her, model the first word, phrase, or sentence. *NOTE:* Setup should have occurred prior to the session. Refer to task setup above.

Step 2:  Ask your client to read the same text in unison with you.

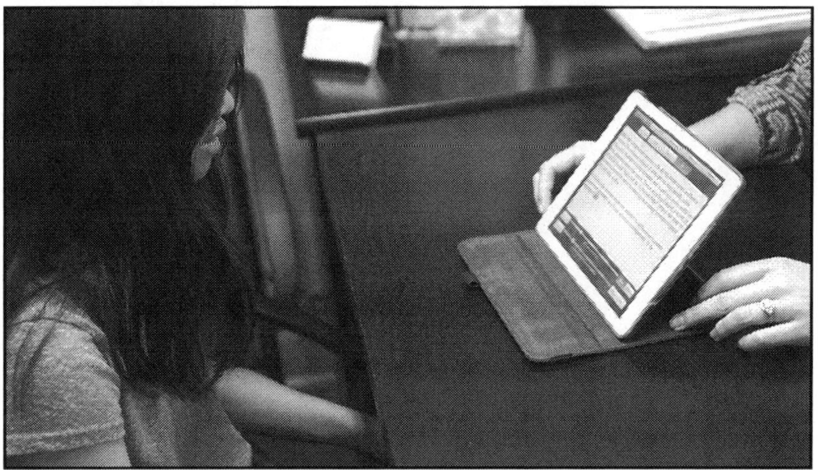

**FIGURE 8–5.** Mae Bissell Pacesetter Granite Bay Speech.

Step 3:  Ask your client to read the word, phrase, or sentence independently only after you have modeled it for him or her and read it in unison. Confirm that the client understands the task. If not, repeat Steps 1 and 2 until he or she is comfortable reading independently.

Step 4:  Practice reading with the Pacesetter app. After each word, phrase, or sentence, tally a plus if it's fluent and a minus if it's not. Calculate the percentage of accuracy and then consult with the supervising SLP to determine next objective. *NOTE:* After your client demonstrates independent reading skills, read each selection only once during a session due to the adaptation effect. It has been noted that most individuals who stutter become more fluent during repeated oral readings of the same material. This adaptation effect may reflect motor learning associated with repeated practice of speech motor sequences (Max & Baldwin, 2010). Max and Baldwin (2010) also suggest that new reading material be introduced during each practice session in order to ensure your clients are improving their fluency skills rather than becoming fluent only on a designated passage.

## Activity 2

Conversation PaceBoard app by Aptus Speech and Language Therapy for all ages working on pacing.

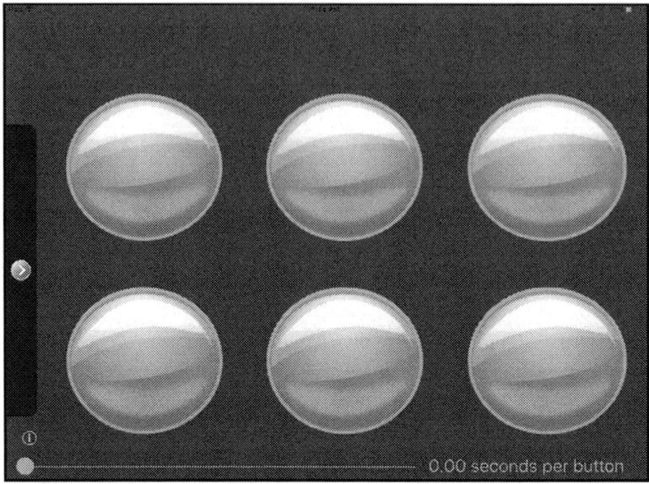


**FIGURE 8–6.** Conversation Paceboard Screenshot. Reproduced with permission of Aptus Speech & Language Therapy.

Conversation Paceboard is designed to help clients with imprecise articulation and a fast speaking rate. It is designed to help them pace their speech and improve their intelligibility during conversation. The visual cues make it a modern pacing board with a motivating difference. The Conversation Paceboard app was originally designed for pacing conversation; however, for the purposes of this activity, we will use it for pacing, vowel prolongation, and fluency.

To download Conversation PaceBoard by Aptus Speech & Language Therapy, visit http://aptus-slt.com

**FIGURE 8–7.** Aptus SLT QR code.

### *Task Setup*

Step 1:  Set the slider bar by moving your finger left to right until it is at the maximum 1.50 seconds per button.

Step 2:  Select objects, words, phrases, and short sentences. For the younger client, objects may be selected from the natural environment, such as toy animals, balls, or food items. The selection of words, phrases, and sentences may be drawn from daily functional language. Conversation Paceboard provides additional conversation topics by pressing the arrow > on the left side of the screen. Scroll through the topics by selecting the < and > buttons.

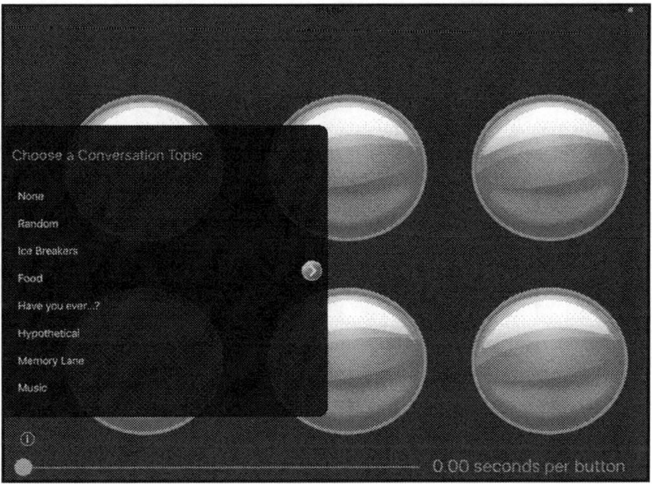


**FIGURE 8–8.** Conversation Paceboard screenshot conversation tab. Reproduced with permission of Aptus Speech & Language Therapy.

### *Individual or Group Session*

Step 1:  For each of the following activities, the clients should hold down the button for the length of time they produce each word, phrase, or sentence. Hold down the button until it fills completely with color and a check mark appears. If the user moves to the next circle too quickly, "Too Quick!" will be displayed. *NOTE:* The SLPA should take initial direction from the supervising SLP in regard to the client's receptive and expressive language skills, reading level, reading speed, frequency of pausing, length of the pause, and other options on the app. The SLP will have determined therapy goals and settings based on the results of a complete fluency evaluation.

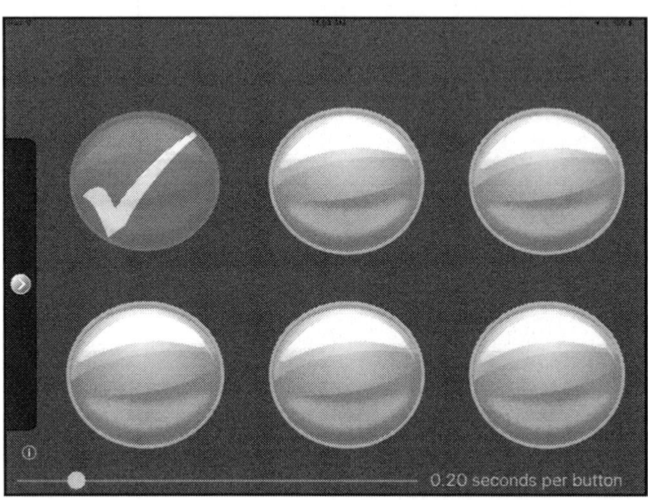


**FIGURE 8–9A.** Conversation paceboard screenshot check mark. Reproduced with permission of Aptus Speech & Language Therapy.

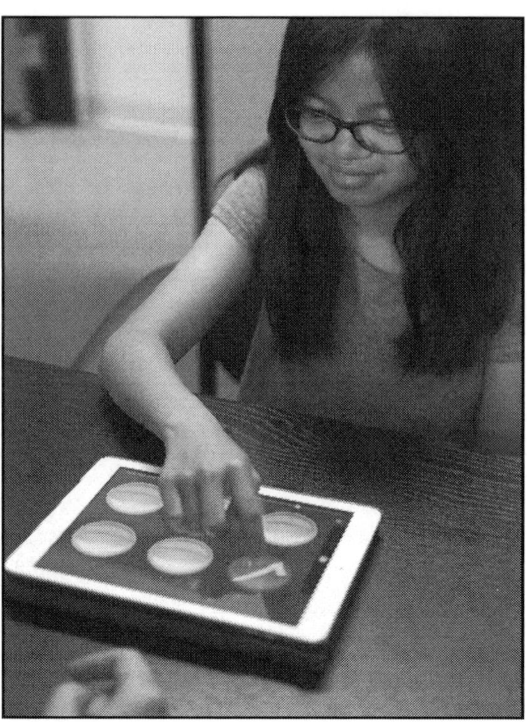

**FIGURE 8–9B.** Mae Bissell Conversation Paceboard GBS.

a. With the client sitting across from you and the app displaying the buttons, model the word, phrase, or sentence.

b. Ask the client to say the selection in unison with you.

c. Instruct the client to repeat the selection independently.

## Activity 3

Fluency shaping, desensitization, and modifying stuttering techniques using Fluency SIS (Smart Intervention Strategy) app for school-age clients.

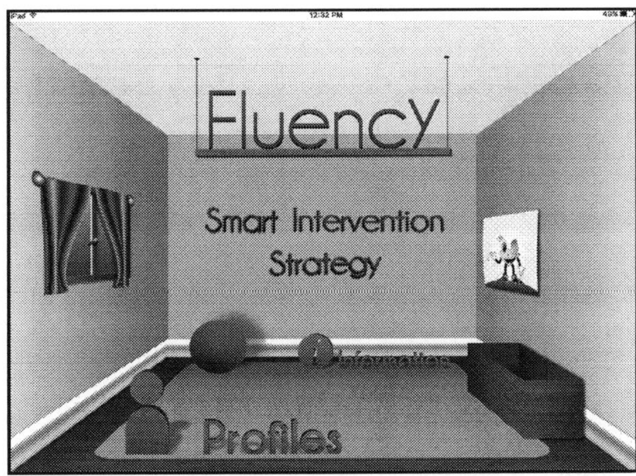


**FIGURE 8–10.** Fluency SIS main screenshot. Reproduced with permission of Joseph Agius. (2013) *Fluency Smart Intervention Strategy*. Developer: Vioside, Malta.

Fluency SIS by Joseph Agius is designed for clients between the ages of 8 and 12, but it may be modified for younger and older clients. There are four activity areas within the Smart Intervention Strategy (SIS). They include:

- Think Smart, Feel Smart using creativity and humor to create a positive attitude toward communication and self

- Cool Speech for fluency shaping, modifying stuttering techniques, and strategies for public speaking skills

- Challenge the Dragons, which identifies feared speaking situations and includes desensitization exercises

- Into the Real World, which supports carryover of skills at home, at school, and in the community

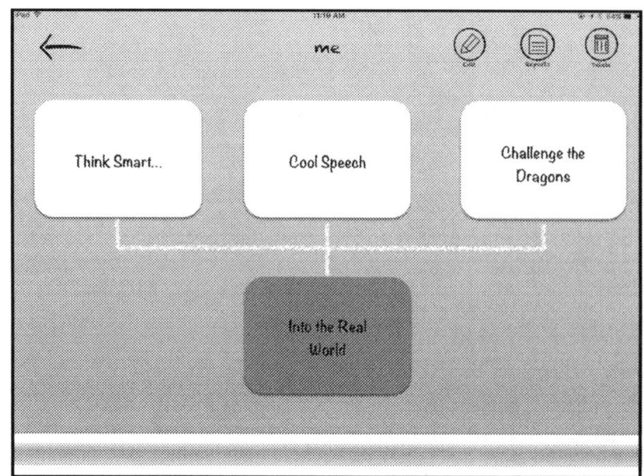


**FIGURE 8–11A.** Fluency SIS four activity areas screenshot. Reproduced with permission of Joseph Agius. (2013) *Fluency Smart Intervention Strategy*. Developer: Vioside, Malta.

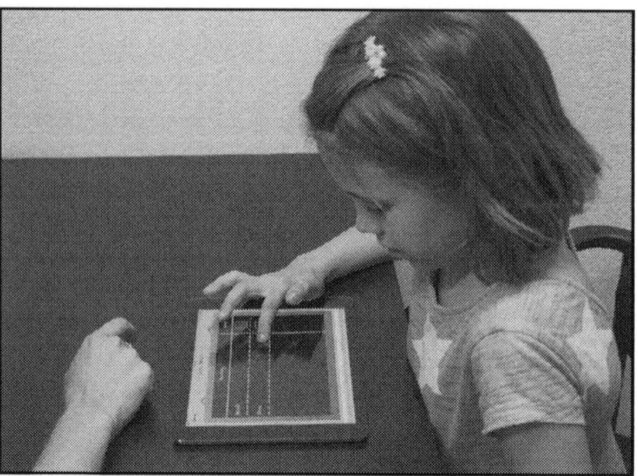

**FIGURE 8–11B.** Payton Ruddy Fluency SIS.

To download the Fluency Smart Intervention Strategy app, visit https://itunes.apple.com/us/app/fluency-sis/id629966836?mt=8

**FIGURE 8–12.** Fluency SIS QR code.

For efficient and effective sessions, create client profiles prior to therapy session.

### *Individual or Small Group Session*

Step 1:  With the client sitting next to or across from you, explain that you will be using the Fluency SIS app to help guide him or her through exercises to work on fluency strategies.

Step 2:  Choose any of the three activity areas (Think Smart/Feel Smart, Cool Speech, or Challenge the Dragons) to reveal a list of suggested exercises. Once your client has completed all the objectives within the first three activities, the "Into the Real World" activity option will be unlocked. *NOTE:* The SLPA should take initial direction from the supervising SLP in regard to client goals.

a.  Think Smart, Feel Smart will display a blackboard with six exercises for using creativity and humor: Shifting Perceptions, Word Play, Exaggeration, Playful Incongruity, Self-Deprecation, and Duchenne Smile.

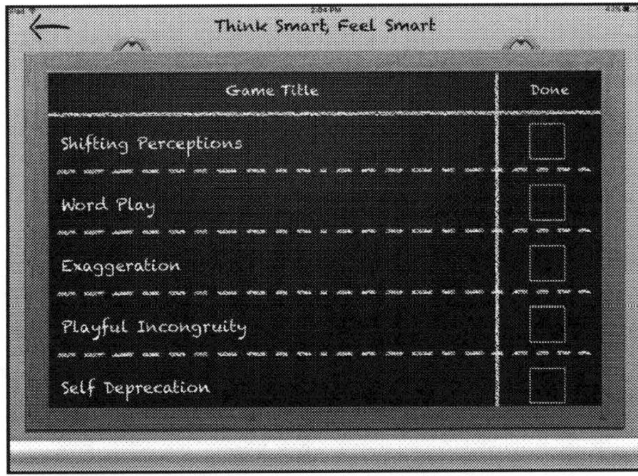


**FIGURE 8–13.** Fluency SIS Think Smart screenshot. Reproduced with permission of Joseph Agius. (2013) *Fluency Smart Intervention Strategy*. Developer: Vioside, Malta.

b.  Cool Speech will display three game areas for fluency shaping and modifying stuttering techniques as well as speaking opportunities: Practice, Reading, and Presenting.

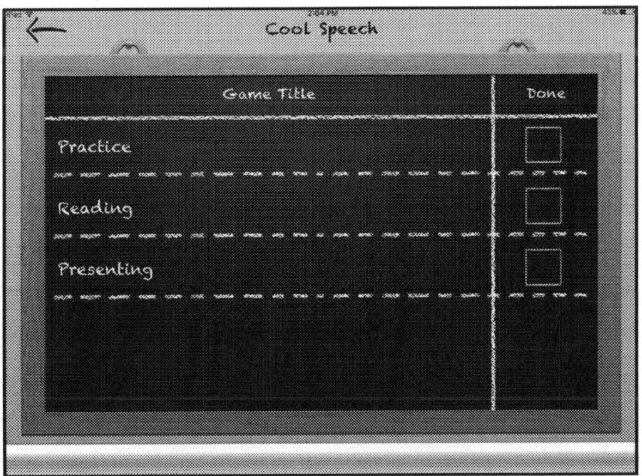


**FIGURE 8–14.** Fluency SIS Cool Speech screenshot. Reproduced with permission of Joseph Agius. (2013) *Fluency Smart Intervention Strategy*. Developer: Vioside, Malta.

c. Challenge the Dragons will display three game areas for desensitization exercises: Phoning, Un-secret Your Secret, and Buying. *NOTE:* Systematic desensitization is a type of behavioral therapy based on the principle of classical conditioning. This therapy aims to remove the fear response gradually by way of counterconditioning (McLeod, 2008). The client creates a hierarchy of triggers for stuttering, starting with the least active triggers at the bottom of the hierarchy and the most active triggers at the top of the hierarchy. The client works in a bottom-up approach in order to desensitize his or her response to stuttering triggers.

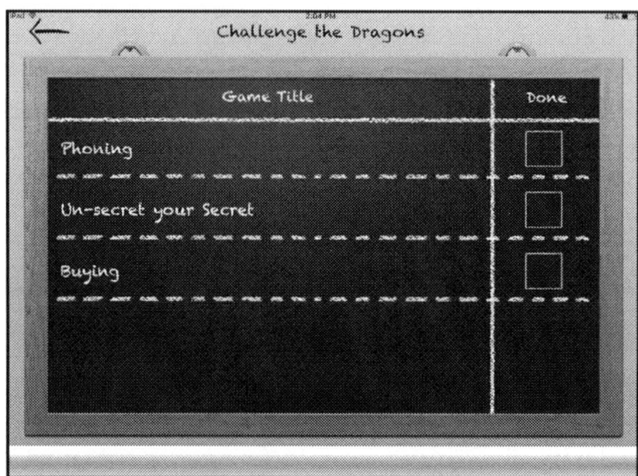


**FIGURE 8–15.** Fluency SIS Challenge of Dragons screenshot. Reproduced with permission of Joseph Agius. (2013) *Fluency Smart Intervention Strategy*. Developer: Vioside, Malta.

d. Upon completing all activity areas, Into the Real World will be unlocked for generalizing techniques at home, at school, and in the community.

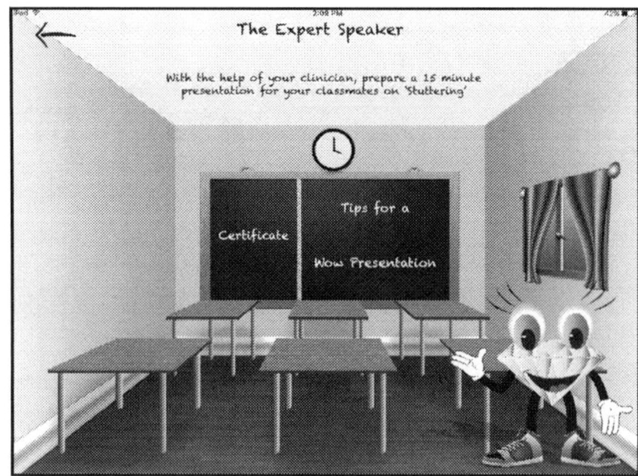


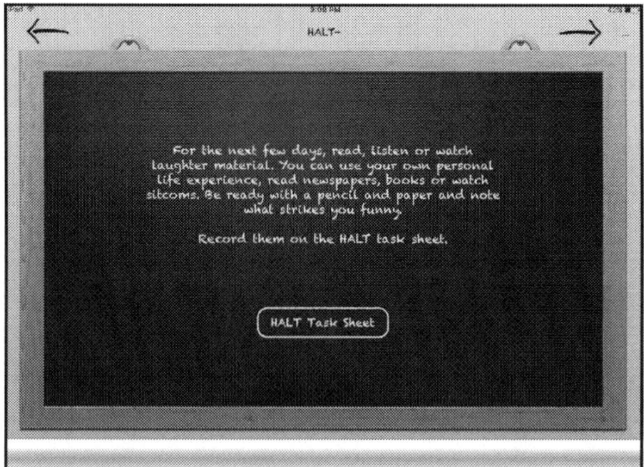


**FIGURE 8–16A.** Fluency SIS WOW presentation screenshot. Reproduced with permission of Joseph Agius. (2013) *Fluency Smart Intervention Strategy*. Developer: Vioside, Malta.

**FIGURE 8–16B.** Fluency SIS HALT screenshot. Reproduced with permission of Joseph Agius. (2013) *Fluency Smart Intervention Strategy*. Developer: Vioside, Malta.

Step 3:  Record data as needed for the client file. Data will be saved to client profiles as exercises are completed and can be printed.

## Activity 4

Syllables Splash app by Smarty Ears for all school-age clients working on easy onset and vowel prolongation.

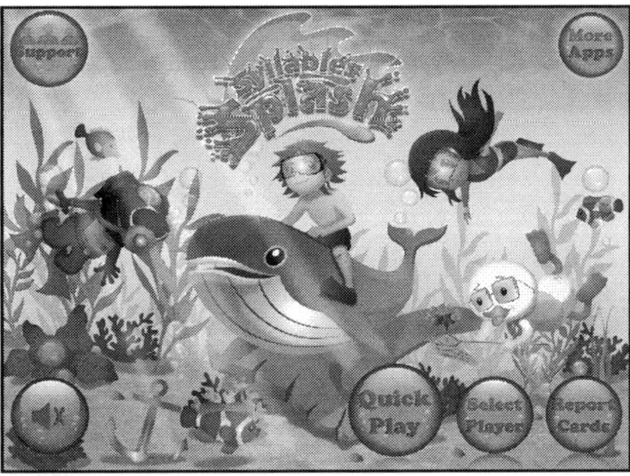

**FIGURE 8–17.** Syllables Splash main screenshot. Reproduced with permission of Smarty Ears, LLC. All rights reserved.

The Syllables Splash app is an engaging way to teach syllable segmentation, as well as easy onset, vowel prolongation, and phrasing. It supports literacy skills and phonologic awareness.

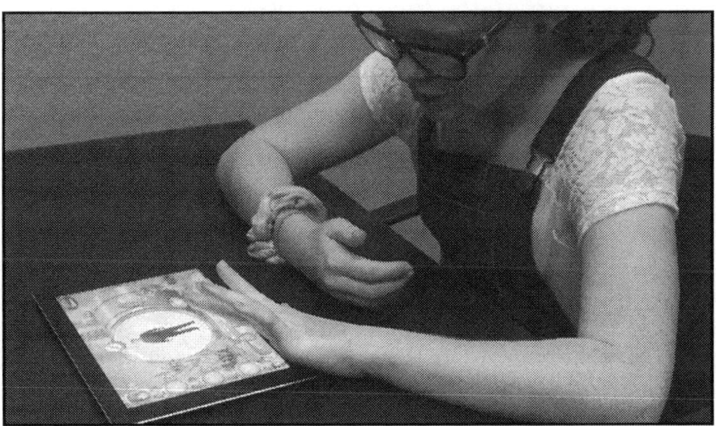

**FIGURE 8–18.** Cameron Tarr Syllables Splash photo.

To download the Syllables Splash by Smarty Ears, visit http://smartyearsapps.com

**FIGURE 8–19.** Smarty Ears QR code.

To create a more efficient and effective therapy session, set up your client and settings prior to therapy sessions.

### Task Setup

Step 1: After opening the app, tap on "Select player."

Step 2: Tap on "Add a Player." Type in the client's name and tap "Done."

Step 3: Tap on the client's name and tap on "Settings."

    a. Set eliminate or buzz settings when the wrong answer is selected.

    b. Set number of wrong options (1, 2, or 3).

    c. Set to automatically increase level if successful (yes/no).

    d. Set syllable length (1, 2, 3, or 4). Increase to more syllables when the client improves.

    e. Set fish and shark animations (yes/no).

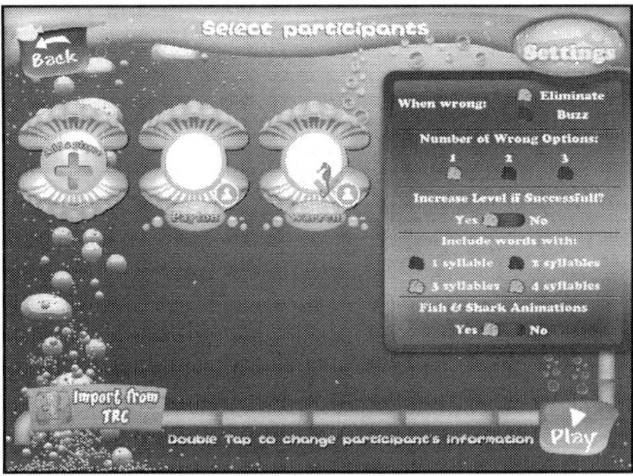


**FIGURE 8–20.** Syllables Splash settings screenshot. Reproduced with permission of Smarty Ears, LLC. All rights reserved.

Step 4:  Activate or deactivate the sound using the speaker icon on the home
screen page.

### *Individual Session or Small Group Session*

Step 1:  With the client sitting across from you and the app displaying the first image or word,
model the single-syllable word using easy onset and vowel prolongation.

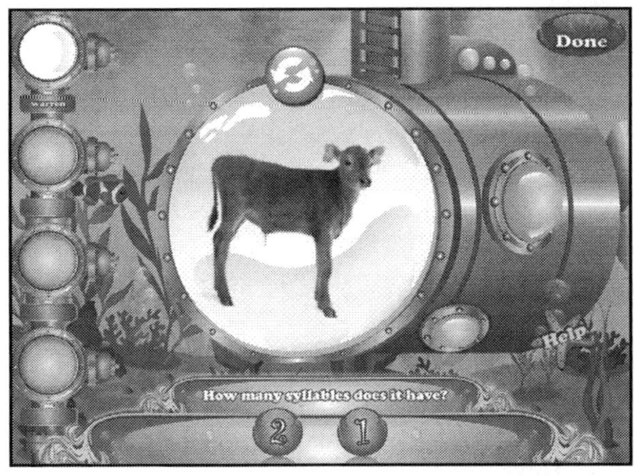


**FIGURE 8–21A.** Syllables Splash picture screenshot. Reproduced with permission of Smarty Ears, LLC. All rights reserved.

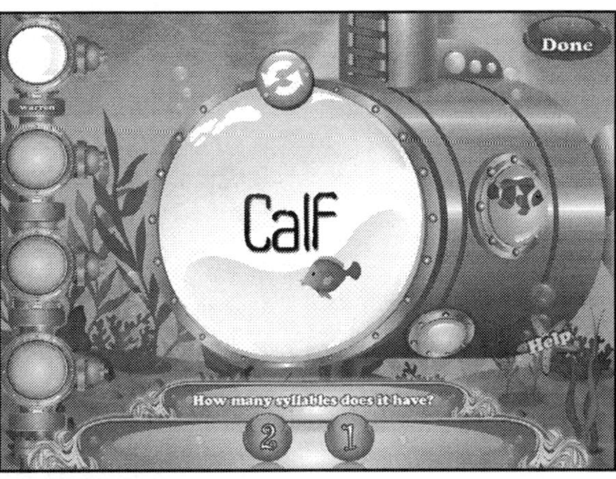


**FIGURE 8–21B.** Syllables Splash word screenshot. Reproduced with permission of Smarty Ears, LLC. All rights reserved.

Step 2:  Open the Syllables Splash app, activate/deactivate the sound as needed, and select
player (client).

Step 3:  Ask your client to repeat the same single-syllable word in unison with you.

Step 4:  Ask your clients to say the single-syllable word independently only after you have
modeled it for them and spoken in unison with them. Confirm that they understand
the task of easy onset and vowel prolongation. If not, repeat Steps 1 and 2 until
objectives are met. After the clients are able to independently demonstrate the
concepts of easy onset and vowel prolongation, proceed to the next picture by having
them tap on the number of syllables (1, 2, 3, or 4). If the clients choose incorrectly, a
mini-animation eliminates the wrong choice.

Step 5:  Tally correct and incorrect productions of easy onset and vowel prolongation to
determine clients' accuracy. *NOTE:* The app does not tally vocal accuracy; it will only
record the number of incorrect or correct syllables chosen.

## Activity 5

Decibel 10th Professional Noise Meter app by SkyPaw for all school-age students and adults working on voice.

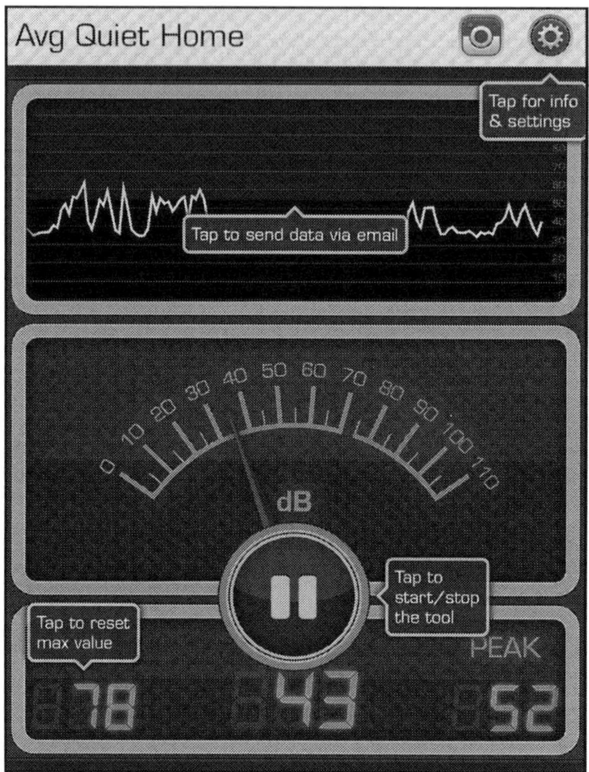


**FIGURE 8–22.** Skypaw Decibel 10th mainscreen shot. Reproduced with permission of SkyPaw.

The Decibel 10th Professional Noise Meter may be used with clients to improve easy onset of vocalization and vowel prolongation to facilitate a healthy voice. Decibel 10th Professional Noise Meter provides a sound meter to measure sound pressure. It displays loudness with a visual graph, as well as a decibel meter. The built-in microphone is sensitive from 0 to approximately 100 decibels.

To download the free Decibel 10th Professional Noise Meter, visit https://itunes.apple.com/us/app/decibel-10th-professional/id448155923?mt=8

**FIGURE 8–23.** Skypaw QR code.

### *Task Setup*

Step 1: Retrieve objects, pictures, words, phrases, and sentences that are appropriate for your client's speech and language skills. *NOTE:* The SLPA should take initial direction from the supervising SLP in regard to the client's voicing status. The SLP will have determined therapy goals and settings based on the results of a complete voice evaluation.

Step 2: Open the Decibel 10th Professional Noise Meter app and proceed.

### *Individual Session or Small Group Session*

Step 1: With the client sitting across from you and the app displaying the graph and decibel meter, model three consonant-vowel-consonant (CVC) words using easy onset and vowel prolongation. Alternate voice on and voice off for 2 seconds each, which will result in a graph displaying three block-like structures.

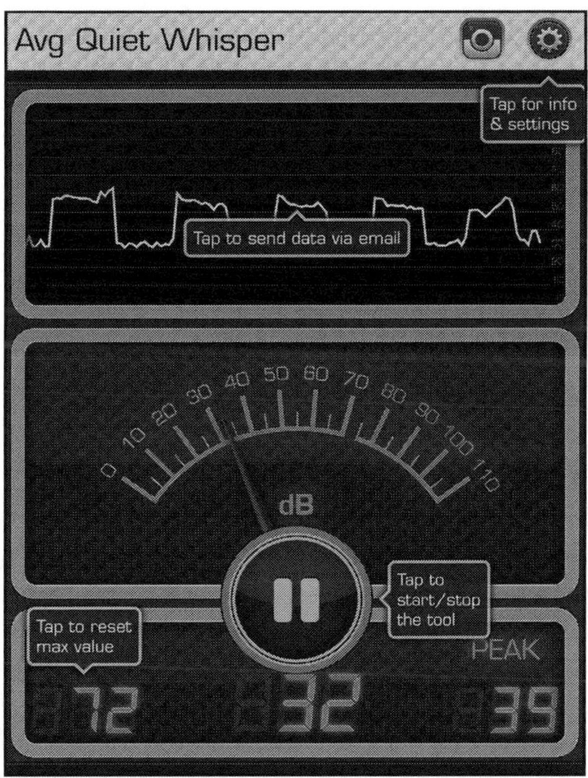


**FIGURE 8–24.** Decibel 10th Graph 1 screenshot. Reproduced with permission of SkyPaw.

The length of the horizontal line will reflect the length of the word, phrase, or sentence targeted.

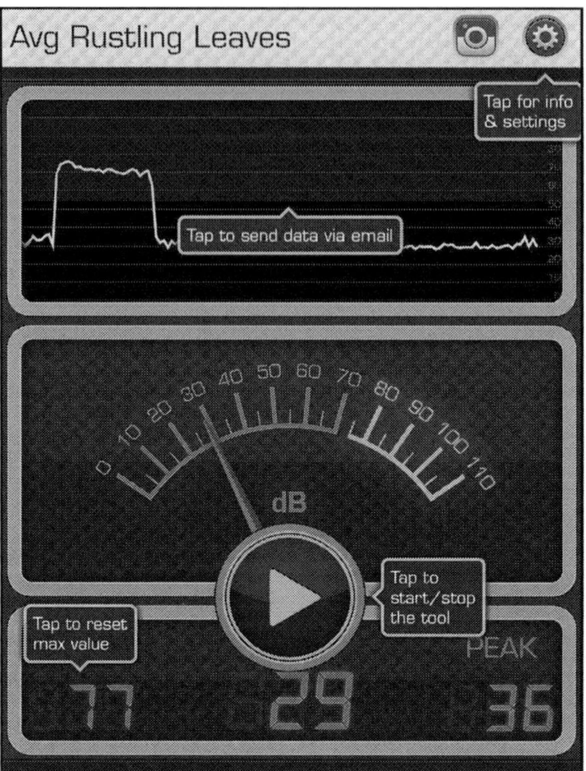


**FIGURE 8–25.** Decibel 10th Graph 2 screenshot. Reproduced with permission of SkyPaw.

Step 2: Ask your clients to repeat the same three CVC words in unison with you.

Step 3: Ask your clients to say the CVC words independently only after you have modeled it for them and spoken in unison with them. Confirm that they understand the task of easy onset and vowel prolongation. If not, repeat Steps 1 and 2 until vocal objectives are achieved.

Step 4: The SLPA should tally correct and incorrect productions of easy onset and vowel prolongation to determine clients' accuracy. *NOTE:* When working on vocal loudness, the Decibel 10th Professional Noise Meter may be used to provide client feedback about appropriate loudness. General conversational levels are approximately 60 decibels.

Step 5: Have the client repeat the phrases independently three times.

## Activity 6

Creating an Interactive Fluency Binder for school-age clients.

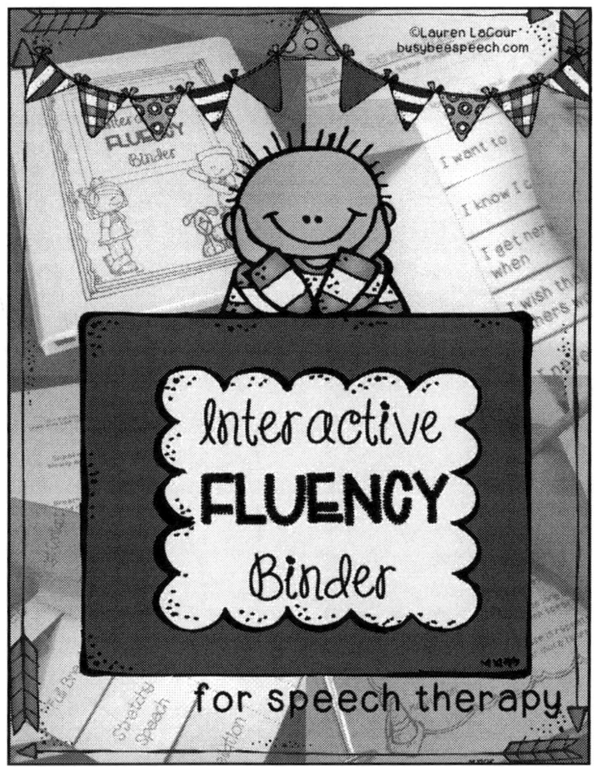


**FIGURE 8–26.** Fluency Binder screenshot. Reproduced with permission of Lauren LaCour, ©Busy Bee Speech.

The Interactive Fluency Binder, created by Lauren LaCour, is a comprehensive packet that can be used to address needed strategies and understanding of stuttering. Some of the aspects related to stuttering are feelings of speech, relaxation, bumpy versus smooth speech, types of disfluencies, types of fluency strategies, and pacing charts. The packet can be used in its entirety with individual fluency students or pick-and-choose activities that best suit client needs.

To download the Interactive Fluency Binder for Speech Therapy, visit https://www.teacherspayteachers.com/Product/Interactive-Fluency-Binder-for-Speech-Therapy-1622099

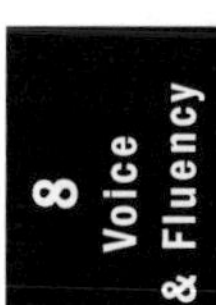

**FIGURE 8–27.** Fluency Binder QR code.

For a more effective and efficient therapy session, this activity can be printed and assembled in notebook fashion for each client prior to the therapy session or copy the appropriate sections that will be needed for the therapy session.

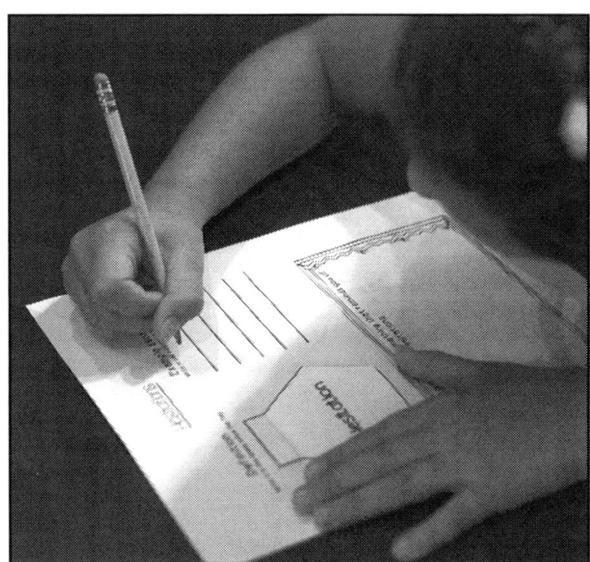

FIGURE 8–28A. Aria Derryberry hesitation worksheet.

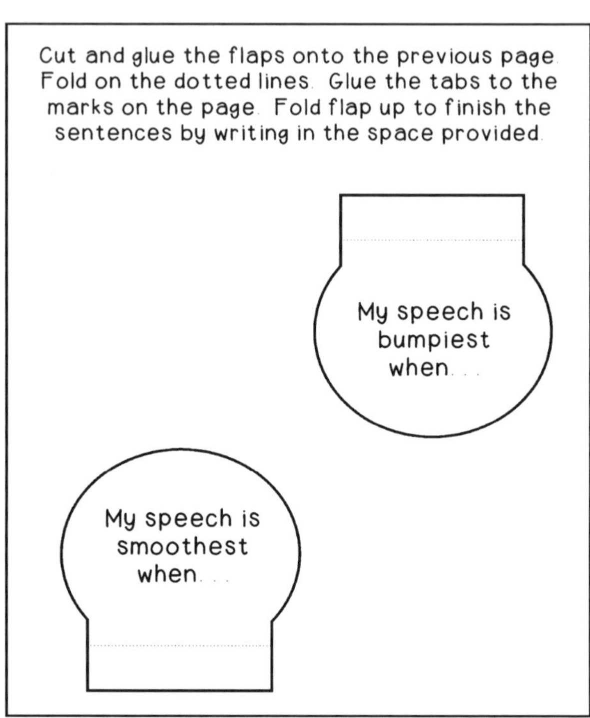


FIGURE 8–28B. Worksheet image. Reproduced with permission of Lauren LaCour, ©Busy Bee Speech.

### Individual or Small Group Session

Step 1:  With the client sitting aside or across from you, give an explanation of what the intended therapy lesson will be (i.e., "Today we will be learning about the different types of disfluencies/bumpy speech."). *NOTE:* The SLPA should take initial direction from the supervising SLP in regard to the client's ability and targeted objectives.

Step 2:  Choose the appropriate activity from the interactive binder to work on for the therapy session (i.e., fluency strategies) or allow your clients to work systematically from the beginning and create their individual interactive binder. For purposes of this lesson, the focus will be on awareness of the Types of Disfluency (i.e., Bumpy Speech).

Step 3:  Proceed to the section of the packet titled Types of Disfluency (Bumpy Speech) and allow clients to work directly in the interactive binder that you have created for them or give the clients the appropriate pages.

Step 4:  Discuss with or ask your clients if they are aware of the types of disfluencies (bumpy speech) that affect them when they speak.

Step 5:  Using the pages from the Interactive Fluency Binder, engage the clients to match, color, cut, and glue definitions. Use this opportunity to have clients give examples (write or say) of the type of disfluency that might affect them.

Step 6:  Record any needed data into the client file and make a note to the continue activity for a future therapy session or begin a new interactive activity with the binder.

### *Essential Resources for Activity*

Visit Lauren LaCour, Busy Bee Speech, at Teacher Pay Teachers to download free and other fluency activities (https://www.teacherspayteachers.com/Product/Fluency-Pinwheels-652191)

**FIGURE 8–29.** Fluency Pinwheel QR code.

## Activity 7

Decreasing stuttering for all ages using the FluencyCoach PRO by SpeechEasy. A microphone headset is needed for this activity.

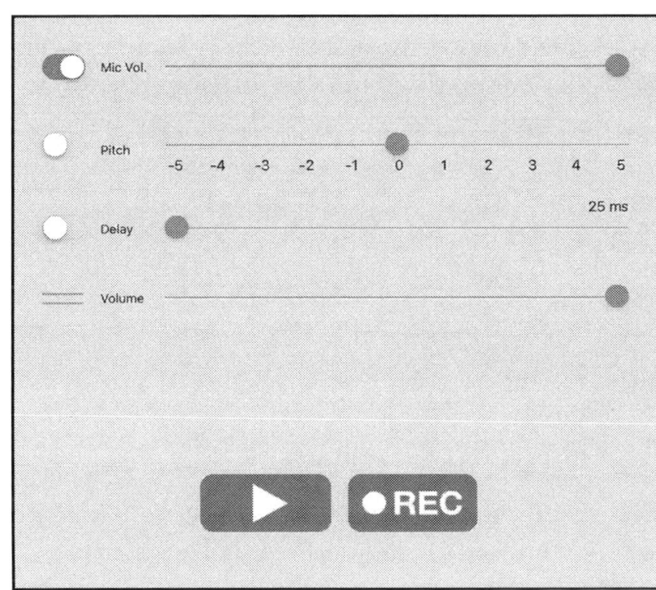



**FIGURE 8–30A.** FluencyCoach screenshot. Reproduced with permission of Janus Development Group, Inc.

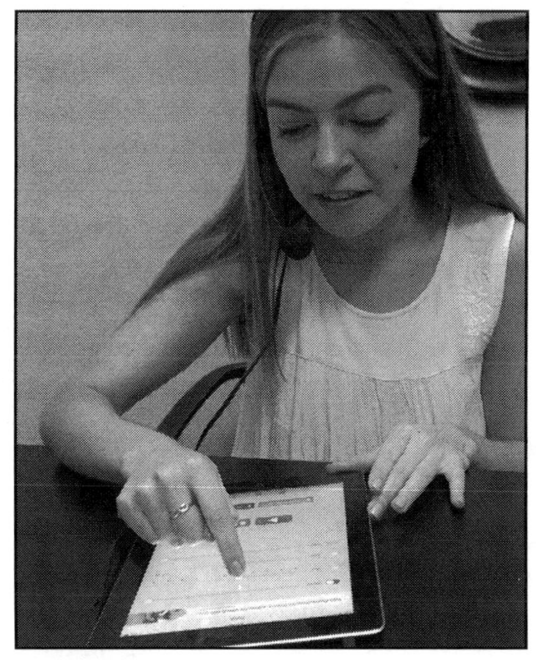

**FIGURE 8–30B.** Christina Chacon FluencyCoach.

The FluencyCoach PRO is used to decrease stuttering by using the fluency-enhancing technique of choral speech (speaking simultaneously with another person). FluencyCoach uses altered auditory feedback (AAF) technology to simulate the effects of choral speech. The feedback can be adjusted in two ways using frequency-altered feedback (FAF) or delayed auditory feedback (DAF).

To download FluencyCoach PRO to an iPad or computer, visit http://fluencycoach.com

**FIGURE 8–31.**
FluencyCoach QR code.

For more effective and efficient therapy sessions, prepare a variety of pictures, words, and sentences based on client needs and objectives prior to the therapy session. Suggestions include rote memory such as counting numbers 1 to 10, stating the days of the week, naming pictures, common conversational phrases (such as "Hello, how are you?" "My name is"), and academic and social language vocabulary.

### *Individual Session*

Step 1: Explain to client that you will be using an app or software program to practice and improve his or her fluency.

Step 2: Open the FluencyCoach PRO app or software program and connect your microphone or headset to your computer or tablet (dependent on download of software or app).

Step 3: With permission, place headset and microphone on the client's head or have client put the headset on.

Step 4: Adjust the microphone sensitivity.

Step 5: Set the pitch on plus 2.

Step 6: Set the delay at 60 ms.

Step 7: Adjust the volume to a comfortable level.

Step 8: Adjust the DAF in 30-ms increments according to client comfort.

Step 9: Instruct your client to use smooth and constant voicing with an appropriately loud vocal volume. The use of additional fluency-enhancing techniques such as gentle onsets and/or prolongations can be used as appropriate.

Step 10:  Practice talking using previously prepared activities. Focus on listening to the altered auditory signal. Increase the DAF in 30-ms increments as appropriate for client and to experience a variety of settings.

Step 11:  Use the recorded speech samples with your supervising SLP to plan future therapy goals and track progress.

## Activity 8

Improving fluency using functional everyday picture and word combinations or sentence completion worksheets for a variety of ages.

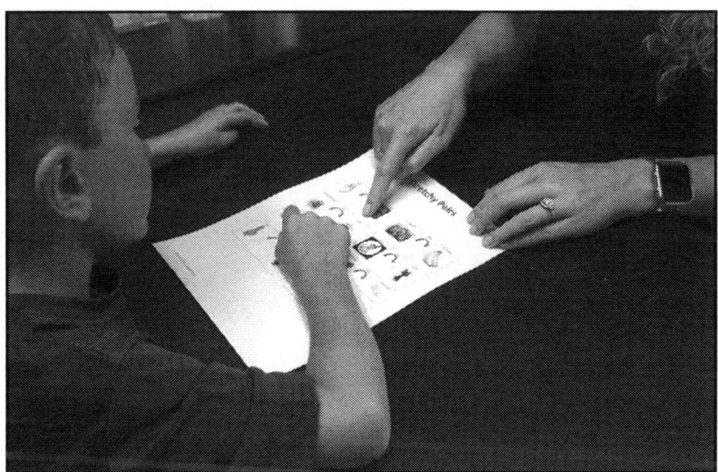

**FIGURE 8–32.** Harrison Boyce GBS.

The use of everyday words and phrases sets the foundation for improved fluency in functional daily activities. Pictures and words may be modified based on your client's maturity level and interests. *NOTE:* The SLPA should take initial direction from the supervising SLP in regard to using the hierarchy to establish long- and short-term goals.

### *Task Setup*

Step 1:  Retrieve color copies of Stretchy Pairs Fluency Activity 1 or Stretchy Pairs Fluency Activity 2 from http://granitebayspeech.com/wordpress/handouts/, copy the PDF within this lesson, or create your own prior to the therapy session.

### *Individual Session or Small Group Session*

Step 1:  With the client sitting across from you:

    a.  Using either of the Fluency activity worksheets, instruct your client to speak in unison with you, prolonging the first vowel of each word. Use continuous voicing as you both move your index finger from the first to the second picture or the sentence completion line.

    b.  Use the visual cue of the green arrow to promote prolonged vocalization of AND between the two pictured items (Activity 1 worksheet) or the sentence completion line (Activity 2 worksheet).

    c.  Allow 3 to 5 seconds to vocalize each pair of words. Repeat each phrase in unison with your client three times.

Step 2:  Repeat Step 1. However, only speak in unison with your client as needed and instruct him or her to produce the phrases independently.

### *Essential Resources for Activity*

To download color copies of worksheets, visit http://granitebayspeech.com/

**FIGURE 8–33.** GBS QR code.

# Stretchy Pairs Activity 1

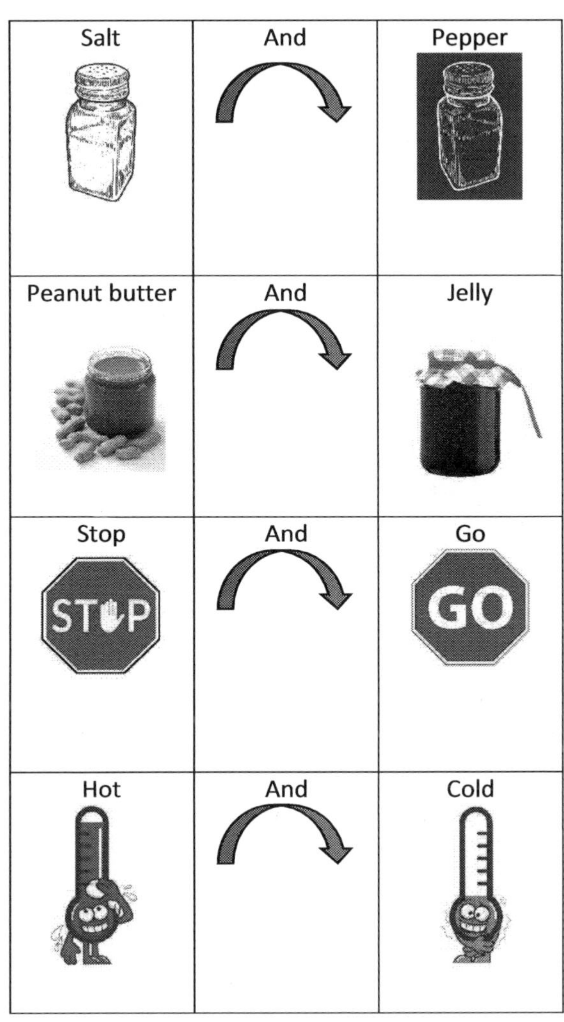


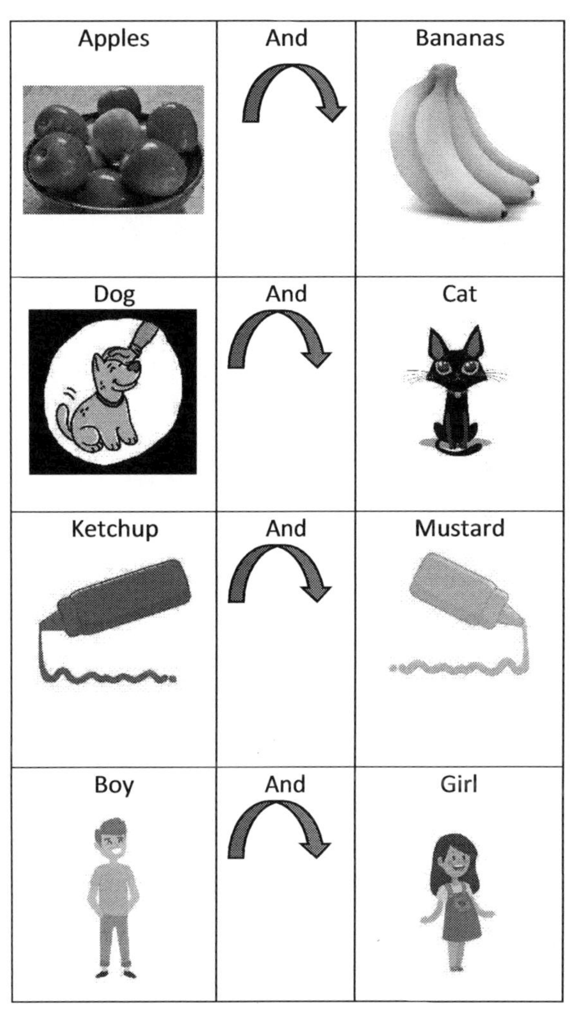


©Granite Bay Speech 2016



**FIGURE 8–34.** PDF Stretchy WORKSHEET Activity 1. Reproduced with permission of Granite Bay Speech.

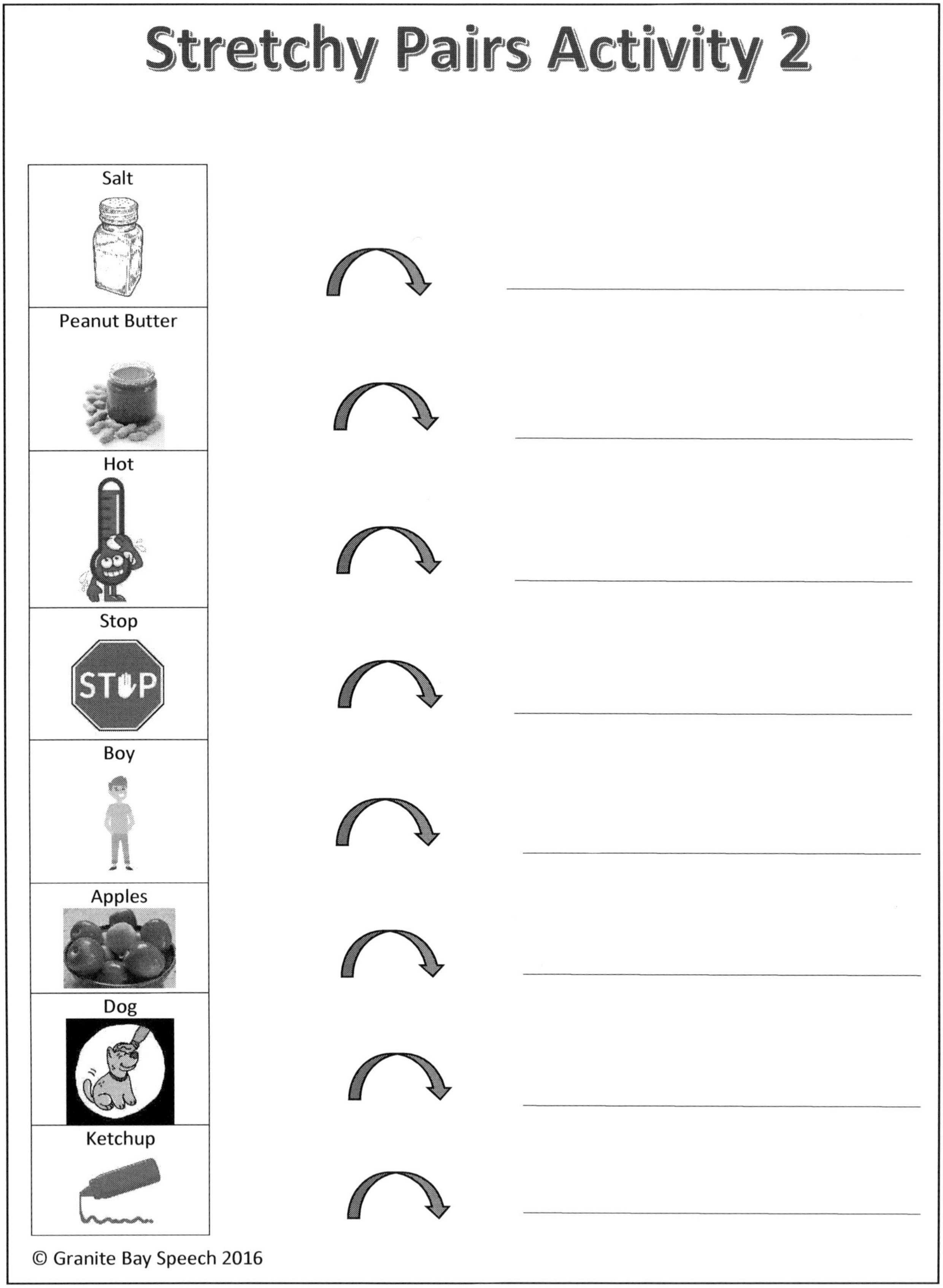

# Stretchy Pairs Activity 2

Salt

Peanut Butter

Hot

Stop

Boy

Apples

Dog

Ketchup



**FIGURE 8–35.** PDF Stretchy WORKSHEET Activity 2. Reproduced with permission of Granite Bay Speech.

## Activity 9

Improving awareness of stuttering triggers using hierarchy worksheets for a variety of ages.

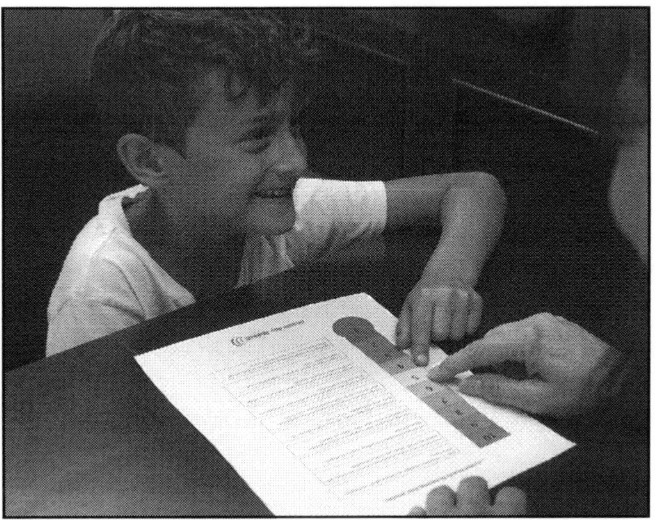

**FIGURE 8–36.** Warren Boyce GBS.

Hierarchies are effective therapy tools utilized to improve clients' awareness of stuttering triggers. Common triggers may include feared situations, people, sounds, or words. As your clients rank the difficulty of triggers, they develop a better understanding of their short-term treatment goals. The use of hierarchies helps to manage clients' expectations. They are an integral component of any therapy program that seeks to treat the whole person, rather than only overt stuttering behaviors. *NOTE:* The SLPA should take initial direction from the supervising SLP in regard to using the hierarchy to establish long- and short-term goals.

### *Task Setup*

Step 1:  Retrieve color copies of hierarchy worksheets (blank thermometer, situational stuttering triggers, or sound and word stuttering triggers) from http://granitebay speech.com/wordpress/handouts/, copy the PDF within this lesson, or create your own prior to the therapy session.

> For more effective and efficient therapy sessions, prepare pictures and printed words of common people, situations, words, and phrases the client may utilize throughout the day prior to the therapy session. Tailor the choices to meet the communication needs of the client. Common pictures and words may include school, home, and social situations.

### *Individual Session or Small Group Session*

Step 1:  With the client sitting across from you, ask your client to choose common situations, people, words, or sounds that commonly trigger his or her stuttering. For younger clients, use photographs or pictures (older clients may write a short description on each line).

Step 2:  Have the client rank each stuttering trigger by placing the word or picture on the line that corresponds with the severity level.

Step 3:  Start working on each trigger utilizing therapy techniques chosen with SLP supervision.

Step 4:  Record data in the client file as needed.

### *Essential Resources for Activity*

To download color copies of hierarchy worksheets, visit http://granitebayspeech.com

**FIGURE 8–37.** GBS QR code.

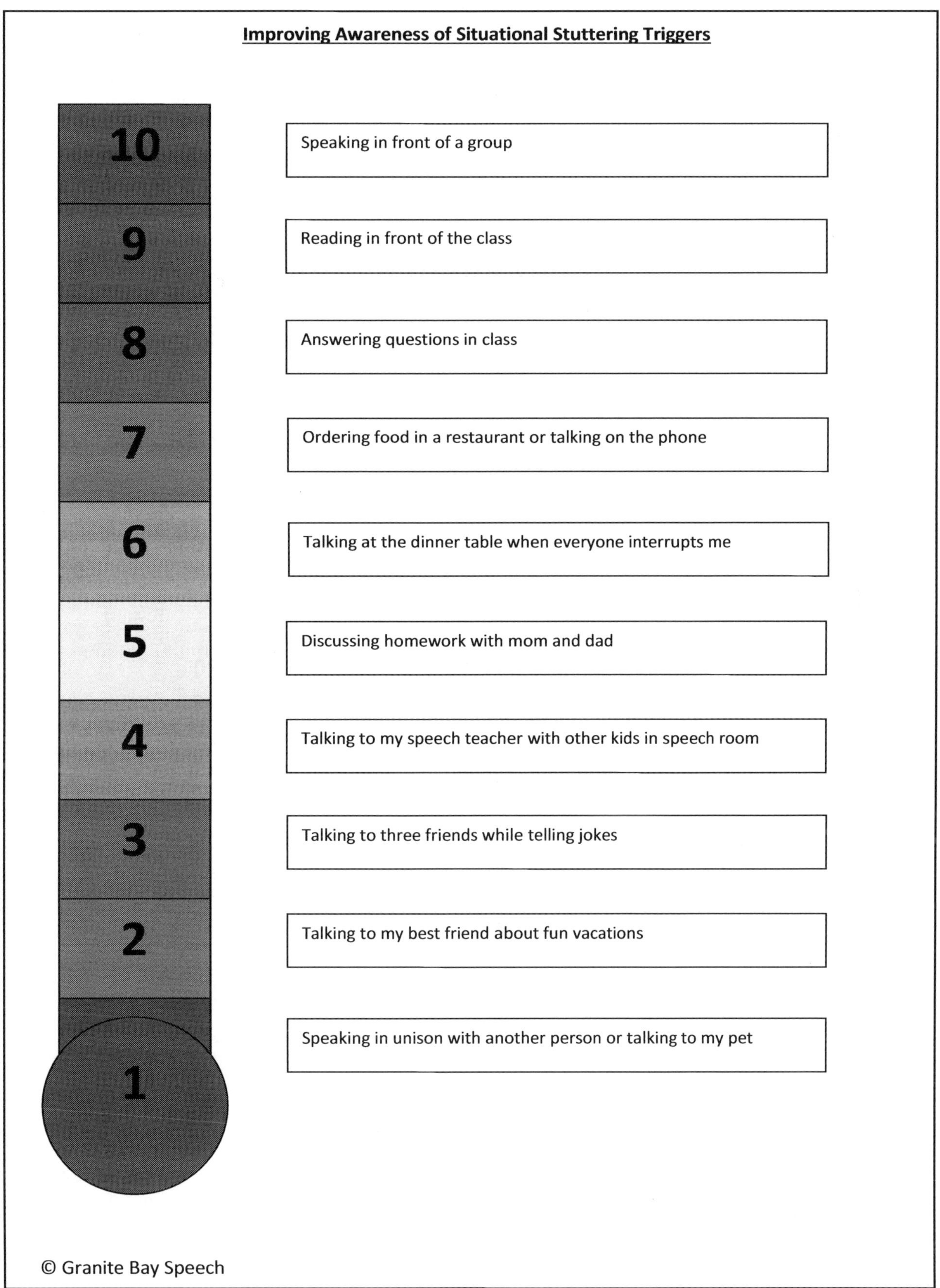



**FIGURE 8–38.** PDF hierarchy worksheet situational. Reproduced with permission of Granite Bay Speech.

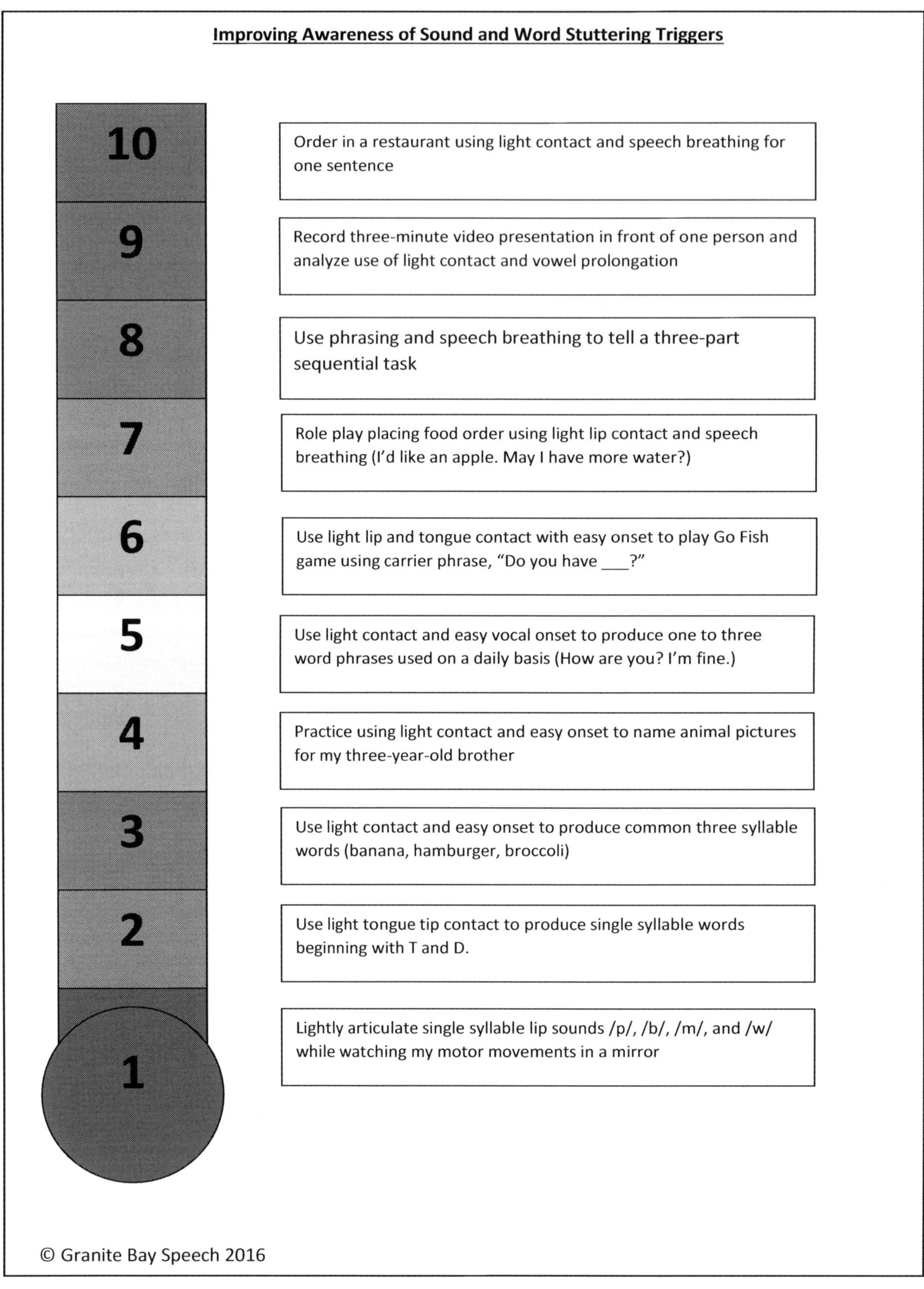


**FIGURE 8–39.** PDF hierarchy worksheet word and sound. Reproduced with permission of Granite Bay Speech.

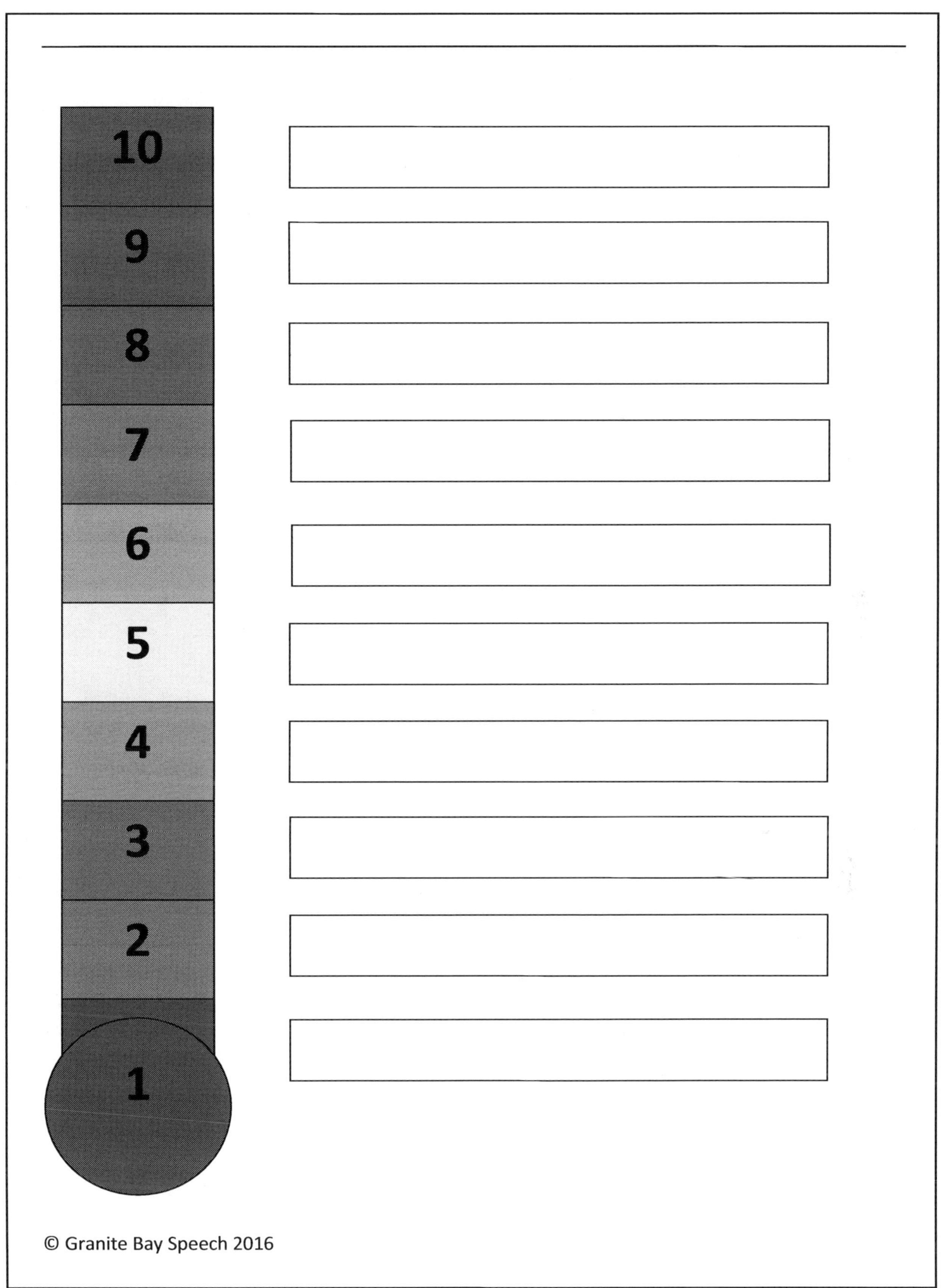





**FIGURE 8–40.** PDF blank hierarchy thermometer. Reproduced with permission of Granite Bay Speech.

# REFERENCES

American Speech-Language-Hearing Association (ASHA). (2016). Communication for life. Retrieved February 4, 2016, from http://www.asha.org/public

Max, L., & Baldwin, C. J. (2010). The role of motor learning in stuttering adaptation: Repeated versus novel utterances in a practice-retention paradigm. *Journal of Fluency Disorders, 35*(1), 33–43.

McLeod, S. (2008). Systematic desensitization. Retrieved April 8, 2016, from http://www.simplypsychology.org/Systematic-Desensitisation.html

Stemple, J. C. (2014). *Clinical voice pathology.* San Diego, CA: Plural.

# 9

# Behavior Management Techniques

The behavior management techniques discussed in this chapter consist of both visual schedules and motivation/rewards.

Visual schedules are useful tools for both child and adult clients. A visual schedule is a physical (or digital) map of the day's activities. They are especially helpful for managing transitions in very young children and those who struggle with transition due to defiance issues, general off-task behaviors, and children on the autism spectrum. Visual schedules are also beneficial for adults with cognitive and language impairments.

Waters, Lerman, and Hovanetz (2009) found that problem behaviors are preserved by access to preferred activities and escaping nonpreferred activities. Therapy is most effective when visual schedules are used in combination with extinction and differential reinforcement techniques. Prompting can be used to transition from one activity to another. A common prompting procedure is the "three-step prompting procedure." Three-step prompting begins with Step 1: The speech-language pathology assistant (SLPA) requests the client perform a certain action. If the client does not comply after 10 seconds, the SLPA would gain eye contact and provide a model of the requested action (Step 2). If the client continues to refuse to comply, the SLPA will repeat the instructions while "guiding" the client to perform the action (Wilder, Myers, Fischetti, Leon, Nicholson, & Allison, 2012).

Social story intervention can also be used to monitor transitions and behavior expectations via verbal and visual stimuli. Social stories must be tailored to the clients' needs in order to optimize effectiveness. When developing a story, consider the target behavior, best times or opportunities for implementing, and the client's ability to focus. Social stories can work in conjunction with visual schedules when using the same picture icons.

Motivation/reinforcement can be intrinsic or extrinsic. Intrinsic motivation is characterized by internal rewards or desire. The opposite is extrinsic motivation, taking action based on outside stimulation whether that is to avoid adverse outcomes or gain a reward.

Examples of intrinsic motivation include:

1. Taking part in an activity because it is fun

2. Solving a problem because it is exciting and challenging

3. Finishing a project because it is satisfying

Examples of external reinforcement include:

1. A sticker for every correct production of /r/

2. Specific vocal affirmation such as, "You correctly used 'she'; I like it when you use the right pronoun."

3. Removal of an object or not doing an activity when negative behavior is presented. For example:
   a. Clinician states, "I want to play with bubbles with you, when you put your toys in the box we can play with bubbles."
   b. Child does not clean up.
   c. Clinician states, "I'm sad we don't get to play with bubbles because you didn't clean up your mess, well maybe next time."
   d. Clinician does not fold if the child starts to clean up after told he or she cannot play with bubbles.

First-time fast-time clean-up method:

1. Set a visual timer for the client.

2. Vocalize how long an activity will go for.

3. Tell the client that when the timer goes off, "we clean up fast."

4. Remind the client during the session "first-time fast-time clean-up."

5. When the timer goes off, vocalize once "first-time fast-time clean-up."

## VISUAL SUPPORTS

### Objectives

The following are some sample objectives for using a visual schedule:

1. Given a portable word/picture schedule with a sequence of tasks or activities, the client will follow the schedule and remove each icon once the activity/task is completed or time is called to move to next activity, in four out of five consecutive opportunities.

2. Given a first/then board and choice of a preferred activity to be earned upon completing a preferred or nonpreferred task, the client will complete the first activity without protesting in four out of five consecutive opportunities.

3. Given calming strategies to self-regulate and use proactively before behavior escalates or the client feels overwhelmed, the client will actively use these strategies and ask for a break as needed in four out of five consecutive opportunities.

### Activity 1

Choiceworks app by Bee Visual for all ages using visual schedules, including short video clips to develop self-control, follow and complete routines.

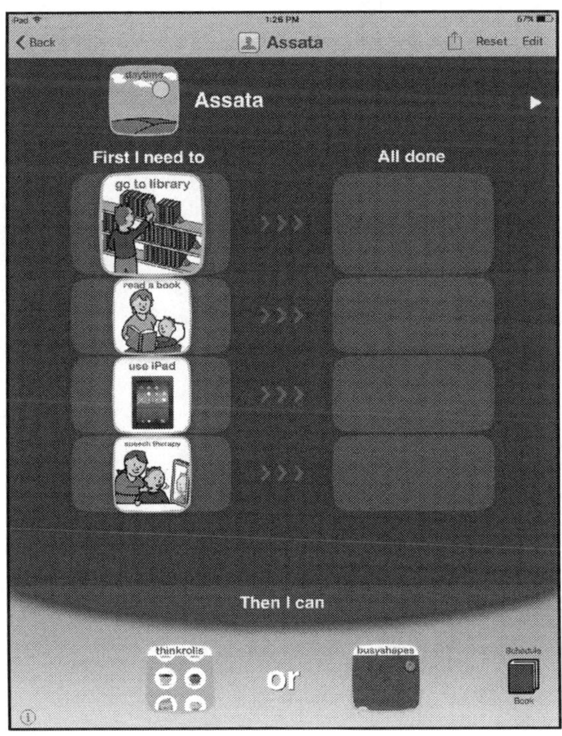

**FIGURE 9–1A.** BeeVisual schedule screenshot. Reproduced with permission of Bee Visual, LLC.

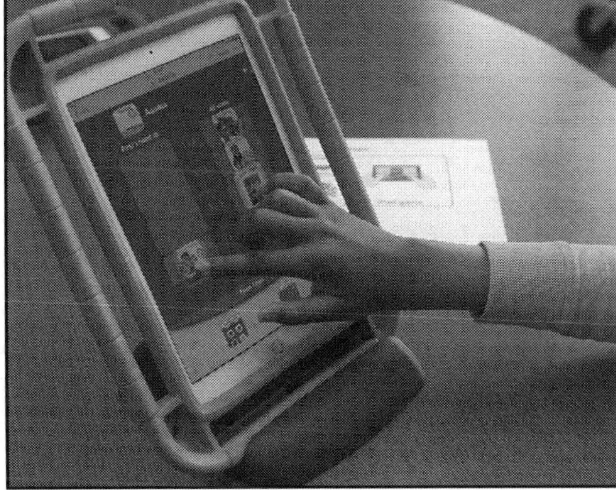

**FIGURE 9–1B.** Assata Shakir.

The Choiceworks app is a tool for helping complete daily routines and tasks as well as to help improve self-regulation. This app features three types of boards: schedule, waiting, and feelings, along with companion social storybooks that support each concept/board. The Choiceworks library contains more than 180 built-in images and professional audio. Adding images from your personal photo library and your own audio narration allows for unlimited customization. Choiceworks has the option to add custom video onto any board image and can be used for multiple clients, and boards can be shared via email, file sharing, and printing.

> To make for more effective and efficient therapy sessions, whenever possible, create and customize the client's board/schedule in the app prior to the therapy session.

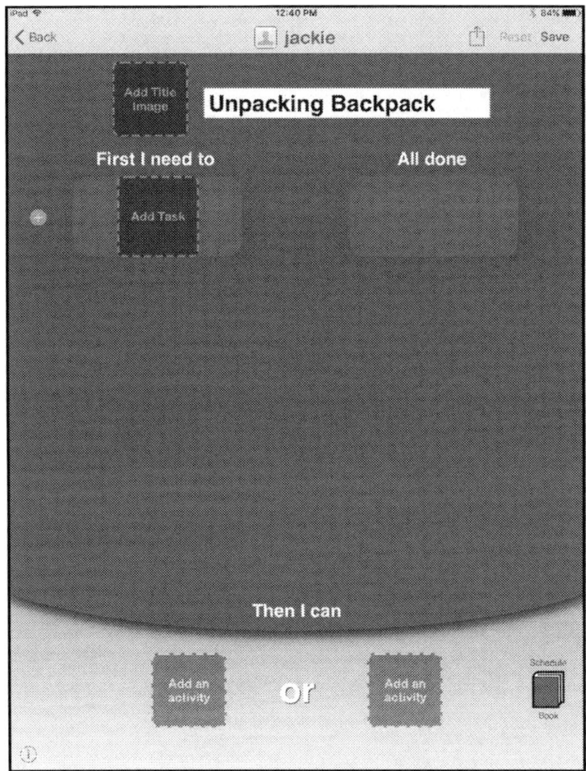


**FIGURE 9–2A.** BeeVisual edit schedule screenshot. Reproduced with permission of Bee Visual, LLC.

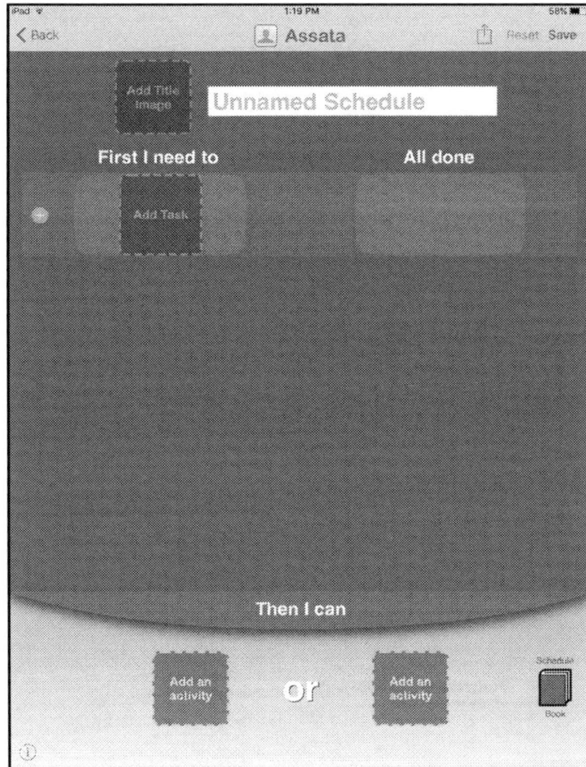


**FIGURE 9–2B.** BeeVisual edit wait screenshot. Reproduced with permission of Bee Visual, LLC.

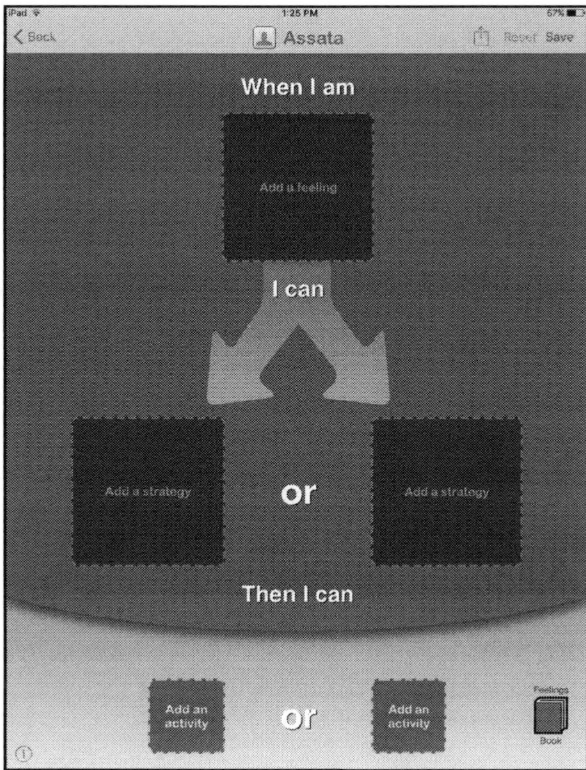


**FIGURE 9–2C.** BeeVisual edit feelings screenshot. Reproduced with permission of Bee Visual, LLC.

To download Choiceworks, visit http://www.beevisual.com

**FIGURE 9–3.** BeeVisual QR code.

### *Task Setup*

Required steps for creating client profiles:

Step 1:   Open the app "Choiceworks" and proceed.

     a. Tap "Profiles" at the top of the screen.

     b. Tap "New" on the profiles popup.
       Type client's name and add the optional photo. *NOTE:* Keep in mind privacy and confidentiality when adding client photos. You may add a favorite image for the client versus an actual client photo OR do nothing and keep the photo area blank. Adding a favorite image can be a fun activity for clients to have some ownership for their boards and schedules.

     c. Tap "Save."

     d. Repeat Steps a through d to add other profiles.

Step 2:   Once your client profiles are set up, tap "Profiles" and choose the appropriate client to begin setting up the board by tapping the "+" on the top of the screen and choose the type of board you would like to create: schedule, waiting, or feelings. For purposes of this activity, we will choose "Schedule."

Step 3:   Name the schedule board by typing the name in the text box and tapping "Done" on the keyboard. For example, Unpacking backpack. A corresponding title image may be added by choosing a preloaded image or adding one from your personal photo library (i.e., a photo of a client with a backpack).

Step 4:   Begin to add the task images to the board by tapping in the "Add Task" box. Choose an image from the Choicworks library, customize a current Choiceworks image as needed, or add an image from your photo library.

Step 4A:  To choose task images within the Choiceworks library:

     1. Tap "Add Task."

     2. Type a word to indicate the type of task you need (i.e., lunch in "Search box" or scroll through the images to choose the task).

     3. Continue to add steps for this schedule and tap "Save."

---

The option to include a time limit for each task can be added by tapping "Add Timer."

Step 4B:  To customize (add, edit, or delete) using available Choiceworks images:

1.  Tap "Back" located in the upper left corner.

2.  Tap "Settings" symbol (gear image) located in the upper left corner.

3.  Tap "Manage Image Library."

4.  Type name of an image that you want to edit in the "search" box (i.e., backpack).

5.  Choose corresponding image and tap "Create a duplicate."

6.  Type a new image caption in text box and tap "Done."

7.  Add customized image audio by tapping the record button to begin and again to end the recording. *NOTE:* Audio cues can be turned off within the settings area as needed.

8.  Tap "Save" in the upper left corner to save your new customized image and return to the saved board within the appropriate profile to add the newly created task image by tapping "Edit" on the board.

Step 4C:  To use an image from your photo library or use the camera on your device:

1.  Tap the "Settings" symbol (gear image) located in the upper left corner.

2.  Tap "Manage Image Library."

3.  Tap the "+" located in the upper right corner.

4.  Tap "Add image" and choose camera or your photo library.

5.  Choose the appropriate photo or take a photo.

6.  Type a new image caption in the text box and tap "Done."

7.  Add image audio by tapping the record button to begin and again to end the recording. *NOTE:* Audio cues can be turned off within the settings area as needed.

8.  Tap "Title, Task or Activity" to place the image in the appropriate area.

9.  Tap "Save" in the upper left corner to save your new customized image and return to the saved board within the appropriate profile to add the newly created task image by tapping "Edit" on the board.

Step 5:  Add one or two activities for reward or motivation in the same manner you added tasks for your schedule.

Step 6:  Use the newly created SAVED schedule/board in combination with your planned lesson to increase task attendance.

## Activity 2

Sticker or stamp charts to record appropriate behavior or correct productions are helpful for clients to visualize their progress.

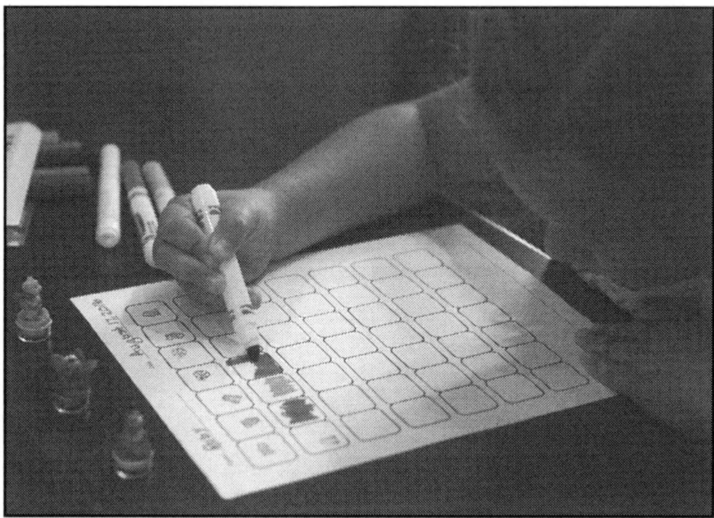

**FIGURE 9–4.** Ruby Derryberry chart.

Using a chart can be helpful for those clients who need a little extra help with motivation and encouraging a job well done. Provide an agreed-upon reward when reaching the "reward" box on the chart (i.e., an extra stamp/mark or choose a reward from a prize box). Allow the client to put a sticker/stamp or other marking on the chart when:

- Client/student arrives to a speech/language session on time without a reminder; helpful for the elementary age clients/students and eliminates the SLPA from calling and disrupting a classroom.
- Client/student returns completed and signed homework by caregiver/parent/ guardian.
- Client/student puts in extra effort during a speech and language session.
- SLPA feels is appropriate (i.e., a kind gesture toward another within a group session).

Step 1:  Copy or create a similar chart for each client and keep in the client work file.

Step 2:  At the end of each session or during the session, allow the client to mark the chart appropriately.

Step 3:  Replace with a new chart when complete.

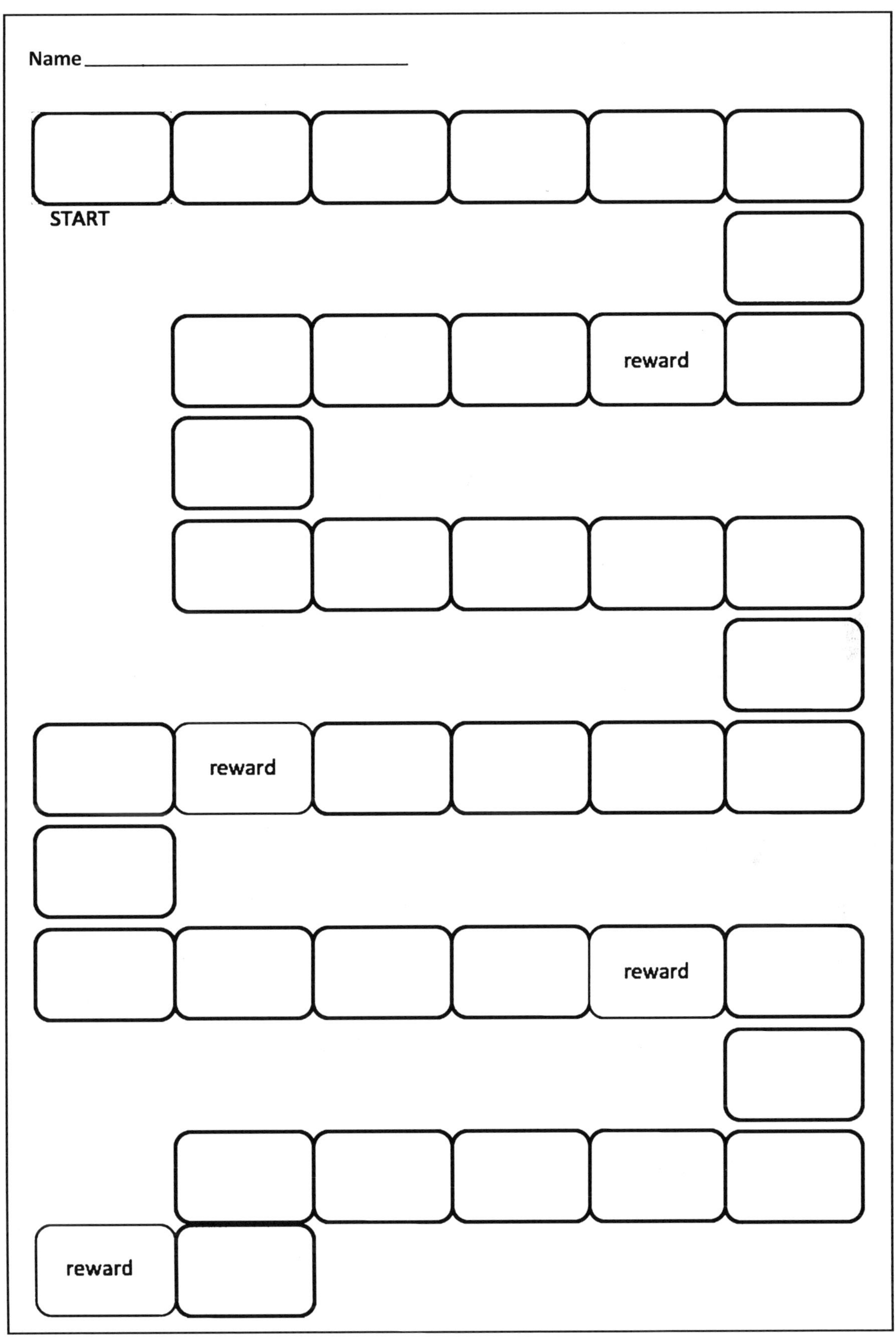


**FIGURE 9–5.** Sticker chart.

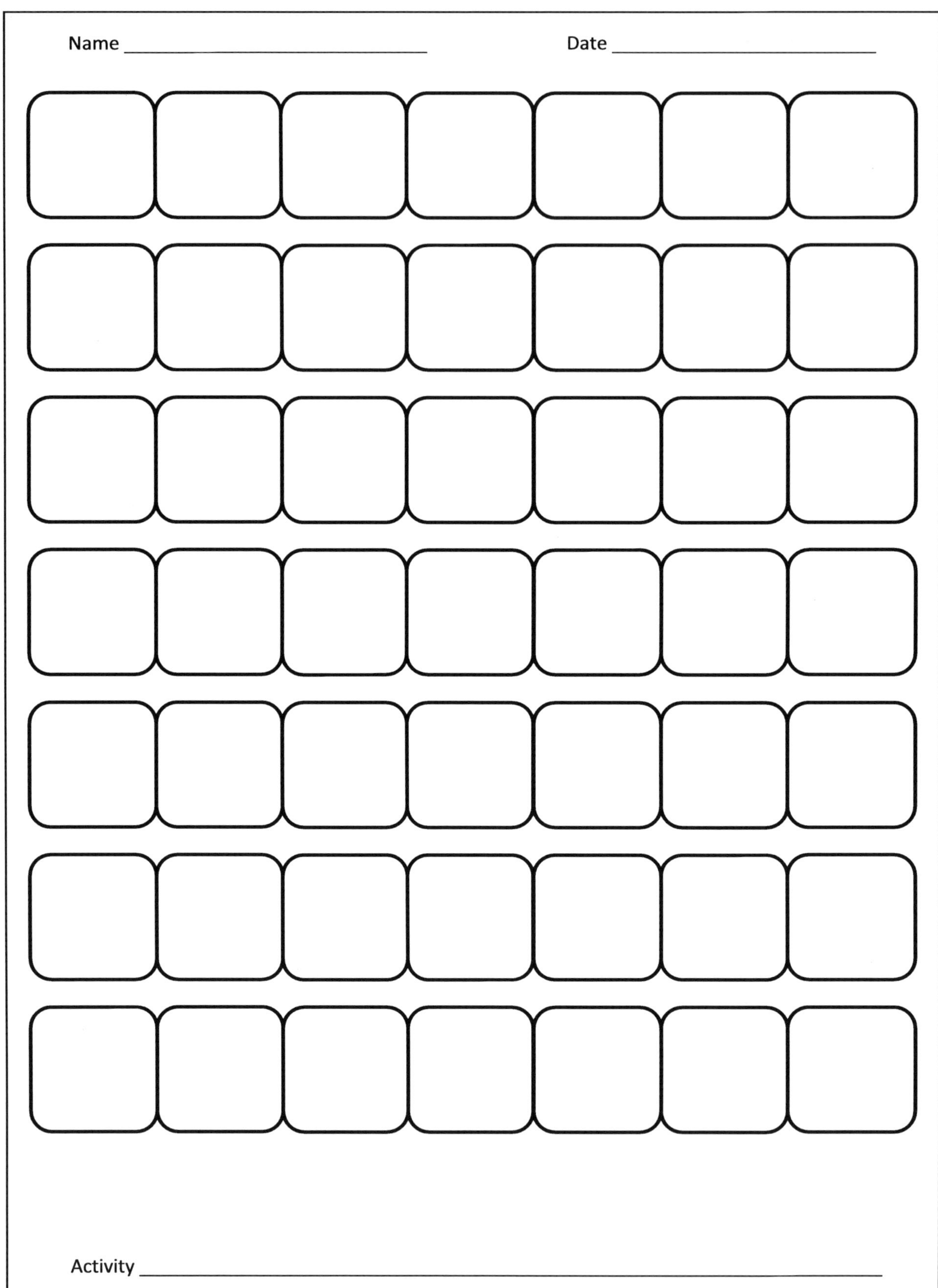



**FIGURE 9–6.** Color block chart.

## Activity 3

First/then boards and other motivational visuals created on the Custom Boards app.

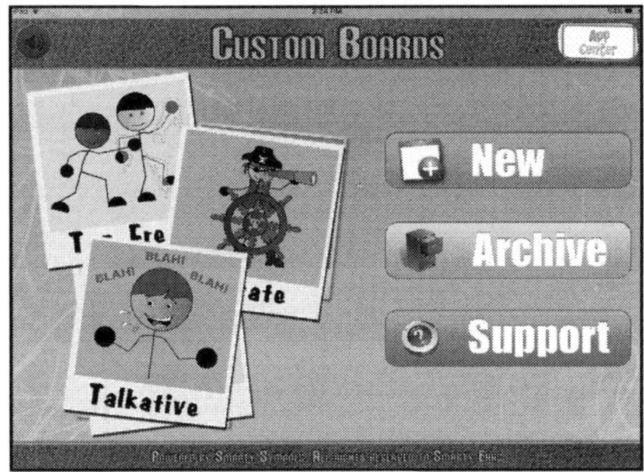

**FIGURE 9–7A.** Smarty Ears Custom Boards screenshot. Reproduced with permission of Smarty Ears, LLC. All rights reserved.

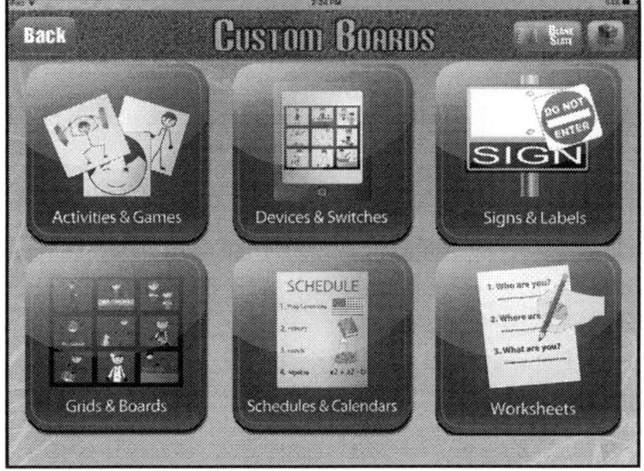

**FIGURE 9–7B.** Smarty Ears Custom Boards main screenshot. Reproduced with permission of Smarty Ears, LLC. All rights reserved.

Custom Boards by Smarty Ears is a board and activity creator to create visuals supports with over 125 templates within six categories: Activities & Games, Devices & Switches, Signs & Labels, Grids & Boards, Schedules & Calendars, and Worksheets. There is an option to create a visual support from either a blank portrait or landscape template. Boards can be shared or printed, or use the visual support directly from the device.

To download Custom Boards by Smarty Ears, visit http://smartyearsapps.com

**FIGURE 9–8.** Smarty Ears QR code.

> To make for more effective and efficient therapy sessions, whenever possible, create and customize the client's board/schedule prior to the therapy session.

### *Individual or Small Group Session*

Step 1: Open the Custom Boards app and tap "New" to create a new visual support or tap "Archive" to choose previously created visuals.

Step 2: Tap one of the categories to display the board template choices or tap "blank slate" to start from scratch.

Step 3: Tap any of the templates to begin adding images to the template.

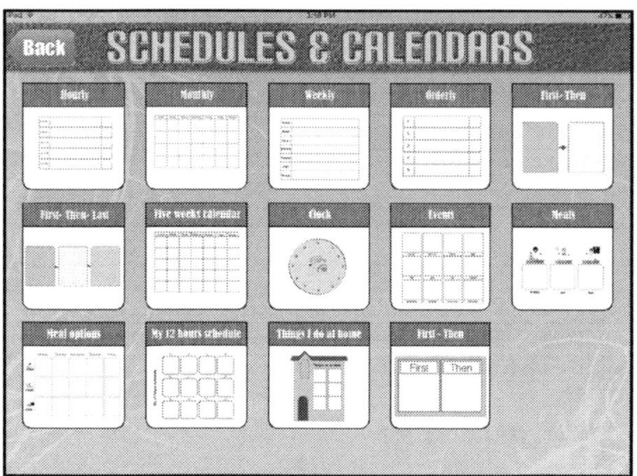

**FIGURE 9–9A.** Smarty Ears schedule choice screenshot. Reproduced with permission of Smarty Ears, LLC. All rights reserved.

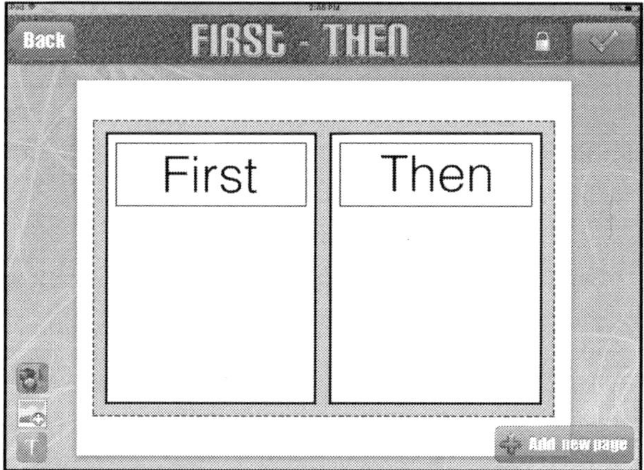

**FIGURE 9–9B.** Smarty Ears First Then template screenshot. Reproduced with permission of Smarty Ears, LLC. All rights reserved.

Step 4: Add images from over 10,000 built-in Smarty Symbols or choose images from your photo library. Customize borders, text placement, and font as needed.

Step 5: Tap "the check mark" at the top of the screen to save the template.

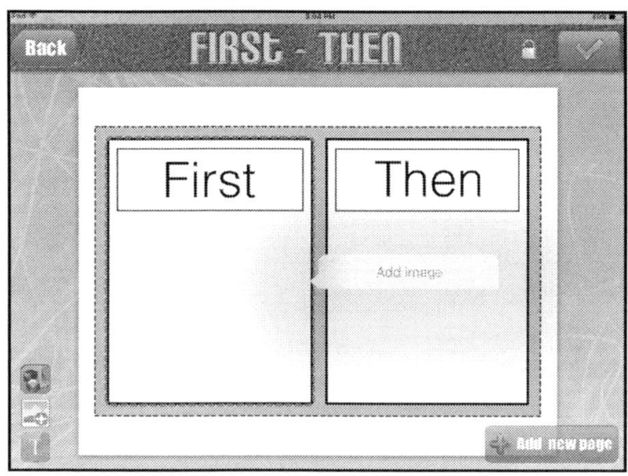

**FIGURE 9–10A.** Smarty Ears image screenshot. Reproduced with permission of Smarty Ears, LLC. All rights reserved.

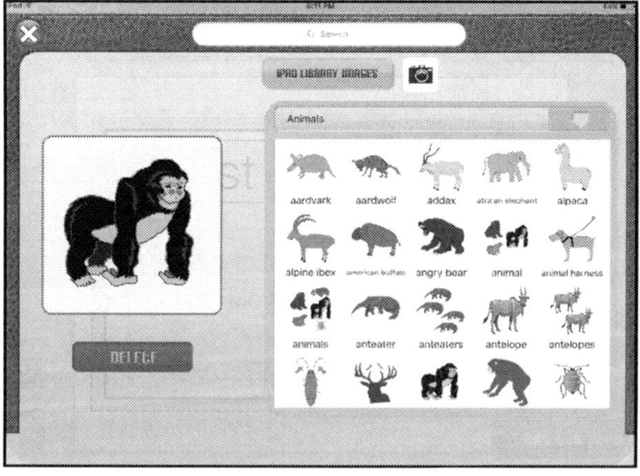

**FIGURE 9–10B.** Smarty Ears image picker screenshot. Reproduced with permission of Smarty Ears, LLC. All rights reserved.

Step 6:  Tap "Save to app" and tap "Share PDF" to print or email the new visual support.

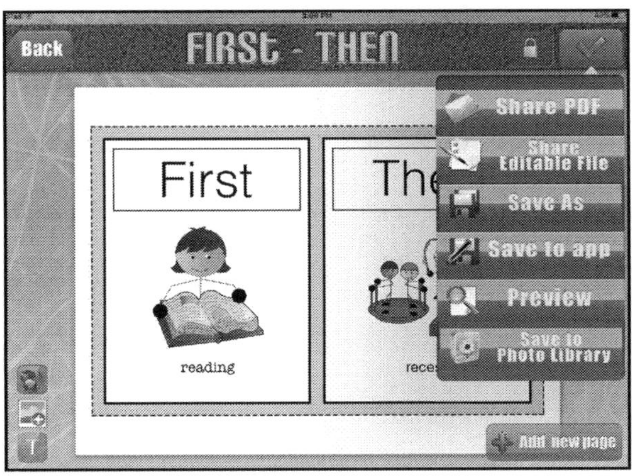

**FIGURE 9–11A.** Smarty Ears save screenshot. Reproduced with permission of Smarty Ears, LLC. All rights reserved.

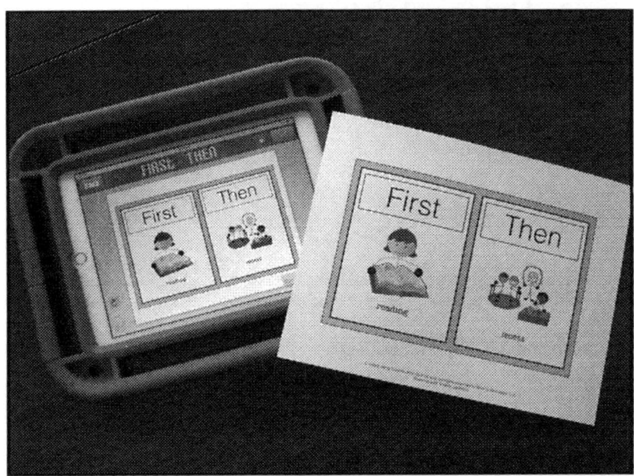

**FIGURE 9–11B.** Visual device display and printed visual. Reproduced with permission of Smarty Ears, LLC. All rights reserved.

Step 7:  If you would prefer to use the visual support directly on the device after saving the template to the app, tap "Archive" and tap the newly created visual support. After it displays, tap the "lock icon" at the top of the screen. You are now ready to use the device to display your visual support.

## Activity 4

Video clips as visual support for learning with WordToob.

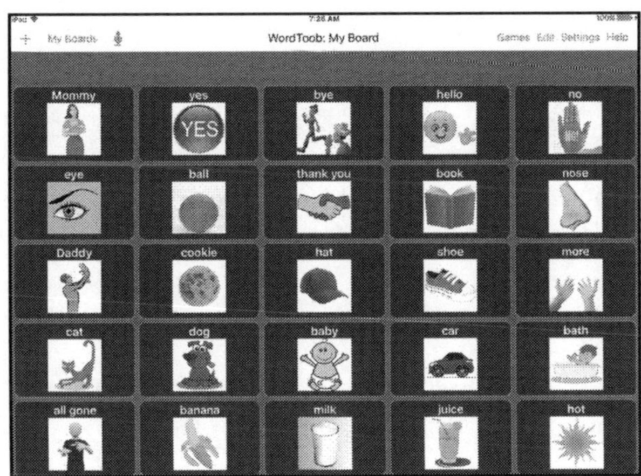

**FIGURE 9–12A.** WordToob board screenshot. Reproduced with permission of WordToob.

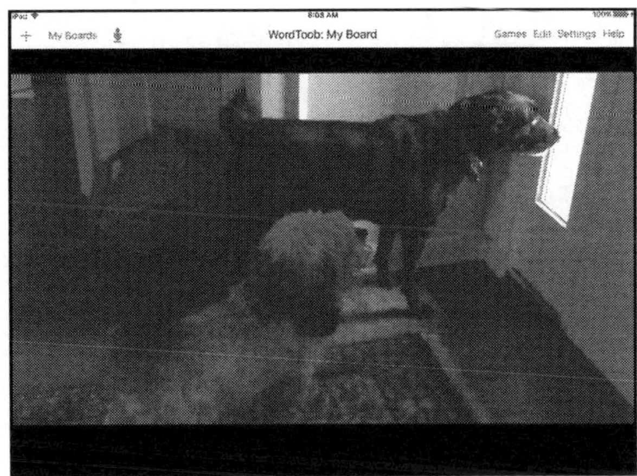

**FIGURE 9–12B.** WordToob video screenshot. Reproduced with permission of WordToob.

WordToob by John Halloran is an app that supports learning vocabulary and new skills in a fun visual manner through images and videos. Build boards with customized images and video clips to engage clients.

To download WordToob or to view a demonstration and ideas for use, visit http://word toob.com

**FIGURE 9–13.**  WordToob QR code.

### *Individual or Small Group Session*

Step 1:  To create a new board, open WordToob.

Step 2:  Tap "My Boards" and choose from a template containing the number of cells (up to 84) you would like to appear on the board (i.e., 2, 15, 60, and 84).

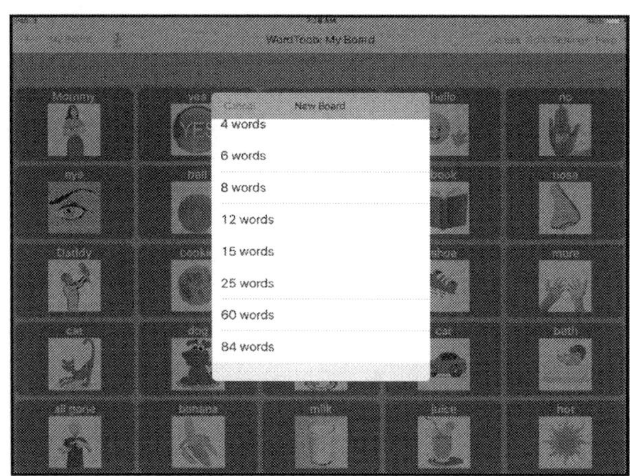

**FIGURE 9–14A.**  WordToob cell screenshot. Reproduced with permission of WordToob.

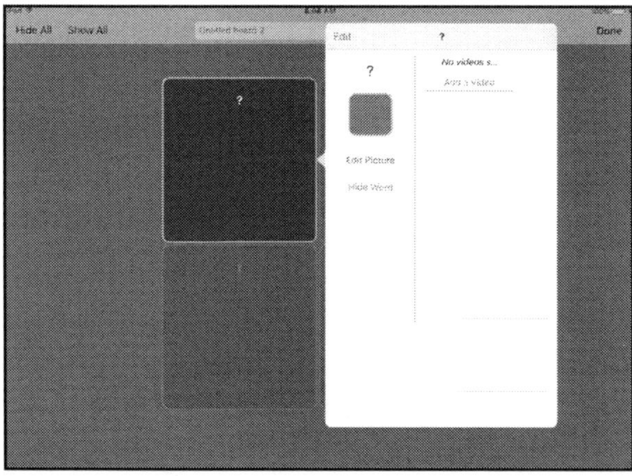

**FIGURE 9–14B.**  WordToob edit screenshot. Reproduced with permission of WordToob.

a.  Tap "Edit" and add name/word for the cell (i.e., wait).

b.  Add an image from your photo library (i.e., image of client waiting) by tapping "Edit Picture." *NOTE:* To save time when creating boards, have your images in your photo library prior to making a new board or take an image as you go through the steps to create your board.

   c. Add a video by tapping "Add a Video" and choose "existing" or "take video."
*NOTE:* To save time when creating boards, have video stored in your photo library prior to making a new board or take a video clip as you go through the steps to create your board (i.e., video of a student a playing game or video that depicts the definition of a word). Keep video clips short (a few seconds) to support just the word or action you want the client to learn.

Step 3:  Repeat Step 2 for all cells on the new board.

Step 4:  Use WordToob to visually support clients with:

- AAC needs
- Visual schedule
- Promote literacy
- Second language
- Social skills with video modeling
- Articulation video modeling

# SUGGESTIONS FOR REINFORCEMENT

Each client is different with his or her own unique interests. It's important to consider those interests when choosing what might be reinforcing for a client. Don't rule out logic puzzles, math, or spelling games as rewards at the end of a therapy session. Giving clients choices is also encouraging and helpful. This section offers ideas that have worked with a variety of clients of all ages.

## Suggestion 1

Feed the Woozle is a game that offers opportunities for body awareness, fine and gross motor skills, counting, taking turns, rolling a die, spinning a spinner, and working cooperatively.

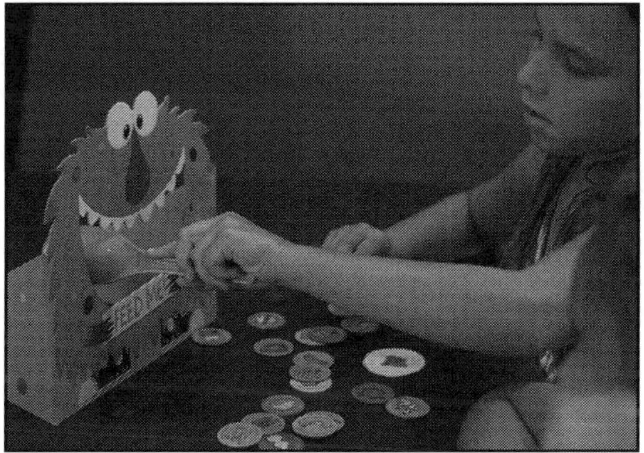

**FIGURE 9–15A.** Aria Derryberry Woozle game.

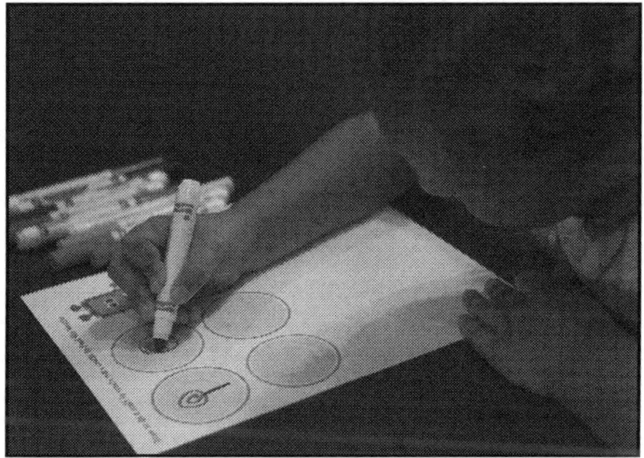

**FIGURE 9–15B.** Ruby Derryberry Woozle activity.

To find out more about Feed the Woozle by Peaceable Kingdom, visit http://www.peaceable kingdom.com

**FIGURE 9–16.** Peaceable Kingdom QR code.

Incorporate this game during the therapy session by:

- Having clients take turns feeding the Woozle after each correct answer they arrive at or at each turn in a small group.

- Using sound cards as the food for the Woozle. A regular articulation card or verb card will fit right into the Woozle's mouth.

- Visit OMazing Kids at https://omazingkidsllc.com for a free pdf to make your own Woozle food and other fun ideas for the game, as well as other free resources. Consider having clients write articulation or category words on the tokens. Each time they use a word with correct production, they can feed the Woozle.

**FIGURE 9–17.** OMazing Kids QR code.

- Brainstorm with your clients on other fun ways to use the Feed the Woozle game.

## Suggestion 2

Use the built-in games in the Articulation Carnival (free version) or Articulation Carnival PRO (full version) if you already own it.

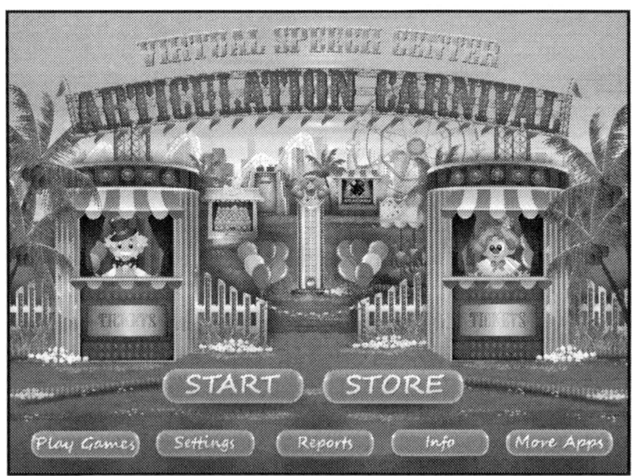


**FIGURE 9–18A.** Virtual Speech Center articulation carnival main screenshot. Reproduced with permission of Virtual Speech Center.

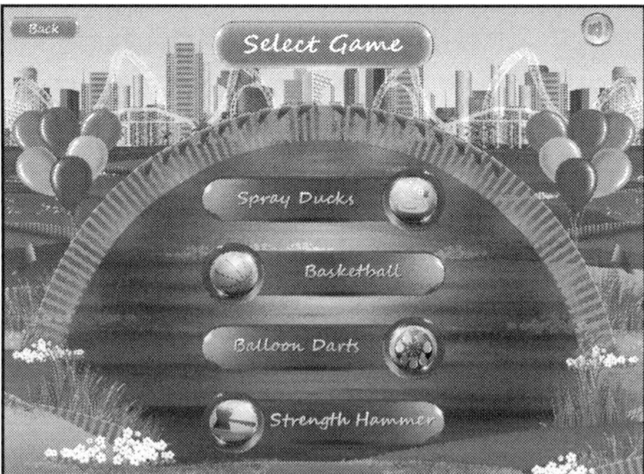


**FIGURE 9–18B.** Virtual Speech Center carnival games screenshot. Reproduced with permission of Virtual Speech Center.

Articulation Carnival free version by Virtual Speech Center is an articulation app that comes with one phoneme /p/ and all four carnival games. The home screen allows for access to the games without using the app for therapy.

To download Articulation Carnival, visit https://www.virtualspeechcenter.com

**FIGURE 9–19.** Virtual Speech Center QR code.

Included are four games that are fun for a variety of ages: Basketball Free Throw, Balloon Dart Throw, Duck Spray Game, and Hammer Game.

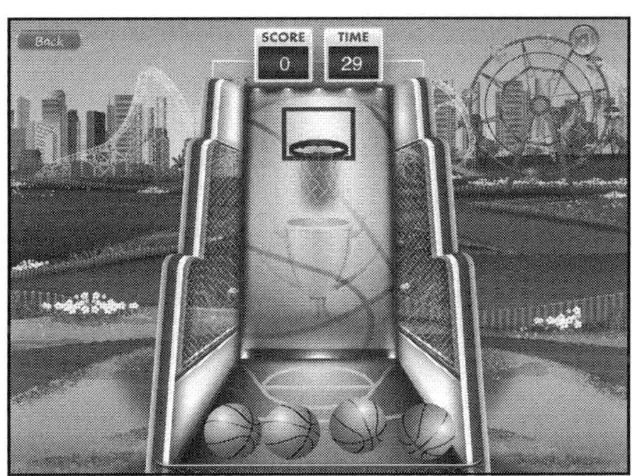


**FIGURE 9–20A.** Virtual Speech Center basketball game screenshot. Reproduced with permission of Virtual Speech Center.

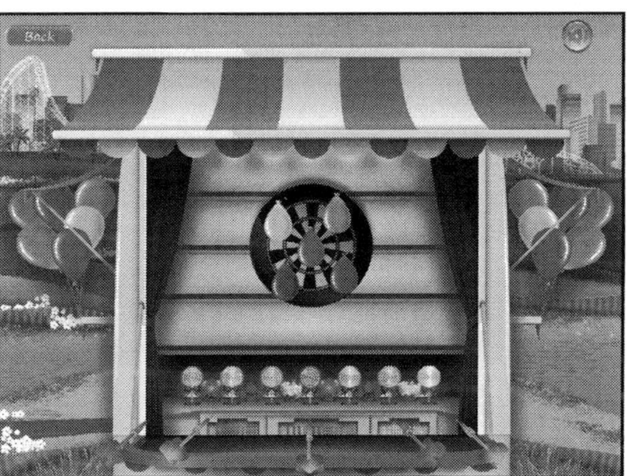


**FIGURE 9–20B.** Virtual Speech Center balloon dart game screenshot. Reproduced with permission of Virtual Speech Center.

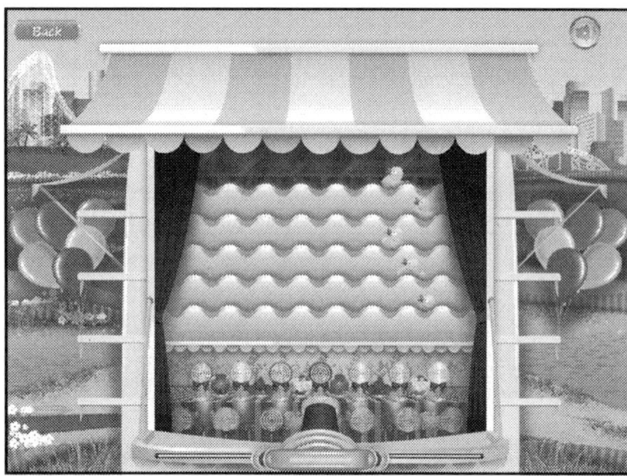

**FIGURE 9–20C.** Virtual Speech Center duck spray game screenshot. Reproduced with permission of Virtual Speech Center.

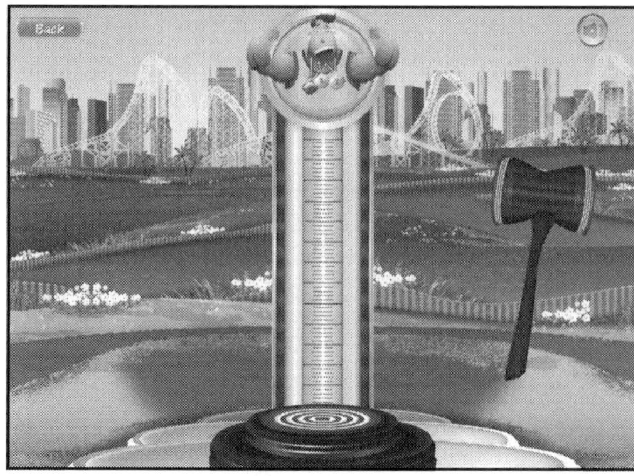

**FIGURE 9–20D.** Virtual Speech Center hammer game screenshot. Reproduced with permission of Virtual Speech Center.

Incorporate these games into therapy by:

- Using for rewards after successful therapy sessions. Save a few minutes for game play at the end.

- Using the games during therapy. Allow clients to use while waiting for their therapy turn or after correction productions.

## Suggestion 3

Use traditional puzzles or interactive app puzzles.

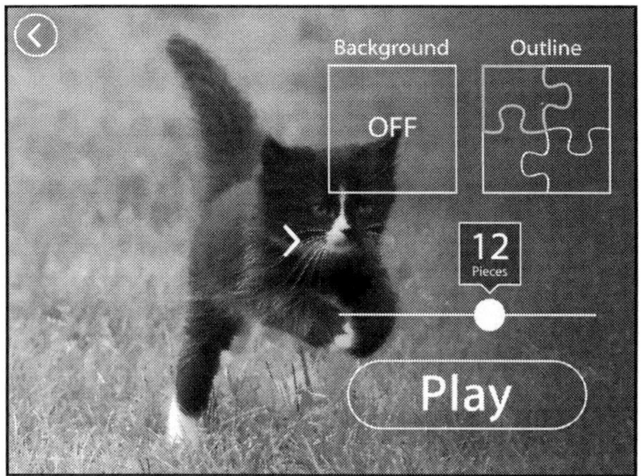


**FIGURE 9–21A.** Eggroll Games kitten screenshot. Reproduced with permission of Eggroll Games, LLC.

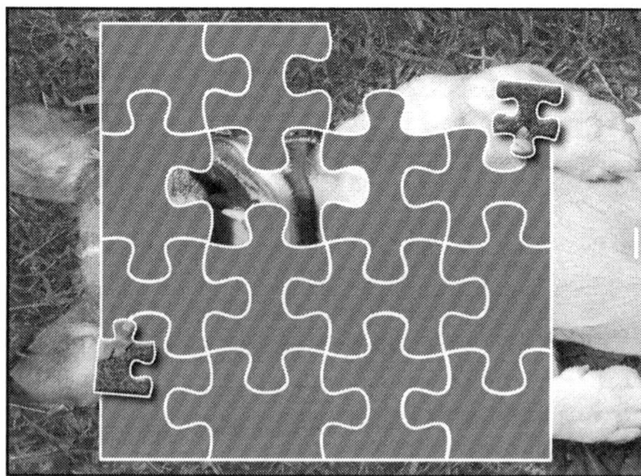

**FIGURE 9–21B.** Eggroll Games puppy piece screenshot. Reproduced with permission of Eggroll Games, LLC.

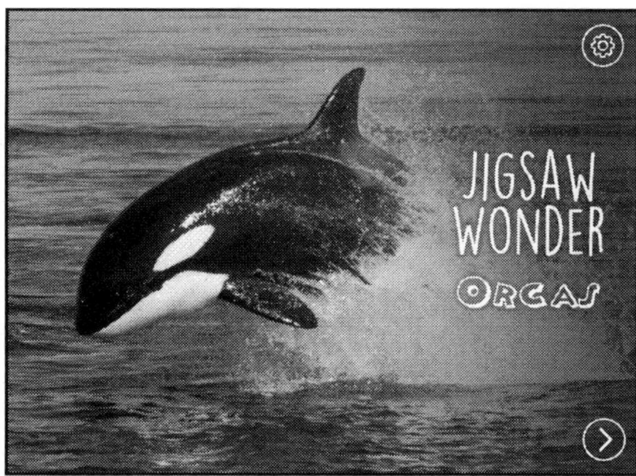


**FIGURE 9–21C.** Eggroll Games orca puzzle screenshot. Reproduced with permission of Eggroll Games, LLC.

Eggroll Games has a number of puzzles containing topics with beautiful graphics (i.e., sharks, kittens, puppies, polar bears, whales). The puzzles are appropriate for a variety of ages, abilities, and interests.

To download Eggroll Games Jigsaw Wonder Puzzles, visit http://eggrollgames.com

**FIGURE 9–22.** Eggroll Games QR code.

Many clients like puzzles, which can be a successful way to reinforce progress or a therapy session.

- With traditional puzzles, give clients puzzle pieces to add to the puzzle as they work through the therapy session. Depending on the size of the puzzle, this can make for a reinforcer that will last for weeks of therapy.

- With interactive app puzzles, allow clients to add pieces to their puzzle as they work through therapy. Pass the tablet around and allow all clients within a small group to add a piece.

## Suggestion 4

Offering opportunities for refocusing when needed and using fidgets (i.e., squeeze balls, feathers, brightly colored fuzzy pipe cleaners).

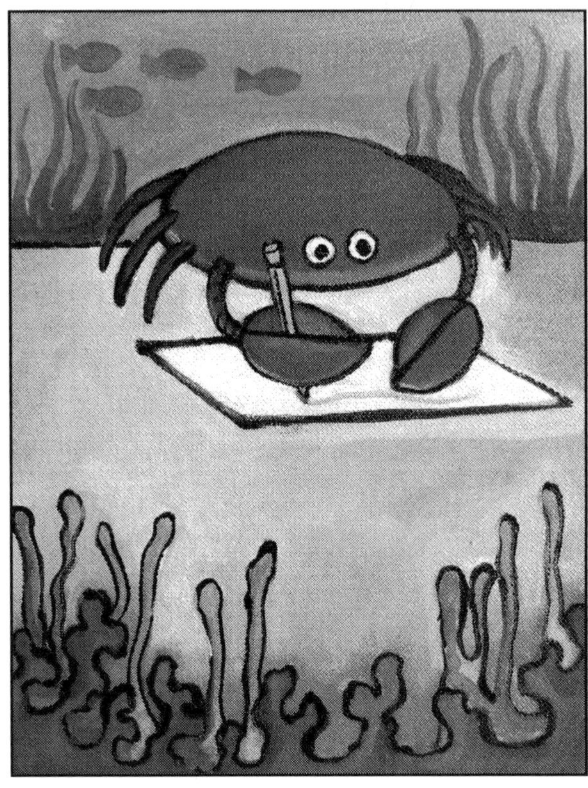

**FIGURE 9–23A.** Wellbeyond focus screenshot. Reproduced with permission of Wellbeyond and Noelle Dass. Copyright 2016. All rights reserved.

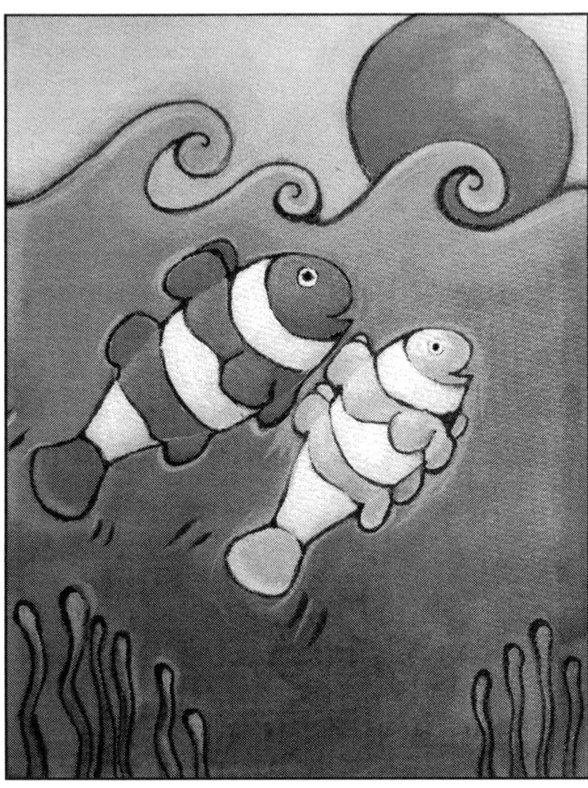

**FIGURE 9–23B.** Wellbeyond kindness screenshot. Reproduced with permission of Wellbeyond and Noelle Dass. Copyright 2016. All rights reserved.

Wellbeyond has created a relaxation and focus app with hand-painted illustrations, gentle music, and guided relaxations (sleep, focus, feelings, centering, and kindness).

To download Wellbeyond Meditation for Kids, visit https://itunes.apple.com/us/app/well beyond-meditation-for/id1082891966?mt=8

**FIGURE 9–24.**
Wellbeyond QR code.

This app can be quite useful for clients who need a bit of time to refocus during a therapy session or at the beginning or end of the session.

## Suggestion 5

Interactive Logic Puzzlers

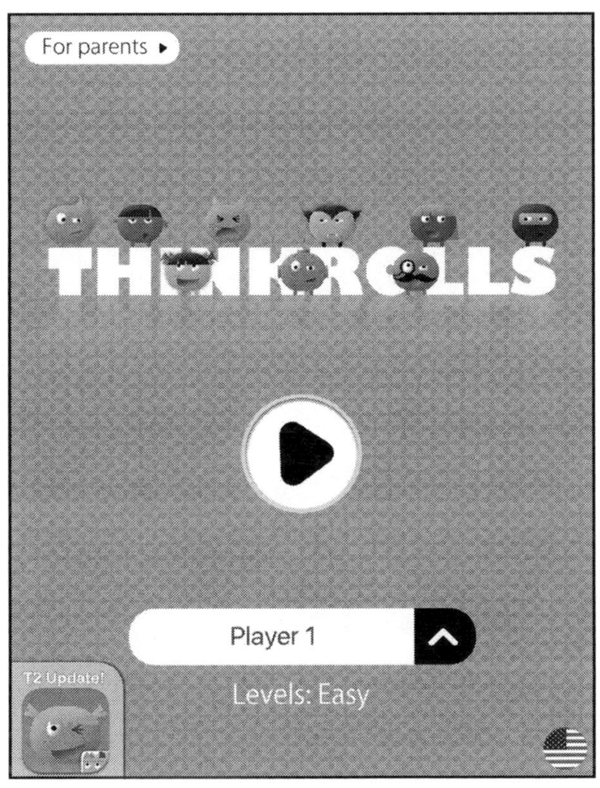

**FIGURE 9–25A.** Avokiddo Thinkrolls screenshot. Reproduced with permission of Avokiddo E.E.

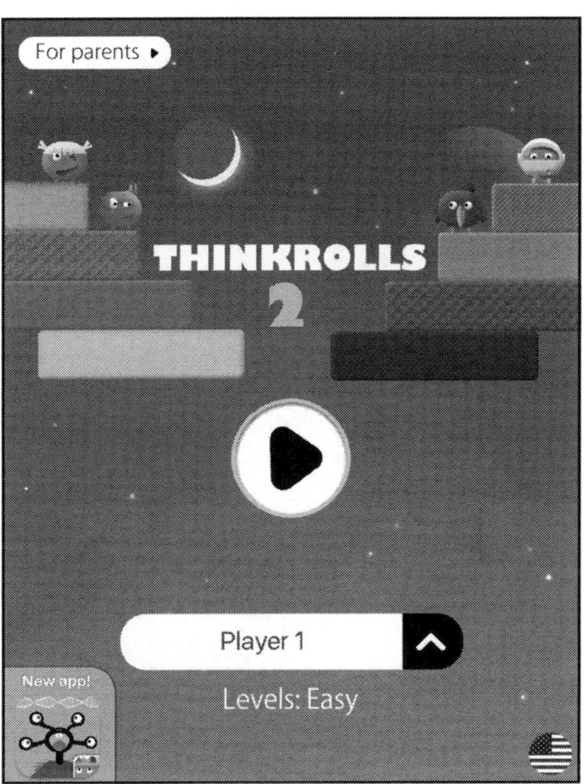

**FIGURE 9–25B.** Avokiddo Thinkrolls 2 screenshot. Reproduced with permission of Avokiddo E.E.

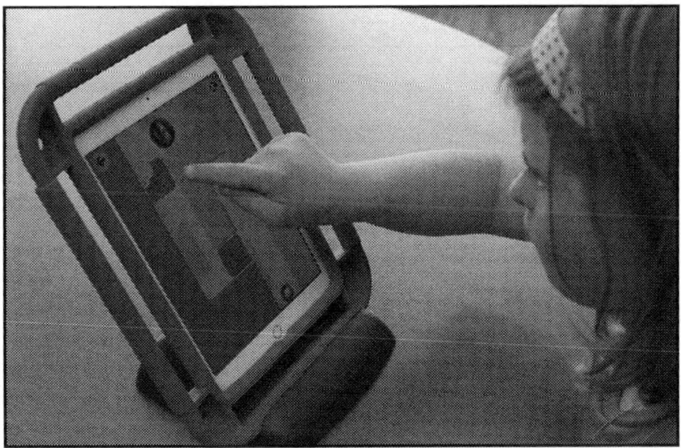

**FIGURE 9–25C.** Elizabeth Giese Avokiddo.

Thinkrolls and Thinkrolls 2 by Avokiddo make for fun critical thinking and interactive rewards at the end of a therapy session. They can also be used for describing, retelling, and sequencing during a therapy session and make for a lesson within itself.

To download Thinkrolls, visit http://avokiddo.com

**FIGURE 9–26.** Avokiddo QR code.

Winky Think by Spinlight Studios is an interactive logic puzzle with 180 puzzles. Offer Winky Think as a reward and clients will have loads of fun while developing problem solving and motor skills with each challenging puzzle. Winky Think is appropriate for all ages. Also use this interactive logic puzzle for turn-taking and cooperative play.

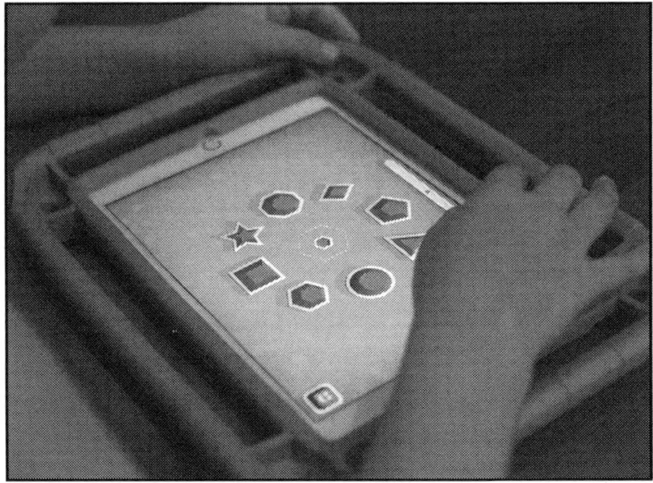

**FIGURE 9–27.** Winky Think game photo.

To download Winky Think, visit http://spinlight.com

**FIGURE 9–28.** Spinlight Studios QR code.

Edoki Academy offers a number of fun logic puzzlers: Busy Shapes, Crazy Gears, and Busy Water. Each of these apps offers high levels of engagement and critical thinking for all ages.

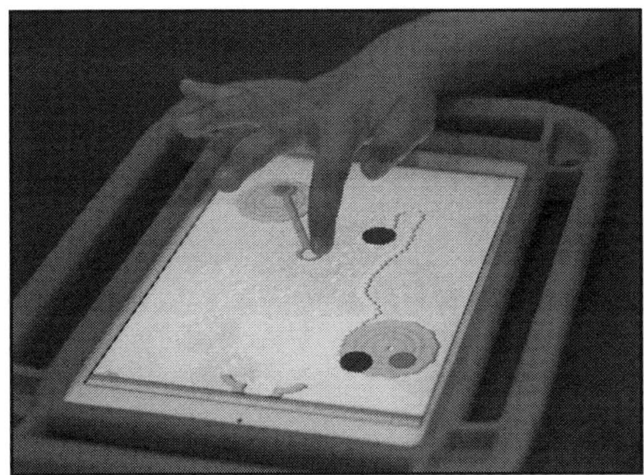

**FIGURE 9–29A.** Crazy Gears example.

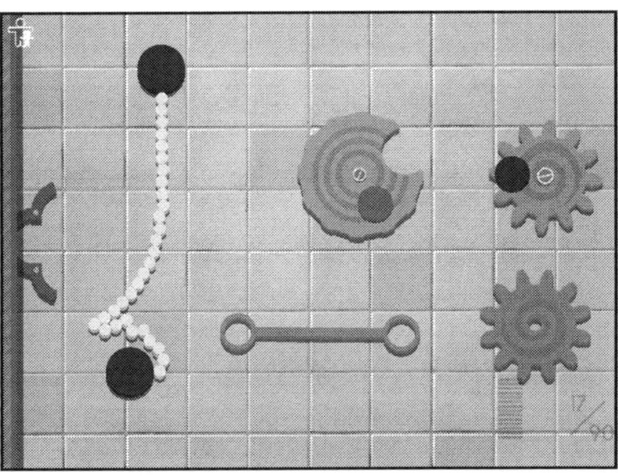

**FIGURE 9–29B.** Crazy Gears screenshot by Edoki Academy. Reproduced with permission of Edoki Academy.

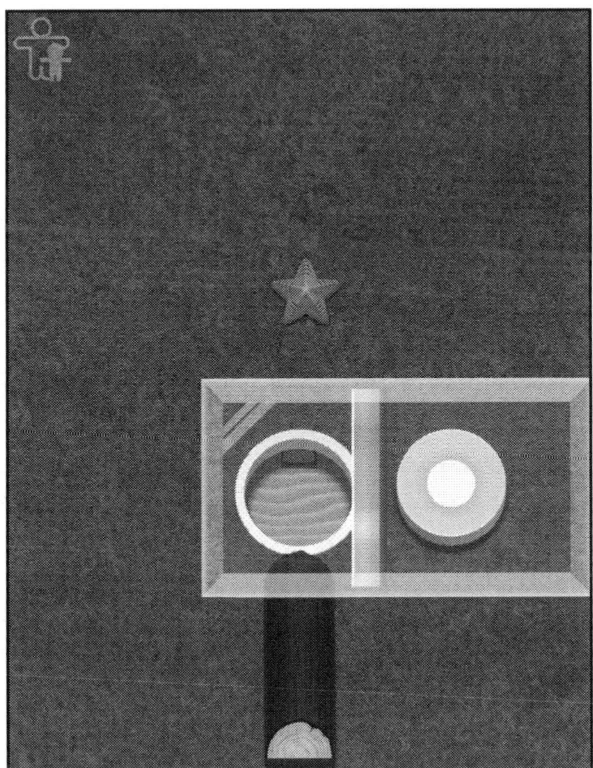

**FIGURE 9–29C.** Busy Shapes screenshot by Edoki Academy. Reproduced with permission of Edoki Academy.

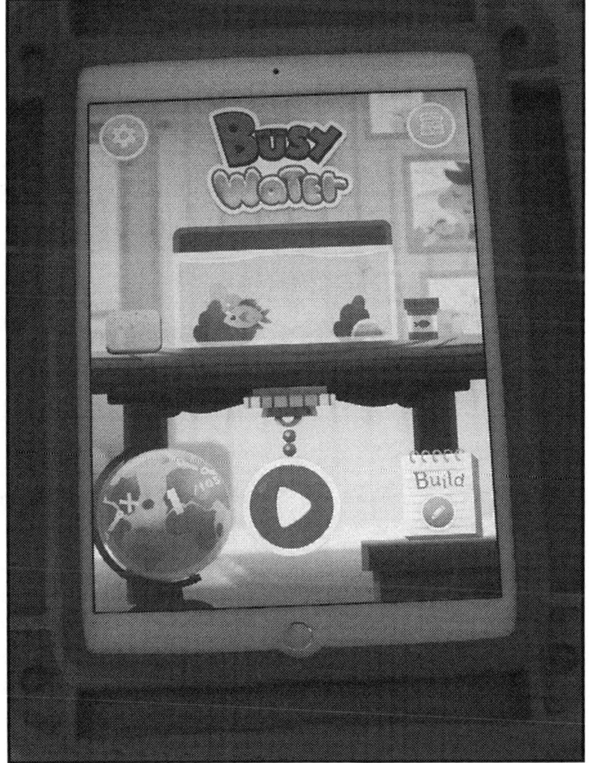

**FIGURE 9–29D.** Busy water example.

To download Busy Shapes, Crazy Gears, or Busy Water by Edoki Academy, visit https://www.edokiacademy.com/en

**FIGURE 9–30.** Edoki Academy QR code.

## Suggestion 6

Open-ended play apps. Apps by Toca Boca, Sago Sago, and FizzBrain are interactive open-ended play apps that offer high engagement for a variety of ages.

Toca Boca has a variety of open-ended apps. Allow clients to earn time after successful therapy. Many of the Toca Boca apps are also useful for following directions and familiarizing with functional vocabulary.

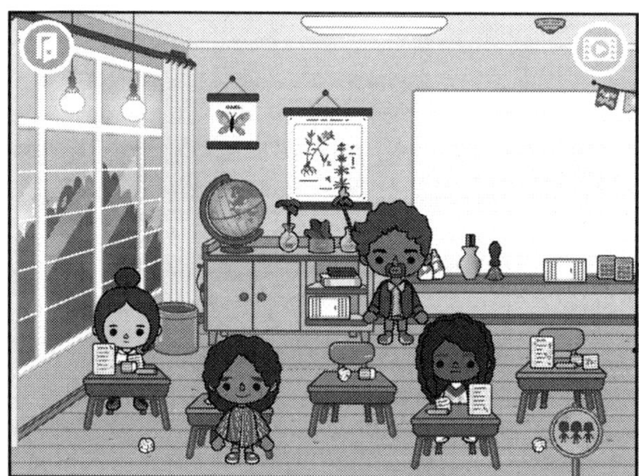

**FIGURE 9–31A.** Toca Boca school screenshot. Reproduced with permission of Toca Boca.

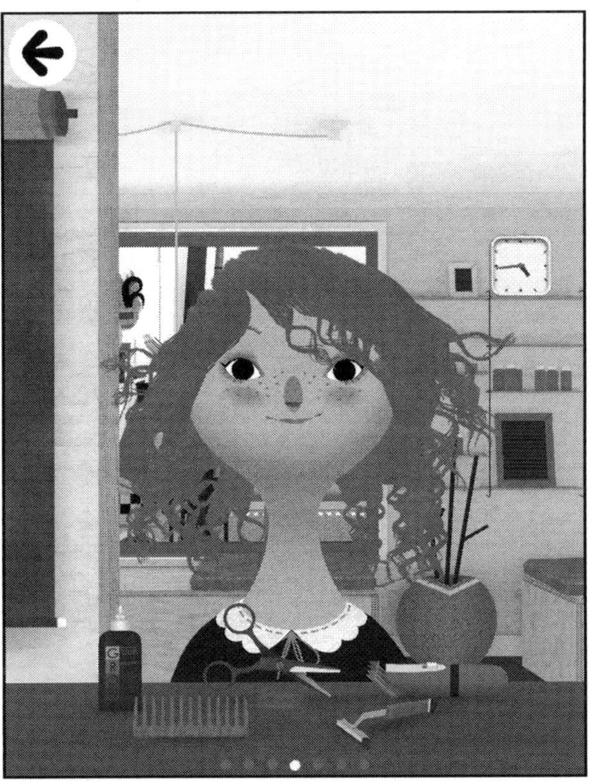

**FIGURE 9–31B.** Toca Boca hair salon screenshot. Reproduced with permission of Toca Boca.

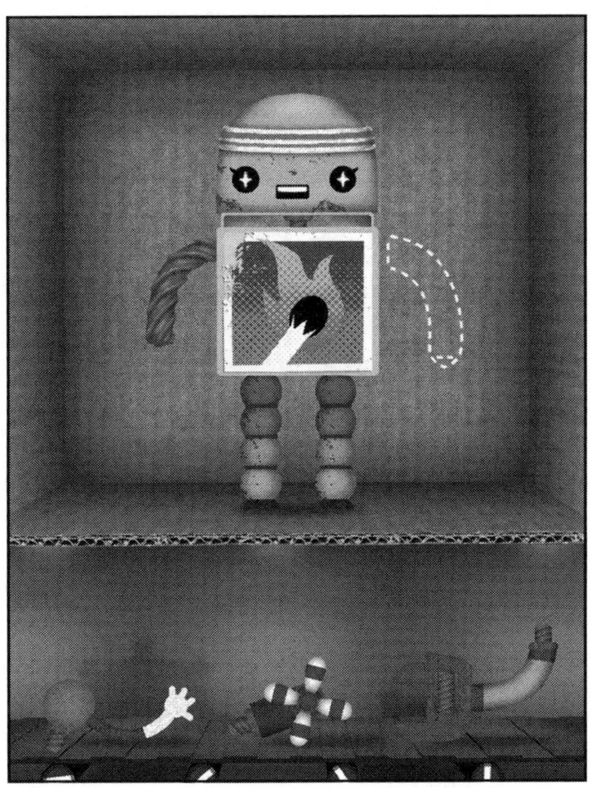

**FIGURE 9–31C.** Toca Boca robot lab screenshot. Reproduced with permission of Toca Boca.

Some client favorites are:

- Toca Life series: School, City, Town, Vacation
- Toca Kitchen 1 and 2
- Toca Hair Salon
- Toca Nature
- Toca Store
- Toca Robot Lab
- Toca Nature

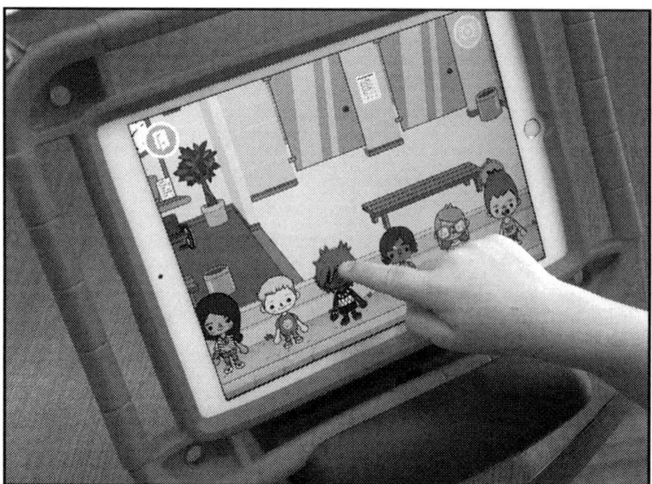

**FIGURE 9–32.** Toca Boca screenshot example.

To download or become familiar with the many Toca Boca apps, visit https://tocaboca.com

**FIGURE 9–33.** Toca Boca QR code.

Sago Sago has a variety of open-ended apps. Allow clients to earn time after successful therapy. Many of the Sago Sago apps are also useful for following directions and familiarizing with functional vocabulary such as up, down, over, under, in, out, and so on. See Chapter 6 for more information.

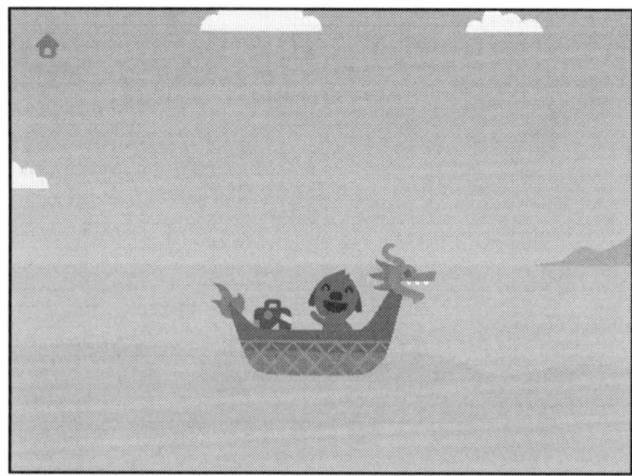

**FIGURE 9–34A.** Sago Sago boat screenshot. Reproduced with permission of Sago Sago.

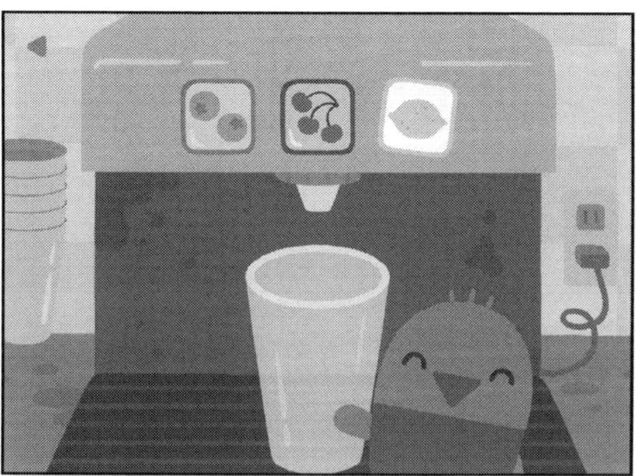

**FIGURE 9–34B.** Sago Sago pet café screenshot. Reproduced with permission of Sago Sago.

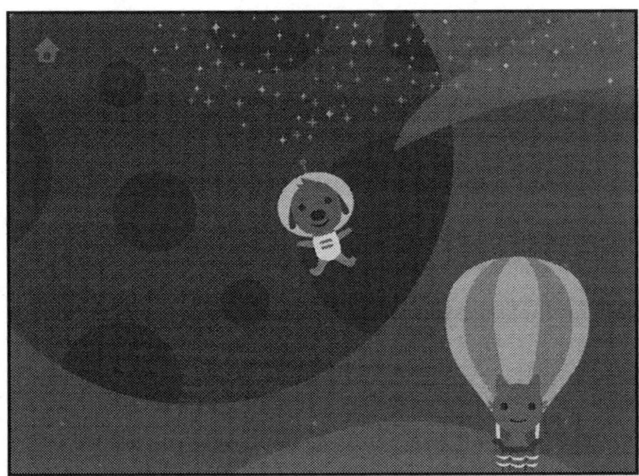

**FIGURE 9–34C.** Sago Sago space explorer screenshot. Reproduced with permission of Sago Sago.

Some client favorites are:

- Pet Café
- Space Explorer
- Fairy Tales
- Tool Box
- Bug Builder
- Ocean Swimmer
- Trucks and Diggers

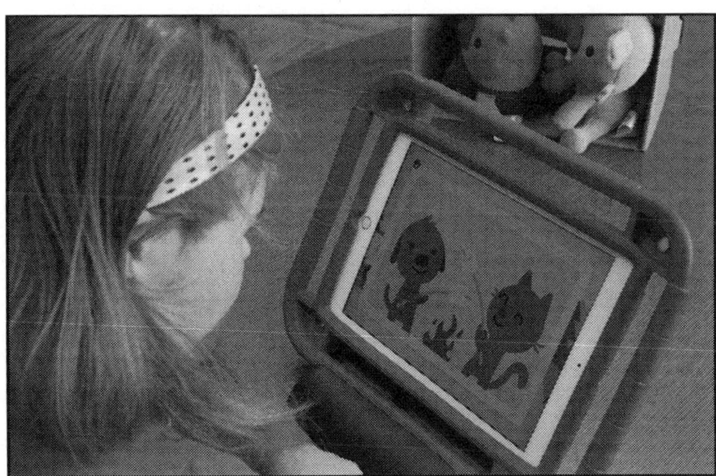

**FIGURE 9–35.** Elizabeth Giese Sago play.

To download or become familiar with Sago Sago apps, visit http://www.sagomini.com

**FIGURE 9–36.** Sago Sago QR code.

FizzBrain apps offer fun creativity with the Touch and Write series: Touch and Write, Cursive Touch and Write, Touch and Write Phonics, and Shapes Touch and Write. Offer any one of these apps for a job well done. Clients love the option to choose their writing medium (i.e., chalk, pudding, ketchup, shaving cream, and more). Consider creating word lists in the custom feature of these apps and use them as the therapy lesson.

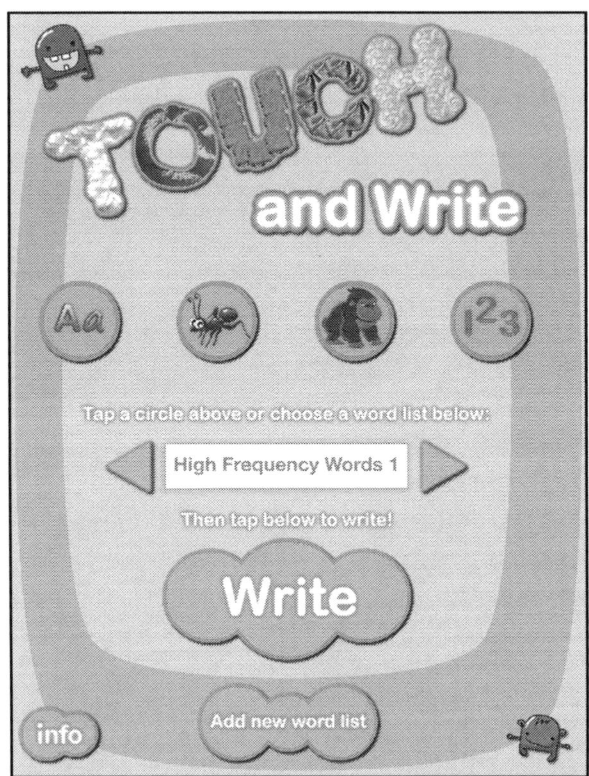


**FIGURE 9–37A.** FizzBrain Touch and Write screenshot. Reproduced with permission of FizzBrain, LLC.

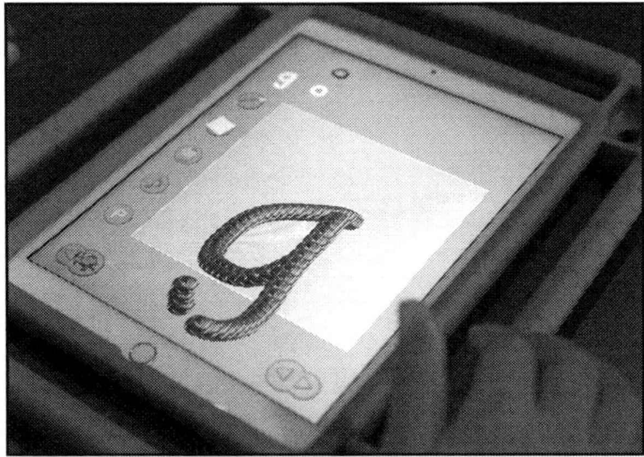

**FIGURE 9–37B.** FizzBrain photo example.

To download any of the FizzBrain Touch and Write series, visit http://www.fizzbrain.com

**FIGURE 9–38.** FizzBrain QR code.

# REFERENCES

Waters, M., Lerman, D., & Hovanetz, A. (2009). Separate and combined effects of visual schedules and extinction plus differential reinforcement on problem behavior occasioned by transitions. *Journal of Applied Behavioral Analysis. 42*(2), 309–313.

Wilder, D., Myers, K., Fischetti, A., Leon, Y., Nicholson, K., & Allison, J. (2012). An analysis of modifications to the three-step guided compliance procedure necessary to achieve compliance among preschool children. *Journal of Applied Behavior Analysis, 45*(1), 121–130.

# INDEX